HEALTH PROMOTION PROGRAMS

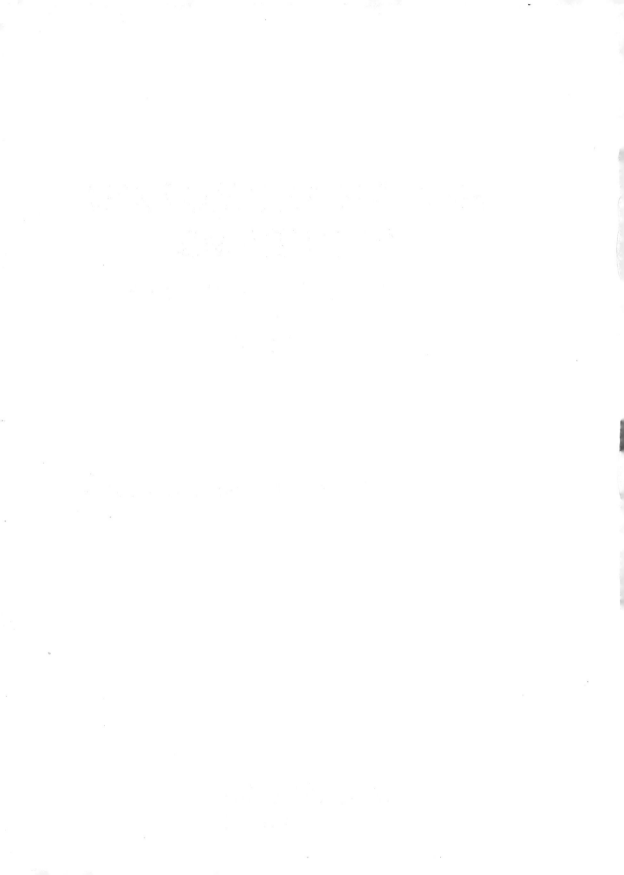

HEALTH PROMOTION PROGRAMS

FROM THEORY TO PRACTICE

Second Edition

Carl I. Fertman
Diane D. Allensworth
Editors

 Society for Public Health Education

JB JOSSEY-BASS™
A Wiley Brand

Published by Jossey-Bass
A Wiley Brand

One Montgomery Street, Suite 1000, San Francisco, CA 94104-4594—www.josseybass.com

Jossey-Bass books and products are available through most bookstores. To contact Jossey-Bass directly call our Customer Care Department within the U.S. at 800-956-7739, outside the U.S. at 317-572-3986, or fax 317-572-4002.

Wiley publishes in a variety of print and electronic formats and by print-on-demand. Some material included with standard print versions of this book may not be included in e-books or in print-on-demand. If this book refers to media such as a CD or DVD that is not included in the version you purchased, you may download this material at http://booksupport.wiley.com. For more information about Wiley products, visit www.wiley.com.

Library of Congress Cataloging-in-Publication Data

Names: Fertman, Carl I., 1950- editor. | Allensworth, Diane DeMuth, editor.
Title: Health promotion programs : from theory to practice / Carl I. Fertman, Diane D. Allensworth, editors.
Description: Second edition. | San Francisco, CA : Jossey-Bass & Pfeiffer Imprints, Wiley, [2017] | Series: The society for public health education | Includes bibliographical references and index.
Identifiers: LCCN 2016016575 (print) | LCCN 2016016877 (ebook) | ISBN 9781119163336 (pbk.) | ISBN 9781119163343 (pdf) | ISBN 9781119163350 (epub)
Subjects: LCSH: Health promotion.
Classification: LCC RA427.8 .H5255 2017 (print) | LCC RA427.8 (ebook) | DDC 362.1—dc23
LC record available at https://lccn.loc.gov/2016016575

Cover design: Wiley
Cover image: © Itana/Shutterstock and © Apostrophe/Shutterstock

Printed in the United States of America

SECOND EDITION

PB Printing 10 9 8 7 6 5 4 3

For my wife, Barbara Murock, promoter of love,
family, health, and biking

—Carl I. Fertman

To my best friend, colleague, and husband, John,
who encouraged and supported my dreams

—Diane D. Allensworth

CONTENTS

Part One: Foundations of Health Promotion Programs   1

Chapter 1   What Are Health Promotion Programs? 3

Carl I. Fertman, Diane D. Allensworth, and M. Elaine Auld

Chapter 2   Advancing Equity and Eliminating Health Disparities . . . 29

*Francisco Soto Mas, Diane D. Allensworth, Camara Phyllis Jones,
and Holly E. Jacobson*

Chapter 3   Theory in Health Promotion Programs 53

Melissa Grim and Brian Hortz

Part Two: Planning Health Promotion Programs   83

Chapter 4   Assessing the Needs of Program Participants 85

James H. Price, Joseph A. Dake, and Britney Ward

**Chapter 16 Promoting Community Health: Local Health
Departments and Community Health Organizations . . . 397**

*Michael T. Hatcher, Diane D. Allensworth,
and Frances D. Butterfoss*

LIST OF FIGURES AND TABLES

Figures

Tables

EDITORS

Carl I. Fertman
Associate Professor
Department of Health and Physical Activity
School of Education
University of Pittsburgh

Diane D. Allensworth
Professor Emeritus
College of Education
Kent State University

THE CONTRIBUTORS

Neyal J. Ammary-Risch
Director
National Eye Health Education Program
National Eye Institute
National Institutes of Health

M. Elaine Auld
Chief Executive Officer
Society for Public Health Education

Kelly Bishop
Health Education Specialist
Centers for Disease Control and Prevention

Jean M. Breny
Professor and Chair
Department of Public Health
Southern Connecticut State University

Frances D. Butterfoss
President, Coalitions Work
Professor
Department of Pediatrics
Eastern Virginia Medical School

Huey-Shys Chen
Professor and Associate Dean of Research and Scholarship
College of Nursing
University of Toledo

W. William Chen
Professor Emeritus
Department of Health Education and Behavior
University of Florida

Sara L. Cole
Adjunct Professor
University of Central Oklahoma

Katherine Crosson
Associate Director
Center for Quality Improvement and Patient Safety
Agency for Healthcare Research and Quality

Joseph A. Dake
Professor
School of Population Health
College of Health and Human Services
University of Toledo

Michael C. Fagen
Associate Professor in Preventive Medicine
Northwestern University

Regina A. Galer-Unti
Faculty Member
Walden University

Cezanne Garcia
Senior Program and Resource Specialist
Institute for Family-Centered Care

Melissa Grim
Professor and Chair
Department of Health and Human Performance
Radford University

Jim Grizzell
Health Educator
California State Polytechnic University

Anna Grummon
Student
Gillings School of Global Public Health
University of North Carolina at Chapel Hill

Michael T. Hatcher
Chief, Environmental Medicine
Division of Toxicology
Agency for Toxic Substances and Disease Registry
Centers for Disease Control and Prevention

Brian Hortz
Associate Professor
Assistant Athletic Director
Director of SportsMedicine
Denison University

Holly E. Jacobson
Associate Professor
Department of Linguistics
University of New Mexico

Camara Phyllis Jones
Senior Fellow
Satcher Health Leadership Institute
Morehouse School of Medicine
Atlanta, Georgia

Timothy R. Jordan
Professor
School of Population Health
College of Health and Human Services
University of Toledo

Ellen Langhans
Technical Information Specialist
HHS Office of Disease Prevention and Health Promotion

Laura Linnan
Professor
Department of Human Behavior and Education
Gillings School of Global Public Health
University of North Carolina at Chapel Hill

Francisco Soto Mas
Associate Professor
College of Population Health
University of New Mexico

Angela D. Mickalide
Health and Safety Researcher and Practitioner
Kensington, MD

James H. Price
Professor Emeritus
School of Population Health
College of Health and Human Services
University of Toledo

Regina McCoy Pulliam
Associate Professor
University of North Carolina-Greensboro

Kathleen M. Roe
Professor
Department of Health Science and Recreation
San Jose State University

Jiunn-Jye Sheu
Associate Professor
School of Population Health
College of Health and Human Services
University of Florida

David A. Sleet
Associate Director for Science
Division of Unintentional Injury Prevention
Centers for Disease Control and Prevention

Karen A. Spiller
Manager, Jump Up & Go Program
Blue Cross Blue Shield of Massachusetts

Beth Stevenson
Principal Consultant
Stevenson Solutions, LLC

Marlene K. Tappe
Professor
Department of Health Science
Minnesota State University, Mankato

Louise Villejo
Executive Director
Patient Education Office
University of Texas
M. D. Anderson Cancer Center

Britney Ward
Director of Community Health Improvement
Hospital Council of Northwest Ohio

Margaret Wielinski
Assistant Director of Community Health Improvement
Hospital Council of Northwest Ohio

Allison Zambon
Health Education Specialist
Fox Chase Cancer Center–Temple
University Health System

The Society for Public Health Education (SOPHE) is a nonprofit professional organization founded in 1950. SOPHE's mission is to provide global leadership to the profession of health education and health promotion and to promote the health of society through advances in health education theory and research, excellence in professional preparation and practice, advocacy for public policies conducive to health, and the achievement of health equity for all. SOPHE is the only independent professional organization devoted exclusively to health education and health promotion.

SOPHE's membership extends health education principles and practices to many settings, including schools; universities; medical and health care settings; work sites; voluntary health agencies; international organizations; and federal, state, and local governments.

Contact SOPHE at 10 G Street N.W., Suite 605, Washington, DC 20002-4242; telephone: (202) 408-9804; website: www.sophe.org

We are pleased to share this second edition of *Health Promotion Programs: From Theory to Practice*. In the short period of time since the first edition was published in 2010, health promotion programs have evolved to be integral to promoting a culture of health and wellness and to health care across the United States and internationally. The Society for Public Health Education (SOPHE) recognized the need for a book to help advance the field. Escalating rates of chronic disease, soaring health care costs, and increasing diversity of the U.S. population, as well as aging of the current health education workforce, all call for training a new generation of health promoters. The SOPHE board of trustees, executive director, and members offer this book, which combines the theoretical and practice base of the field with step-by-step practical sections on how to develop, implement, and evaluate health promotion programs. SOPHE hopes that this book, read in its entirety or in part, will help not only students who choose to major or minor in health education, health promotion, community health, public health, or health-related fields (e.g., environmental health, physical fitness allied health, nursing, or medicine) but also professionals already working who want to acquire the technical knowledge and skills to develop successful health promotion programs. Acquiring the competencies to effectively plan, implement, and evaluate health promotion programs can improve health outcomes, promote behavioral and social change, and contribute to eliminating health disparities. This book offers a concise summary of the many years of research in the fields of health education and health promotion, along with the expertise of many SOPHE members working in diverse contemporary settings and programs. The book also reflects SOPHE's mission and its commitment to professional preparation and continuing education for the purpose of improving the quantity and quality of the lives of individuals and communities.

Undergraduate and graduate programs that prepare professionals to work in public health, health education, and health promotion and wellness have been flourishing in the United States and throughout the world for more than half a century. Thousands of students graduate every year with a baccalaureate or advanced degree in health promotion and get jobs in schools, colleges, businesses, health care facilities and systems, community organizations, and government.

We are enormously grateful to the many SOPHE members who wrote this book. Their expertise in many fields, including health education, public health, sociology, anthropology, psychology, nursing, medicine, physical education, nutrition, allied health, and many others, have been braided into this health promotion anthology. They have shared the foundations of the field as well as their own practical experiences in health promotion planning. May this book help teach, guide, inspire, catalyze, and transform students and professionals in their quest to develop successful health promotion programs that address the health challenges of both today and tomorrow.

About the Second Edition

The main purpose of the second edition is the same as the first edition's: to provide a comprehensive introduction to health promotion programs by combining the theory and practice with a hands-on guide to program planning, implementation, and evaluation. One of the fundamental premises of this book is the importance of using an approach based in both research and practice to guide and inform planning, implementation, and evaluation of health promotion programs. A secondary goal is to present the widespread opportunities to implement health promotion programs in schools, communities, workplaces, and health care organizations and systems. This text addresses the needs of students and professionals who are pursuing careers in health education as well as nursing, medicine, public health, and allied health.

The second edition presents the new opportunities for health promotion programs with the passage of the Affordable Care and Patient Protection Act 2010, commonly called the Affordable Care Act (ACA). This edition includes an enhanced focus on the application of health theories and health program planning models for diverse populations and settings. Reflecting social change, the book has moved from the first edition's focus on eliminating health disparities to promoting health equity in this edition. As new information and communication technologies have created an unprecedented range of strategies for health promotion, this edition integrates coverage of eHealth into health promotion program examples throughout the book. We have added a new chapter on big data and its application to understanding and improving health. These issues that are broad and of growing importance are integrated in all of the chapters and in particular highlighted in the chapters that address health promotion in schools, the workplace, health care organizations, and communities. We believe that these additions strengthen the book and increase its appropriateness for use with students and in settings around the world.

Who Should Read This Book

This book is aimed at three audiences. The first audience is students pursuing a major or minor in health education, health promotion, community health, public health, or health-related fields such as environmental health, physical activity and education, allied health, nursing, or medicine. The second audience is young and mid-career practitioners, practicing managers, researchers, and instructors who for the first time are responsible for teaching, designing, or leading health promotion programs. The third audience is colleagues and professionals not trained in the health fields but working in settings where health promotion programs are increasingly prevalent and might be under their supervision (for example, school superintendents and principals, human resource directors working in business and health care, college deans of student affairs, faculty members, board members of nonprofit organizations, community members, and employers and staff members in businesses and health care organizations).

Overview of the Contents

This volume presents an up-to-date understanding of health promotion program planning, implementation, and evaluation in a variety of settings. The book is divided into five parts. Part One presents the foundations of health promotion programs: what health and health promotion are, the history of health promotion, sites of health promotion programs, and the key people (stakeholders) involved in programs. Highlighted and explored are the two guiding forces in planning, implementing, and evaluating health promotion programs. The first is promoting health equity. The second is the use of health theories and planning models.

Parts Two (planning), Three (implementation), and Four (evaluation) provide a step-by-step guide to planning, implementing, and evaluating a health promotion program. Each chapter within these parts covers specific phases of health promotion program planning, implementation, and evaluation. Practical tips and specific examples aim to facilitate readers' understanding of the phases as well as to build technical skills in designing and leading evidence-based health promotion programs.

Part Five presents health promotion programs across four settings: schools (preschool through college), health care organizations, workplaces, and communities. Each chapter presents keys for effective site-specific programs to promote health.

At the beginning of each chapter the Learning Objectives give a framework and guide to the chapter topics. The key terms at the end of each chapter can be used as a reference while reading this book as well as a way to recap key definitions in planning, implementation, and evaluation of health promotion programs. At the end of the text, all the key terms are listed and defined in a glossary.

Practical examples throughout the book reinforce the need for health promotion programs to be based on in-depth understanding of the intended audiences' perceptions, beliefs, attitudes, behaviors, and barriers to change as well as the cultural, social, and environmental context in which they live. By referring to current theories and models of health promotion, the book also reinforces the need for health promotion practitioners to base their programs on theories, models, and approaches that guide and inform health promotion program design, implementation, and evaluation.

Each chapter ends with practice and discussion questions that help the reader to reflect upon as well as utilize key terms. Finally, all chapters are interconnected but are also designed to stand alone and provide a comprehensive overview of the topic they cover.

Features

- Learning objectives
- Practice and discussion questions
- Lists of key terms
- Glossary of key terms

Editors' Note

As editors, we hope that we contribute to preventing disease and promoting health. We believe that understanding the theory and practice of health promotion program planning, implementation, and evaluation will allow more individuals and groups to enjoy the benefits of good health and will encourage more schools, workplaces, health care organizations, and communities to be designated as health-promoting sites. We are grateful to the SOPHE members who have authored chapters in this text and admire their commitment and dedication to making a difference in the health outcomes of the individuals, communities, groups, and organizations they serve.

Health Promotion Programs: From Theory to Practice has been established as a widely used text and reference book both in the United States and internationally. It is our hope that the second edition will continue to be relevant and useful and stimulate readers' interest and knowledge in health promotion programs that utilize health theory to promote health equity. We aspire to provide readers with information and skills to ask critical questions, think conceptually, and stretch their thinking to promote health across diverse populations and settings.

We appreciate the opportunity to plan and edit this text, which the SOPHE board of trustees, executive director, staff, and members provided to us. SOPHE provides leadership and works to contribute to the health of all people and the elimination of disparities through advances in health promotion theory and research, excellence in professional preparation and practice, and advocacy for public policies conducive to health. SOPHE and its members advocate for and support the work of thousands of professionals who are committed to improving people's health where they live, work, worship, or play. We hope that this book helps advance these goals and helps guide and inspire a healthier world.

To the Instructor

An instructor's supplement is available at www.wiley.com/go/hpp2e. Additional materials such as videos, podcasts, and readings can be found at www.josseybasspublichealth.com. Comments about this book are invited and can be sent to publichealth@wiley.com.

ACKNOWLEDGMENTS

Health Promotion Programs: From Theory to Practice, Second Edition is a team effort. We acknowledge and thank Seth Schwartz, editor, and Melinda Noack, senior editorial assistant, at Jossey-Bass for their support, as well as Patricia (Tisha) Rossi, editor at John Wiley & Sons. We recognize and remember our friend Andy Pasternack (1955–2013), senior editor at Jossey-Bass's Public Health & Health Series, who fought cancer with the intelligence, passion, and humor that he brought to everything he did. Andy championed and supported the book's initial development and publication. We miss him.

We thank the chapter authors as well as their supporting organizations and families. We also recognize the staff of the Maximizing Adolescent Potentials Program in the Department of Health and Physical Activity, School of Education, University of Pittsburgh, for their support and effort on behalf of the text. We thank Dr. John Jakicic, chair of the Department of Health and Physical Activity, for his support, and we thank the Allegheny (Pennsylvania) Department of Human Services staff for their support and insights.

In addition, we appreciate and acknowledge the hundreds of SOPHE members and the SOPHE staff and board members who work to promote people's health worldwide. Thank you.

September 2016

Carl I. Fertman
Pittsburgh, Pennsylvania

Diane D. Allensworth
Snellville, Georgia

HEALTH PROMOTION PROGRAMS

PART ONE

FOUNDATIONS OF HEALTH PROMOTION PROGRAMS

CHAPTER 1

WHAT ARE HEALTH PROMOTION PROGRAMS?

Carl I. Fertman, Diane D. Allensworth, and M. Elaine Auld

Health, Health Promotion, and Health Promotion Programs

The World Health Organization (WHO, 1947) defined *health* as "a state of complete physical, mental and social well-being, and not merely the absence of disease or infirmity." While most of us can identify when we are sick or have some infirmity, identifying the characteristics of complete physical, mental, and social well-being is often a bit more difficult. What does complete physical, mental, and social well-being look like? How will we know when or if we arrive at that state? If it is achieved, does it mean that we will not succumb to any disease, from the common cold to cancer?

In 1986, the first International Conference of Health Promotion, held in Ottawa, Canada, issued the *Ottawa Charter for Health Promotion*, which defined health in a broader perspective: "health has been considered less as an abstract state and more as a means to an end which is expressed in functional terms as a resource which permits people to lead an individually, socially, and economically productive life" (WHO, 1986). Accordingly, health in this view is a resource for everyday life, not the object of living. It is a positive concept emphasizing social and personal resources as well as physical capabilities.

Arnold and Breen (2006) identified the characteristics of health not only as well-being but also as a balanced state, growth, functionality, wholeness, transcendence, and empowerment, and as a resource. Perhaps the view of

LEARNING OBJECTIVES

- Define *health* and *health promotion*, and describe the role of health promotion in fostering good health and quality of life.

- Summarize the key historical developments in health promotion over the past century.

- Describe the impact of Healthy People 2020 and the Patient Protection and Affordable Care Act of 2010 on health promotion.

- Compare and contrast health education and health promotion.

- Describe the nature and advantages of each health promotion program setting and identify health promotion program stakeholders.

- Explain how the evolving U.S. health care system and health technology create opportunities and challenges for health promotion programs.

health as a balanced state between the individual (host), agents (such as bacteria, viruses, and toxins), and the environment is one of the most familiar. Most individuals can readily understand that occasionally the host-agent interaction becomes unbalanced and the host (the individual) no longer is able to ward off the agent (for example, when bacteria overcome a person's natural defenses, making the individual sick).

Clearly, good health doesn't just happen; it's more than just luck. Although being born with good genes and having access to health care are important, they do not provide a guaranteed ticket to wellness. The food we eat, levels of physical activity, exposure to tobacco smoke, social interactions, the environment in which we live, and many other factors ultimately influence our health or lack thereof. The health of individuals and the health of our communities reflect the unique combination of biological, psychological, social, intellectual, and spiritual components as well as the cultural, economic, and political environments in which we live. Exploration of the interaction between individuals and their environment in regard to health has been a hallmark in the progress of nations in promoting and improving the health of individuals and the community at large. This ecological perspective on health emphasizes the interaction between and interdependence of factors within and across levels of a health problem. The *ecological perspective* highlights people's interaction with their physical and sociocultural environments. McLeroy, Bibeau, Steckler, and Glanz (1988) identified three levels of influence for health-related behaviors and conditions: (1) the *intrapersonal or individual level*, (2) the *interpersonal level*, and (3) the *population level*. The population level encompasses three types of factors: institutional or organizational factors, social capital factors, and public policy factors (Table 1.1).

Table 1.1   Ecological Health Perspective: Levels of Influence

Concept	Definition
Intrapersonal level	Individual characteristics that influence behavior, such as knowledge, attitudes, beliefs, and personality traits
Interpersonal level	Interpersonal processes and primary groups, including family, friends, and peers, that provide social identity, support, and role definition
Population level	
Institutional factors	Rules, regulations, policies, and informal structures that may constrain or promote recommended behaviors
Social capital factors	Social networks and norms or standards that is formal or informal among individuals, groups, or organizations
Public policy factors	Local, state, and federal policies and laws that regulate or support healthy actions and practices for prevention, early detection, control, and management of disease

Source: Adapted from McLeroy, Bibeau, Steckler, and Glanz, 1988.

The ecological health perspective helps to elucidate multiple levels of influence on individuals' behavior and recognizes that individual behavior both shapes and is shaped by the environment. Using the ecological perspective as a point of reference, health promotion is viewed as planned change of health-related lifestyles and life conditions through a variety of individual, interpersonal, and population-level changes.

Health promotion programs provide planned, organized, and structured activities and events over time that focus on helping individuals make informed decisions about their health. In addition, health promotion programs promote policy, environmental, regulatory, organizational, and legislative changes at various levels of government and organizations. These two complementary types of interventions are designed to achieve specific objectives that will improve the health of individuals as well as, potentially, all individuals at a site. Health promotion programs are now designed to take advantage of the pivotal position of their setting within schools, workplaces, *health care organizations*, or communities to reach children, adults, and families by combining interventions in an integrated, systemic manner.

This focus on planned change in health promotion is applied among individuals in varied settings and at any stage in the natural history of an illness or health problem. Using a framework proposed by Leavell and Clark (1965), health promotion programs can help prevent new cases or incidents of a health problem (for example, preventing falls among the elderly, smoking and drug abuse among middle school and high school students, or risky drinking among college students). These are programs that take action prior to the onset of a health problem to intercept its causation or to modify its course before people are involved. This level of health promotion is called *primary prevention*. Health promotion programs can interrupt problematic behaviors among those who are engaged in unhealthy decision making and perhaps showing early signs of disease or disability. This type of health promotion is called *secondary prevention*. Examples of this type of health promotion program include smoking cessation programs for tobacco users and physical activity and nutrition programs for overweight and sedentary individuals. Health promotion programs can improve the life of individuals with chronic illness (*tertiary prevention*). Examples are programs that work to improve the quality of life for cancer survivors or individuals with HIV/AIDS. Collectively, health promotion programs are a bridge between medicine and health and are part of an ongoing dialogue about how to improve the health and well-being of individuals across settings. Following are some examples of strategies for primary, secondary, and tertiary prevention applied in health promotion and disease prevention.

✳ Primary health promotion and disease prevention strategies include

- Identifying and strengthening protective ecological conditions that are conducive to health

- Identifying and reducing various health risks

✳ Secondary health promotion and disease prevention strategies address low-risk factors and high protective factors through

- Identifying, adopting, and reinforcing specific protective behaviors

- Early detection and reduction of existing health problems

✳ Tertiary health promotion and disease prevention strategies include

- Improving the quality of life of individuals affected by health problems

- Avoiding deterioration, reducing complications from specific disorders, and preventing relapse into risky behaviors

Health promotion programs are designed to work with a priority population (in the past called a target population)—a defined group of individuals who share some common characteristics related to the health concern being addressed. Programs are planned, implemented, and evaluated to influence the health of a priority population. The foundation of any successful program lies in gathering information about a priority population's health concerns, needs, knowledge, attitudes, skills, and desires related to the disease focus. At the planning stage, it is also important to engage schools, workplaces, health care organizations, and communities where the priority population lives and interacts to seek their cooperation and collaboration.

Finally, health promotion programs are concerned with prevention of the root causes of poor health and lack of well-being resulting from discrimination, racism, or environmental assaults—in other words, the social determinants of health. Addressing root causes of health problems is often linked to the concept of social justice. Social justice is the belief that every individual and group is entitled to fair and equal rights and equal participation in social, educational, and economic opportunities. Health promotion programs have a role in increasing understanding of oppression and inequality and taking action to improve the quality of life for everyone.

Historical Context for Health Promotion

Kickbush and Payne (2003) identified three major revolutionary steps in the quest to promote healthy individuals and healthy communities. The first step, which focused on addressing sanitary conditions and infectious diseases, occurred in the mid-19th century. The second step was a shift in community health practices that occurred in 1974 with the release of the *Lalonde report*, which identified evidence that an unhealthy lifestyle contributed more to premature illness and death than lack of health care access (Lalonde, 1974). This report set the stage for health promotion efforts. The third and current revolutionary step in promoting health for everyone challenges us to identify the various combinations of forces that influence the health of a population—the social determinants to health.

In the mid-19th century, John Snow, a physician in London, traced the source of cholera in a community to the source of water for that community. By removing the pump handle on the community's water supply, he prevented the agent (cholera bacteria) from invading community members (hosts). This discovery not only led to the development of the modern science of epidemiology but also helped governments recognize the need to combat infectious diseases. Initially, governmental efforts focused only on preventing the spread of infectious diseases across borders by implementing quarantine regulations (Fidler, 2003), but ultimately, additional ordinances and regulations governing sanitation and urban infrastructure were instituted at the community level. As an outgrowth of the New Deal in the United States, water and sewer systems were constructed across the nation. By the 1940s, the regulatory focus had expanded to include dairy and meat sanitation, control of venereal disease, and promotion of prenatal care and childhood vaccinations (Perdue, Gostin, & Stone, 2003).

As environmental supports for addressing infectious diseases were initiated (for example, potable water and vaccinations), deaths from infectious diseases were reduced. Compared with people who lived a century ago, most people in our nation and other developed nations are living longer and have a better quality of life—and better health. While new infectious diseases (e.g., HIV/AIDS, bird flu, MRSA, Ebola, Zika virus) have emerged since the end of the 20th century and continue to demand the attention of health workers, the emphasis of health promotion shifted in the last quarter of the 20th century to focus on the prevention and treatment of chronic diseases and injury, which are the leading causes of illness and death. This change was stimulated, in part, by the Lalonde report, which observed in 1974 that health was determined more by lifestyle than by human biology or genetics, environmental toxins, or access to appropriate health care. It was estimated that one's lifestyle—specifically, those health risk behaviors practiced by individuals—could account for up to 50% of premature illness and death. Substituting healthy behaviors, such as avoiding tobacco use, choosing a diet that was not high in sugar or calories, and engaging in regular physical activity, for high-risk behaviors (tobacco use, poor diet, and a sedentary lifestyle) could prevent the development of most chronic diseases, including heart disease, diabetes, and cancer (Breslow, 1999). With recognition of the importance of one's lifestyle in the ultimate manifestations of disease, a shift in the understanding of disease causation occurred, making *health status* the responsibility not only of the physician, who ensures health with curative treatments, but also of the individual, whose choice of lifestyle plays an important role in preventing disease.

The Lalonde report set the stage for the WHO meeting in which the *Ottawa Charter for Health Promotion* (WHO, 1986) was developed. This pivotal report was a milestone in international recognition of the value of health promotion. The report outlined five specific strategies (actions) for health promotion:

1. Develop healthy public policy.

2. Develop personal skills.

3. Strengthen community action.

4. Create supportive environments.

5. Reorient health services.

In the United States, the Lalonde report formed the foundation for *Healthy People: The Surgeon General's Report on Health Promotion and Disease Prevention* (U.S. Department of Health and Human Services, 1979), which sets national goals for reducing premature deaths. *Healthy People* is a public-private initiative, which has been updated every 10 years since its first release in 1980. (*Healthy People* is discussed in the next chapter section). In the subsequent 40 years since the first *Healthy People* report, the focus on the root causes of premature illness and death now include an understanding of the social determinants of health. Choices individuals make about individual health behaviors are determined not only by personal choice but also by opportunities or lack thereof in the places that they live, work, and play. This was also documented by the HHS Secretary's Task Force Report on Black and Minority Health (Heckler Report) in 1985, which revealed the existence of health disparities among racial and ethnic minorities in the United States.

In 1997, the *Jakarta Declaration on Leading Health Promotion into the 21st Century* (WHO, 1997) added to and refined the strategies of the *Ottawa Charter* by articulating the following priorities:

- Promote social responsibility for health.

- Increase investment for health developments in all sectors.

- Consolidate and expand partnerships for health.

- Increase community capacity and empower individuals.
- Secure an infrastructure for health promotion.

The *Jakarta Declaration* gave new prominence to the concept of the health setting as the place or social context in which people engage in daily activities in which environmental, organizational, and personal factors interact to affect health and well-being. No longer were health programs the sole province of the community or school. Various settings were to be used to promote health by reaching people who work in them, by allowing people to gain access to health services, and through the interaction of different settings. Most prominently, workplaces and health care organizations as well as schools and communities were now seen as sites for action in health promotion (WHO, 1998).

The third and current stage of health promotion started at the beginning of the 21st century with the realization that even within high-income countries there could a difference of almost 20 years in life expectancy—even in those countries that had a well-developed health care system providing care to all citizens (Kaplan, Spittel, & David, 2015). Individual decisions about health behaviors were rooted in the social environment in which people are born, live, work, and play (Marmot, 2005). The social institutions (economic systems, housing, health care system, transportation system, educational system), the surrounding environment, social relationships, and civic engagement all provide opportunities for individuals to make healthy choices—or not. One's opportunities for a healthy lifestyle are severely limited if there is no affordable low-income housing, no transportation infrastructure that allows individuals to pursue employment outside of their neighborhood, no supermarkets in the neighborhood with fresh fruits and vegetables, no safe parks in which to play or exercise, or no schools that provide a quality education in the neighborhood.

Today, health promotion is a specialized area in the health fields that involves the planned change of health-related lifestyles and life conditions through a variety of individual and environmental changes. Figure 1.1 illustrates the dynamic interaction between individual strategies and strategies for the entire population. In actuality, the distinction is somewhat artificial in that individuals constitute the population. Nonetheless, certain health promotion strategies are needed to effect changes in knowledge and skill so that population-based or environmental strategies is enacted. Although there is no question that regulatory and legislative actions generate the broadest potential behavioral changes within a population, these actions are difficult to enact and cannot be achieved without support from key stakeholders and individuals who are willing to contact their legislators to urge support for the proposed policy changes.

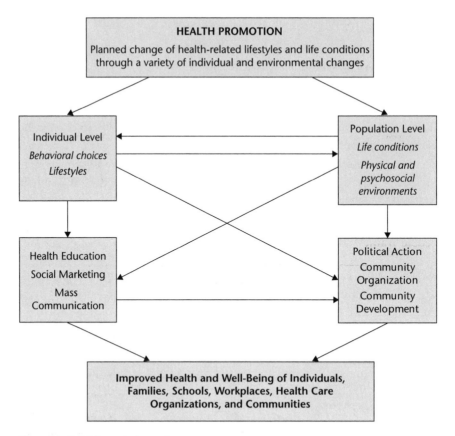

Figure 1.1   Health Promotion Interactions
Source: Adapted from Rootman and O'Neill, 2007.

Healthy People: A National Public-Private Partnership to Promote Health

Every decade since 1980, the U.S. Department of Health and Human Services has reinstituted the same public-private process and released an updated version of *Healthy People* that provides the overarching goals and objectives that will guide and direct the health promotion actions of federal agencies; local and state health departments; and practitioners, academics, and health workers at all levels of government. At the turn of the 21st century, *Healthy People* 2010 issued a comprehensive, nationwide health promotion and disease prevention agenda, which included for the first time the elimination of health disparities as a major goal.

Healthy People 2020, which was released in 2010 to be achieved by 2020, has the following goals:

◆ Eliminate preventable disease, disability, injury, and premature death.

◆ Achieve health equity, eliminate disparities, and improve the health of all groups.

◆ Create social and physical environments that promote good health for all.

◆ Promote healthy development and healthy behaviors across every stage of life.

For individuals engaged in health promotion, one value of the Healthy People framework is access to national data and resources. Because the initiative addresses such a broad range of health and disease topics, health promotion program staff can usually find objectives that are similar to those they are planning to address in their locales. Using Healthy People information allows program staff to compare their local population data with national data and to use resources that have been generated nationally in order to achieve the national objectives.

Like its predecessors, *Healthy People 2020* reflects continuing efforts on the part of national and various other health promotion program sites (see Figure 1.2). It helps set programming initiatives by federal public health agencies, as well as provides a framework for state and local public health departments to address risk factors, diseases, and disorders and also the determinants of health that affect the health of individuals across health settings. Furthermore, many other national nongovernmental health and educational organizations, philanthropies, and public and private universities consult the *Healthy People 2020* objectives when setting the direction for their respective health promotion programs. This decade's initiative engages nontraditional sectors such as businesses, faith-based organizations, state and local elected officials, policy organizations, health care organizations, and all others whose actions have significant health consequences. Health promotion is not just an activity for public health workers but an endeavor that requires the collaboration of traditional and nontraditional partners, particularly because understanding of the root factors of disease has expanded to include the social determinants of health (The Secretary's Advisory Committee on National Health Promotion and Disease Prevention Objectives for 2020, 2008).

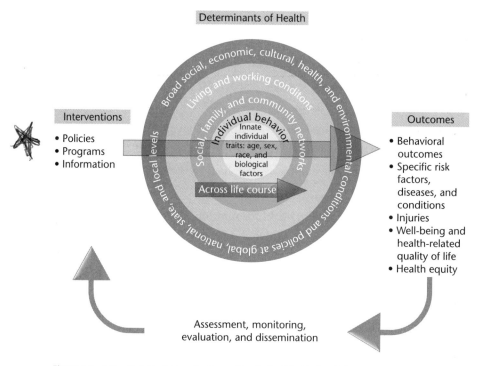

Figure 1.2   Action Model to Achieve the Overarching Goals of *Healthy People 2020*

Impact of the Patient Protection and Affordable Care Act on Health Promotion

The *Patient Protection and Affordable Care Act*, commonly known as the *Affordable Care Act* (ACA) passed in 2010, aims primarily to decrease the number of uninsured Americans (i.e., 47 million), making our country more equitable in its approach as well as reduce the overall costs of health care. The ACA provides a number of mechanisms—including mandates, subsidies, and tax credits—to employers and individuals in order to increase the coverage rate. Additional reforms are aimed at improving health care outcomes, reducing hospital readmissions, coordinating the delivery of health care, and emphasizing prevention—all to help reduce the overall cost of health care in the United States. The ACA requires insurance companies to cover all applicants and offer the same rates regardless of preexisting conditions or gender.

The ACA has a number of provisions that support a broad culture of health and health promotion across the United States. For example Section 1302 of the ACA provides for the establishment of an Employee Health Benefit (EHB) package. The law directs that the EHB be equal in scope to the benefits covered by a typical employer plan and cover at least the following 10 general categories: ambulatory patient services; emergency services; hospitalization; maternity and newborn care; mental health and substance use disorder services, including behavioral health treatment; prescription drugs; rehabilitative and habilitative services and devices; laboratory services; preventive and wellness services and chronic disease management; and pediatric services, including oral and vision care. Furthermore individuals can no longer be denied health insurance due to a preexisting health condition. And finally children up until the age of 26 can remain on their parents' health insurance. Previously it was age 21, if they were in college.

One significant element of the ACA is the creation and participation of patient centered medical homes (PCMHs) and accountable care organizations (ACOs), which relate to how we pay for health care. An ACO and PCMH are similar in that they are health care organizations characterized by a payment and coordinated care delivery model that seeks to tie provider reimbursements to quality metrics and reductions in the total cost of care for an assigned population of individuals. A group of coordinated health care providers forms an ACO, which then provides care to a group of individuals (i.e., employees). The ACO is accountable to the individuals and the third-party payer for the quality, appropriateness, and efficiency of the health care provider (McClellan, McKethan, Lewis, Roski, & Fisher, 2010).

The significance of PCMHs and ACOs for health promotion programs is a higher degree of accountability for program quality, appropriateness, and efficiency, as well as a focus on improved program outcomes. The expectations are now for health promotion programs (as well as all health care providers and services) to use evidence-based interventions and practices; reduce variability in strategies, methods, and resources use that cannot be clinically justified; increase coordination of programs through the use of information technology and team-based initiatives, while emphasizing prevention and disease management; and give individuals (employees) a stronger voice in their own health and health care and in defining what matters (McClellan et al., 2010). The ACO's utilization of case management and care stratification lend further support to fitting and tailoring health promotion programs to different populations of individuals at varied sites (Peels et al., 2014).

The ACA provides a variety of opportunities for health education (promotion) specialists (Society for Public Health Education [SOPHE], 2013). They can apply theories and models of behavior change to improve health behaviors; assist individuals to evaluate and select a health exchange, outreach to health providers, complete the enrollment process, and navigate the health system; and help connect patients who are being discharged from the hospital to locate community resources to help manage their condition. Health education specialists can develop health communication materials and strategies that are culturally/linguistically appropriate for populations; help develop coalitions and direct prevention grants/funding opportunities, e.g., tobacco, chronic disease, reastfeeding; and plan/conduct staff development and training, including recruitment, management, and supervision of community health workers. They can support individuals and ACO's that are required to have patient engagement and feedback (Figure 1.3). The ACA regulations require nonprofit hospitals to conduct community health needs assessments (CHNAs) every three years to maintain their nonprofit status. Health education specialists are being called up to develop and implement the CHNA surveys, as well as work with hospitals to ensure the community needs are addressed.

Health education specialists are an integral part of the health care team as their efforts help people to manage their health and prevent disease. However, since their work is not a distinct clinical service, it is not always recognized as reimbursable by third-party payers. In January 2014, the Centers for Medicaid and Medicare Services enacted a rule that allows state Medicaid programs to provide reimbursement of community

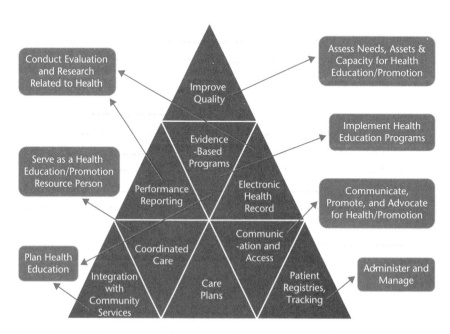

Figure 1.3 Health Educator Competencies that support ACOs
Source: SOPHE, 2013.

prevention services provided by nonlicensed practitioners (e.g., health education specialists). To be implemented, each state must amend its health plan to incorporate this rule. This represents exciting new opportunities for health education specialists in primary care, ACOs, and other settings. In summary, the ACA in its development and implementation provides a broader context and opportunities for promoting the health of individuals, families, communities, and workplaces that can help our nation achieve its health goals. Despite significant legislative and regulatory challenges that have occurred since the law was first enacted in 2010, ACA is moving forward in transforming the health care and health promotion.

Health Education and Health Promotion

Health promotion has its roots in *health education* (Chen, 2001). In the United States, health education has been in existence for more than a century. The first academic programs trained health educators to work in schools, but the role of health educators working within communities became increasingly popular in the 1940s and 1950s. Health education promotes a variety of learning experiences to facilitate voluntary action that is conducive to health (Green, Kreuter, Deeds, & Partridge, 1980). These educational experiences facilitate gaining new knowledge, adjusting attitudes, and acquiring and practicing new skills and behaviors that could change health status. The educational strategies are delivered through individual (one-to-one) or group instruction or interactive electronic media in order to promote changes in individuals, groups of individuals, or the general population. Mass communication strategies that might be used include public service announcements, webinars, social marketing techniques, and other new strategies from text messaging to blogging.

Health education as a discipline has a distinct body of knowledge, a code of ethics, a skill-based set of competencies, a rigorous system of quality assurance, and a system for credentialing health education professionals (Livingood & Auld, 2001). Approximately 250 professional preparation programs offer degrees in health education at the baccalaureate, master's, or doctoral levels. Health education was one of the first disciplines to engage in rigorous, scientific role delineation, a process that resulted in verified competencies for health education practice. The distinct occupation of health educator is recognized and tracked by the U.S. Department of Labor, which estimated that there were some 115,700 health educators in the workforce in 2014 (U.S. Department of Labor, Bureau of Labor Statistics, 2015). When health educators working in schools and businesses are added, the number is even greater. Employment of health educators is projected

Table 1.2   Components of Health Promotion Programs

Health Education to Improve	Environmental Actions to Promote
Health knowledge	• Advocacy
Health attitudes	• Environmental change
Health skills	• Legislation
Health behaviors	• Policy mandates, regulations
Health indicators	• Resource development
Health status	• Social support
	• Financial support
	• Community development
	• Organizational development

to grow 13 percent from 2014 to 2024, faster than the average for all occupations. Growth will be driven by efforts to improve health outcomes and to reduce healthcare costs by teaching people healthy habits and behaviors and explaining how to use available healthcare services. (U.S. Department of Labor, 2015).

Health promotion has been defined as the combination of two levels of action: (1) health education and (2) environmental actions to support the conditions for healthy living (Green & Kreuter, 1999). Environmental actions include strategies and interventions to promote political, economic, social, organizational, regulatory, and legislative changes that can improve the health of a population of people (Table 1.2). As noted earlier, the priorities for health promotion programs identified by WHO (1997) were promoting social responsibility for health, the empowerment of individuals, and an increase in community capacity, which requires consolidating and expanding partnerships for health within the community, securing an infrastructure for health promotion, and increasing investments for health developments in all sectors. Health promotion uses complementary strategies at both personal and population levels. In the past, *health education* was used as a term to encompass the wider range of environmental actions. These methods are now encompassed in the term *health promotion*, and a narrower definition of health education is used to emphasize the distinction.

Settings for Health Promotion Programs

Earlier in this chapter, we discussed the impact of the *Jakarta Declaration* in giving prominence to the concept of the health setting as the place or social context in which people engage in daily activities and in which environmental, organizational, and personal factors interact to affect health and well-being. Health is promoted through interactions with people who work in various settings, through people's use of settings to gain access to health services, and through the interaction of different settings.

Schools

Schools are pivotal to the growth and development of healthy children, adolescents, and young adults. School settings include child care; preschool; kindergarten; elementary, middle, and high schools; 2-year and 4-year colleges; universities; and vocational-technical programs. Young people spend large portions of their lives in schools. Increasingly, postsecondary institutions are sites where one can find nontraditional students (for example, adults seeking a career change or retired individuals seeking enrichment). The correlation between learning and health has been documented. Graduation from high school is associated with an increase in average life span of 6 to 9 years (Wong, Shapiro, Boscardin, & Ettner, 2002). It has been noted that as a nation, we could save an annual amount of more than $17 billion in Medicaid and expenditures for health care for the uninsured if all students were to graduate (Alliance for Excellent Education, 2006).

Health Care Organizations

Health care organizations provide services and treatment to reduce the impact and burden of illness, injury, and disability and to improve the health and functioning of individuals. Health care practitioners work with individuals in community hospitals, specialty hospitals, community health centers, physician offices, clinics, rehabilitation centers, skilled nursing and long-term care facilities, and home health and other health-related entities. Traditionally, these sites are thought of as being part of the health care industry, which is one of the largest industries in the United States and provides 13.5 million jobs. The U.S. Department of Labor (2015) reports that nine of the 20 occupations projected to grow the fastest are in health care. The roughly 545,000 establishments that make up the health care industry vary greatly in size, staffing patterns, and organizational structures. About 76% of health care establishments are offices of physicians, dentists, or other health practitioners. Although hospitals constitute only 2% of all health care establishments, they employ 40% of all health care workers (Reese, 2009). While health promotion programs might seem out of place in a treatment facility, in fact, much work is done in such facilities to reduce the negative consequences associated with disease.

✳Communities

Communities are usually defined as places where people live—for example, neighborhoods, towns, villages, cities, and suburbs. However, communities are more than physical settings. They are also groups of people who come together for a common purpose. The people do not need to live near each other. People are members of many different communities at the same time (families, cultural and racial groups, faith organizations, sports team fans, hobby enthusiasts, motorcycle riders, hunger awareness groups, environmental organizations, animal rights groups, and so on). These community groups often have their own physical locations (for example, community recreation centers, golf, swimming, and tennis clubs; temples, churches, and mosques; or parks). These affinity groups all exist within communities, as part of communities, and at the same time, they are their own community. Health promotion programs frequently seek out people both in the physical environment of the neighborhood where they live and within the affinity groups that they form and call their community.

Within a community, the local health department and community health organizations work to improve health, prolong life, and improve the quality of life among all populations within the community. Local and state health departments are part of the government's efforts to support healthy lifestyles and create supportive environments for health by addressing such issues as sanitation, disease surveillance, environmental risks (e.g., lead or asbestos poisoning), and ecological risks (e.g., destruction of the ozone layer or air and water pollution). The staff at a local health department includes a wide variety of professionals who are responsible for promoting health in the community: public health physicians, nurses, public health educators, community health workers, epidemiologists, sanitarians, and biostatisticians.

Community health organizations have their roots in local community members' health concerns, issues, and problems. These organizations work at the grassroots level, frequently operating a range of health promotion programs for community members. In this text, the term *community health organization* is synonymous with the terms *community agency*, *program, initiative, human services*, and *project*. Some community health organizations do not choose to use these terms in their names, deciding to use a name that reflects those whom they serve, the health issue they address, or their mission—for example, the American Cancer Society, Caring Place, Compass Mark, Youth Center, Maximizing Adolescent Potentials, Bright Beginnings, Strength and Courage, Healthy Hearts, or Drug Free Youth. Regardless of their names, the common bond for community health organizations is their shared health focus.

✳ Workplaces

Workplaces are anywhere that people are employed—business and industry (small, large, and multinational) as well as governmental offices (local, state, and federal). Workplaces are schools, universities, community-based organizations, and health care organizations. And increasingly it is clear regardless if an organization is for profit or nonprofit, art museum or hospital, it makes financial sense to encourage and support employees' healthy practices. Employers, both on their own initiative and because of the Affordable Care Act and federal regulations administered by the Occupational Safety and Health Administration, have been active in creating healthy and safe workplaces. As employers become aware that behaviors such as smoking, lack of physical activity, and poor nutritional habits adversely affect the health and productivity of their employees, they are providing their employees with a variety of workplace-based health promotion programs. These programs have been shown to improve employee health, increase productivity, and yield a significant value for employers (Fertman, 2015; National Institute for Occupational Safety and Health, 2009).

Stakeholders in Health Promotion Programs

Stakeholders are the people and organizations that have an interest in the health of a specific group or population of people. Stakeholders are people or organizations that have a legitimate interest (a stake) in what kind of health promotion program is implemented. First and foremost are the program participants, also called the *priority population* (for example, students, employees, community members, patients). The program is for their benefit and works to address their health concerns and problems. Although the authors of this book believe that the audience of any health promotion initiative is be regarded as the primary stakeholders, the term *stakeholders* traditionally has referred to other stakeholder groups that also have an interest in a program—for example, top civic, business, or health leaders in the community. The term *stakeholders* may also be used to describe the sponsoring organization's executives, administrators, and supervisors; funding agencies; or government officials. In other words, stakeholders in a health promotion program are people who are directly or indirectly involved in the program.

Involving Stakeholders

Involving the stakeholders in a health promotion program is essential for its success. Involvement creates value and meaning for the stakeholders—for example, enlisting stakeholders to assist in identifying a program's approaches and strategies in order to ensure congruence with stakeholders' values and beliefs will strengthen stakeholders' commitment to the program. Different stakeholders have different roles. Some stakeholders might help to define what is addressed in a program by sharing their personal health needs and concerns (a process called *needs assessment,* which is discussed in Chapter 4). Other stakeholders might offer services and activities in conjunction with the program (service collaborators). Stakeholders might serve as members of a program's advisory board or as program *champions* or advocates, roles that are often essential in creating successful health promotion programs.

Advisory Boards

Most health promotion programs form some type of *advisory board* or advisory group (also sometimes called a *team, task force, planning committee, coalition,* or *ad hoc committee*) to provide program support, guidance, and oversight. These groups look different across settings. Some are formal, with bylaws, regular meeting schedules, member responsibilities, and budgets. Others are informal, perhaps without any meetings but acting instead as a loose network of individuals who will offer advice and information when called upon by program staff.

Advisory boards play important roles at different points of planning, implementing, and evaluating a program. For example, during planning, advisory board members are involved with determining program priorities as part of the needs assessment, developing program goals and objectives, and selecting program interventions (Chapters 4 and 5). During implementation, they might participate in the initial program offering, program participant recruitment, material development, advocacy, and grant writing (Chapters 6, 7, 8, and 9). During evaluation they often review reports and give feedback on how best to disseminate and use the evaluation results and findings (Chapters 10, 11, and 12).

Who serves as a member of an advisory group? People with a genuine interest in the setting or program and who communicate well with others. Likewise, it is important to have a diverse group of individuals and organizations represented. Always consider the gender, ethnic, socioeconomic, language, and racial composition of the setting, organization, and community when selecting your membership. In addition, things like geographical boundaries, program representation, and community profile are key factors in the selection process.

Champions and Advocates

Health promotion programs often have champions whose advocacy provides leadership and passion for the program. The *champion* typically knows the setting, the health problems, and the individuals, families, and communities affected by the health problem. In the process of planning, implementing, and evaluating a program, champions provide insight into how the organization operates, who will be supportive, and potential challenges to implementing a health promotion program. They know the history of the health problem and what has worked before in solving it as well as what has not worked. (Frequently, champions are also called *key informants* because they know this important or key information about an organization.) Champions are the people who have initiated the effort to start the program, identify the health problem, or try to solve the problem (often volunteering their time and energy). They fight for resources, funding, and space for the program operations. Building a trusting and honest relationship with program champions, advocates, and key informants builds the foundation for the work of planning, implementing, and evaluating a health promotion program.

Health Promotion, Health Care, and eHealth

Health promotion programs exist within an evolving and complex health care system as well as a world of growing health technology. Going forward, changes and decisions made about health care and health technology is expected to impact health promotion programs across the many sites where they operate creating opportunities and challenges.

Today's health care system is dominated by large commercial interests driven by investors' demand for profit, by nonprofits almost equally focused on revenues, and by government policy decisions that are sometimes shaped by larger ideological, political, and budgetary concerns. For better or worse, health care has become big money and big politics. As a result, for the foreseeable future the structure and cost of health care in the United States will continue to be a problem. Over the last few decades health care spending has risen at rapid rates for both the government and the private sector. In 1970, it accounted for 7.2% of the nation's gross domestic product; by 2010, that had increased to 17.9% (Centers for Medicare & Medicaid Services, 2016). Fueling the boom are expensive new drugs and technologies, plus an increase in chronic conditions such as diabetes, asthma, and heart disease, which are costly to treat. Experts also cite unnecessary spending, with some estimating that 20% or more of total spending is tied to forms of waste, including overtreatment, failure to coordinate a patient's care among providers, and fraud. The consequences are higher costs and lower quality (Berwick & Hackbarth, 2012). Likewise for even the most sophisticated consumer the health care system is overwhelming. In the midst of rapid expansion of medical knowledge intended to benefit many, exists the concern that most individuals do not actually understand medical and health information and cannot navigate the health care system well enough to take advantage of health promotion programs and innovations to improve their health (Koh, 2015; Gawande, 2015).

eHealth is a relatively recent term connected with health promotion and health care practice supported by electronic processes and communication (Table 1.3). Usage of the term varies: some would argue it is interchangeable with health informatics with a broad definition covering electronic/digital processes in health, while others use it in the narrower sense of health care practice using the Internet. It can also include health applications and links on mobile phones, referred to as m-Health. Since about 2011, the increasing recognition of the need for better cybersecurity and regulation may result in the need for these specialized resources to develop safer eHealth solutions that can withstand these growing threats. The term eHealth can encompass a range of services or systems that are at the edge of health, medicine, health care, and information technology.

Table 1.3   What Is eHealth?

What is eHealth? eHealth is the use of digital information and communication technologies to improve people's health and health care. The increasing use of technologies, especially the Internet and mobile devices, to manage health highlights the potential of eHealth tools to improve population health. There are numerous tools and resources that fall under eHealth, including:

- Online communities and support groups
- Online health information
- Online health self-management tools
- Online communication with health care providers
- Online access to personal health records

Why is eHealth important? eHealth tools and resources enable health care consumers and their caregivers to improve health in a number of ways including:

- Real-time monitoring of health vital signs and indicators
- Managing chronic conditions
- Gathering information to make informed medical decisions
- Communicating with health care providers

Source: U.S. DHHS, 2014.

eHealth has the potential to be transformative for promoting the health of individuals, families, and communities. No longer are health promotion programs just at a given site (i.e., school, workplace, hospital) but rather can support individuals' engagement and full participation in promoting their health as well as being decision makers in their health care. eHealth is not limited to a physical place, and therefore health promotion programs are not limited to a particular site. They can and do exist in homes, schools, communities, and workplaces, thereby involving family, colleagues, peers, co-workers, and friends.

Summary

Health promotion programs are the product of deliberate effort and work by many people and organizations to address a health concern in a community, school, health care organization, or workplace. And even though individuals across these sites may share broad categories of health concerns focused on diseases and human behavior, each setting is unique. Effective health promotion programs reflect the individual needs of a priority population as well as their political, social, ethnic, economic, religious, and cultural backgrounds.

Health promotion programs represent an evolution that has passed through three revolutionary steps in the quest to promote health. Today, health promotion programs use both health education and environmental actions to promote good health and quality of life for all. The *Healthy People* initiative is a public-private partnership that allows local health promotion programs to link their health promotion programming with national data and information. Likewise, despite significant legislative and regulatory challenges that have occurred since the law was first enacted in 2010, ACA is moving forward in transforming the health care and health promotion.

Health promotion programs involve stakeholders, advisory boards, champions, and advocates in program planning, implementation, and evaluation in order to ensure effective programming. At the same time the evolution and complexity of the health care system and eHealth create both opportunities and challenges for health promotion programs.

For Practice and Discussion

1. What preliminary ideas did you have about the definition and role of health promotion programs prior to reading this chapter? How do these compare with what you have learned in this chapter?

2. Visit the *Healthy People 2020* website (http://www.healthypeople.gov/ HP2020). Pick a chapter and explore the objectives. As you explore the chapter think of your school and how you might use the Healthy People 2020 information for a specific objective to build a case for implementing a health promotion program to address the identified health concern on your campus. Prepare a brief (250-word) statement to use to support your argument for a program.

3. How has the ACA impacted your life and the lives of your family and friends? What ACA provisions promote health? How is the ACA and U.S. health care system related?

4. What do you think it would be like to work in a health promotion program? This chapter talks about health promotion programs in four different settings—schools, workplaces, health care organizations, and communities. Which setting would be of most interest for you in regard to working in a health promotion program? What is attractive about this setting and the people in the setting? Who would be the stakeholders in this setting?

5. What role does technology play in how you, family members, and friends promote your own health? When is the last time you used the Internet to find health information. What wearable health technologies (e.g., personal health devices) and apps do you use?

KEY TERMS

Advisory boards

Champion

Communities

ecological perspective

eHealth

Health

Health care organizations

Health education

Health promotion

Health promotion programs

Health status

Healthy People 2020

Interpersonal level

Intrapersonal level

Jakarta Declaration

Key informant

Lalonde report

Ottawa Charter

Patient Protection and Affordable Care Act or Affordable Care Act (ACA)

Population level

Priority population	Social determinants of health
Schools	Tertiary prevention
Secondary prevention	Workplaces
Settings	World Health Organization
Stakeholders	

References

Alliance for Excellent Education. (2006, November). *Healthier and wealthier: Decreasing health care costs by increasing educational attainment.* Retrieved from http://all4ed.org/reports-factsheets/healthier-and-wealthier-decreasing-health-care-costs-by-increasing-educational-attainment/

Arnold, J., & Breen, L. J. (2006). Images of health. In M. O'Neill, S. Dupéré, A. Pederson, & I. Rootman (Eds.), *Health promotion in Canada* (2nd ed., pp. 3–20). Toronto, Canada: Canadian Scholars' Press.

Berwick, D. M., & Hackbarth, A. D. (2012). Eliminating waste in U.S. health care. National Institutes of Health. Retrieved from https://www.icsi.org/_asset/y74drr/BerwickWedges2012.pdf

Breslow, L. (1999). From disease prevention to health promotion. *Journal of the American Medical Association, 281*(11), 1030–1033.

Centers for Medicare & Medicaid Services. (2016). The Medicare and Medicaid Statistical Supplement. Retrieved from https://www.cms.gov/research-statistics-data-and-systems/statistics-trends-and-reports/medicaremedicaidstatsupp/2013.html

Chen, W. (2001). The relationship between health education and health promotion: A personal perspective. *American Journal of Health Education, 32*(6), 369–370.

Fertman, C. (2015). *Workplace health promotion programs: Planning, implementation, and evaluation.* San Francisco, CA: Wiley.

Fidler, D. P. (2003). SARS: Political pathology of the first post-Westphalian pathogen. *Journal of Law, Medicine and Ethics, 31*(4), 485–505.

Green, L., & Kreuter, M. (1999). *Health promotion planning: An educational and ecological approach* (3rd ed.). Mountain View, CA: Mayfield.

Green, L. W., Kreuter, M. W., Deeds, S. G., & Partridge, K. B. (1980). *Health promotion planning: A diagnostic approach.* Palo Alto, CA: Mayfield.

Gawande, A. (2015, May). Overkill: An avalanche of unnecessary medical care is harming patients physically and financially. What can we do about it? *The New Yorker.* Retrieved from www.newyorker.com/magazine/2015/05/11/overkill-atul-gawande

Kaplan, R., Spittel, M., & David, D. (Eds.). (2015). *Population health: Behavioral and social science insights.* AHRQ Publication No. 15-0002. Rockville,

MD: Agency for Healthcare Research and Quality and Office of Behavioral and Social Sciences Research, National Institutes of Health.

Kickbush, I., & Payne, L. (2003). Twenty-first century health promotion: The public health revolution meets the wellness revolution. *Health Promotion International, 18*(4), 275–278.

Koh, H. K. (2015). The arc of health literacy. *Journal of the American Medical Association, 14*(12), 1225–1226.

Lalonde, M. (1974). *A new perspective on the health of Canadians.* Ottawa: Health and Welfare Canada.

Leavell, H. R., & Clark, E. G. (1965). *Preventive medicine for the doctor in his community* (3rd ed.). New York, NY: McGraw-Hill.

Livingood, W. C., & Auld, M. E. (2001). The credentialing of population-based health professions: Lessons learned from health education certification. *Journal of Public Health Management and Practice, 7*, 38–45.

Marmot, M. (2005). Social determinants of health inequalities. *Lancet, 365*, 1099–1104. Retrieved from http://www.who.int/social_determinants/strategy/Marmot-Social%20determinants%20of%20health%20inqualities.pdf

McCellan, M., McKethan, A. N., Lewis, J. L., Roski, J., & Fisher, E. S. (2010). A national strategy to put accountable care into practice. *Health Affiliation, 29*(5), 982–90.

McLeroy, K. R., Bibeau, D., Steckler, A., & Glanz, K. (1988). An ecological perspective on health promotion programs. *Health Education Quarterly, 15*, 351–377.

National Institute for Occupational Safety and Health. (2009). *Delivering on the nation's investment in worker safety and health.* Washington, DC: Author. Retrieved from http://www.cdc.gov/niosh/docs/2009-144/pdfs/2009-144.pdf

Peels, D., van Stralen, M., Bolman, C., Golsteijn, R., de Vries, H., Mudde, A., & Lechner, L. (2014). The differentiated effectiveness of a printed versus a Web-based tailored physical activity intervention among adults aged over 50. *Health Education Research, 29*(5), 870–882.

Perdue, W. C., Gostin, L. O., & Stone L. A. (2003). Public health and the built environment: Historical, empirical and theoretical foundations for an expanded role. *Journal of Law, Medicine and Ethics, 31*(4), 557–566.

Reese, C. D. (2009). *Industrial safety and health for people oriented services.* Boca Raton, FL: Taylor & Francis Group.

Rootman, I., & O'Neill, M. (2007). Key Concepts in Health Promotion. In I. Rootman, S. Dupere, A., Pederson, & M. O'Neil (editions) Health Promotion in Canada Critical Perspectives on Practice (3rd ed.). Toronto, Canadian Scholars' Press.

Secretary's Advisory Committee on National Health Promotion and Disease Prevention Objectives for 2020. (2008, October 28). *Phase I report: Recommendations for the framework and format of Healthy People 2020.* Retrieved from https://www.healthypeople.gov/sites/default/files/PhaseI_0.pdf

Society of Public Health Education. (2013). *Affordable Care Act: Opportunities and challenges for health education specialists.* Washington, DC: Society of Public Health Education.

U.S. Department of Health and Human Services. (1979). *Healthy People: The Surgeon General's report on health promotion and disease prevention.* Washington, DC: Author.

U.S. DHHS, Office of Disease Prevention and Health Promotion. (2014). What is e-Health? Retrieved May 15, 2016 from http://www.health.gov/communication/ehealth/

U.S. Department of Labor, Bureau of Labor Statistics. (2015). *Occupational outlook handbook, 2014–15 edition, health educators and community health workers.* Retrieved from http://www.bls.gov/ooh/community-and-social-service/health-educators.htm

Wong, M., Shapiro, M., Boscardin, W., & Ettner, S. (2002). Contribution of major diseases to disparities in mortality. *New England Journal of Medicine, 347,* 1585–1592.

World Health Organization. (1947). Constitution of the World Health Organization. *Chronicle of the World Health Organization, 1*(1–2), 29–43.

World Health Organization. (1986). *The Ottawa charter for health promotion.* Ottawa: Canadian Public Health Association.

World Health Organization. (1997, July 21–25). *Jakarta declaration on leading health promotion into the 21st century.* Fourth International Conference on Health Promotion: New Players for a New Era—Leading Health Promotion into the 21st Century, Jakarta, Indonesia.

World Health Organization. (1998). *Health promotion glossary.* Retrieved February from http://www.who.int/healthpromotion/about/HPR%20Glossary%201998.pdf

CHAPTER 2

ADVANCING EQUITY AND ELIMINATING HEALTH DISPARITIES

Francisco Soto Mas, Diane D. Allensworth,
Camara Phyllis Jones, and Holly E. Jacobson

Population Groups Experiencing Health Inequities and Disparities

Effective health promotion programs strive to promote health *equity* and reduce *health disparities*. Differences in health status among groups within a community are most often related to economic status, *race* and *ethnicity*, *gender*, *education*, *disability*, *geographic location*, or *sexual orientation*. Although genes, behavior, and medical care play a role in how well we feel and how long we live, the social conditions in which we are born, live, and work have the most significant impact on health and longevity. Similarly, the way we organize our communities, the "social structure," affects how we feel about ourselves and the role we play in the society. These social conditions that impact an individual's health status are known collectively as the *social determinants of health*, and they include the human and social capital as well as opportunities for equality in individual development and participation in community life.

Living in poverty is one of the major factors associated with poorer health status as well as lack of *access* to health care. Because more minority individuals live in poverty, they also experience difficulties not only in accessing basic health care but also in finding opportunities for quality education and fair employment conditions. These limit their individual development and the contribution they

LEARNING OBJECTIVES

- Define *health equity, health disparities,* and *social determinants of health* and explain their relevance to planning, implementing, and evaluating a health promotion program.

- Explain the connection between health inequities and health disparities.

- Discuss how society may contribute to health inequities.

- Define health literacy and explain how low health literacy may contribute to health inequities.

- Describe each of the four major categories for racial and ethnic disparities (societal, environmental, individual/behavioral, and medical).

- Discuss the term *race* as it relates to the distribution of health risks and opportunities in society.

- Discuss five strategies health promotion programs can use to reduce health disparities and increase health equity.

make to society. As a consequence, minority and ethnic groups experience more difficulties in maintaining their health and accessing quality health care and suffer disproportionately from diseases and conditions that otherwise could be prevented. If health promotion programs are to be effective, then it is essential that they identify the social conditions that relate to the problem and address the factors that contribute to health disparities among those individuals served by the programs. Elimination of health disparities constitutes an absolute priority in increasing life expectancy and improving quality of life in the United States. Thus, addressing social determinants of health and eliminating health disparities is essential in planning, implementing, and evaluating health promotion programs across all settings. Achieving health equity would occur when all individuals and groups have the opportunity to attain their full health potential regardless of their social position or other socially determined circumstance.

The foundation of any health promotion program is matching the program to people's health needs. Critical to making the match is recognizing that health status and health care vary among individuals and groups of people within the same community. Health professionals when planning programs need to consider how to address disparities (differences) in health status and health care as they consider the race, ethnicity, gender, age, income, education, disability, geographic location, and/or sexual orientation of the population of the recipients of their program.

Gender

It is obvious that some differences in health between men and women are biological, such as incidence and prevalence of cervical and prostate cancer. However, other differences are more difficult to explain. For instance, the reason why women live longer than men has not fully been explained. The World Health Organization noted that a baby girl born in 2012 can expect to live an average of 72.7 years, while a baby boy will only live to an average of 68.1 years. Similarly, women are more likely to be diagnosed with depression, while men tend to have more mental health issues with substance abuse or antisocial disorders (American Psychological Association, 2011).

Income and Education

In the United States, disparities in income and education levels have been associated with differences in the occurrence of many conditions related to ill health, including heart disease, diabetes, obesity, elevated level of lead in the blood, and low birth weight. National data also indicate that income inequality has increased over the past four decades (Stone, Trisi, Sherman, & Brandon, 2015). There are evident demographic differences in poverty by race and ethnicity (Table 2.1) as well as differences in educational (Figure 2.1).

Low education and income levels are associated with health illiteracy which has been identified as a critical factor contributing to health disparities (Paasche-Orlow & Wolf, 2010), and national data confirm that health disparities are exacerbated by the prevalence and severity of limited health literacy (U.S. Department of Education, 2006; U.S. Department of Health and Human Services, Office of Disease Prevention and Health Promotion, 2010). Health literacy is generally referred to as the ability to apply language skills to health situations at home, work, and the community. Ratzan and Parker (2000) defined health literacy as "the degree to which individuals have the capacity to obtain, process, and understand basic health information and services needed to make appropriate health

Table 2.1   Poverty by Race and Ethnicity, 2010

Population	Number of People Below Poverty Level and Below 125 Percent of Poverty Level	Percentage
All Races	43,569,000	14.3
Afro American	9,944,000	25.8
Hispanic (Any race)	9,243,000	25.3
White	29,830,000	12.3
Asian & Pacific Islanders	1,746,000	12.5

Source: U.S. Census Bureau, Current Population Survey, 2012a.

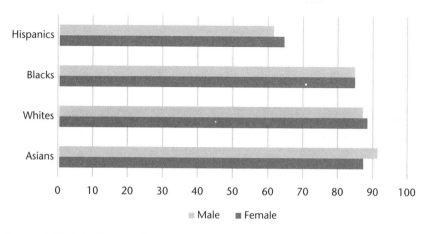

Figure 2.1   High School Educational Attainment by Race and Sex: 2010
Source: U.S. Census Bureau, Current Population Survey, 2012b.

decisions." Nutbeam (2000) divided health literacy into three levels: Level I, Functional Health Literacy; Level II, Communicative or Interactive Health Literacy; and Level III, Critical Health Literacy. These three sequential levels include not only basic reading, writing, and literacy abilities but also communication and social skills needed to critically analyze information and, ultimately, gain greater control over life events through individual and collective action.

Healthy People 2010 identified limited health literacy as a public health problem and recommended collaborations with adult educators and other community partners to facilitate the dissemination of health related information to the community. Healthy People 2020 continued this focus on reducing health illiteracy with another objective to "improve the health literacy of the population" (https://www.healthypeople.gov).

Disability

The Americans with Disability Act (ADA) of 1990 prohibits discrimination against people with disabilities in employment, transportation, public accommodation, communications, and governmental activities. ADA's nondiscrimination standards apply to people who have a physical or mental impairment that substantially limits one or more major life activities. Disabilities are categorized into communicative (vision, hearing, speech), physical (musculoskeletal and neuro-motor systems), and mental (learning, intellectual, degenerative) domains.

Nearly 57 million people in the civilian noninstitutionalized population in 2010 had a disability (Brault, 2012). There are disparities in the prevalence of disability among U.S. adults: from 11.6% among Asians to 29.9% among American Indians and Alaska Natives. Similarly, there are ethnic/racial differences on the self-perception of health for those with a disability: 55.2% of Hispanic adults with a disability report fair or poor health compared to 37% of non-Hispanic Whites and 25% of Asians (Centers for Disease Control and Prevention, 2008).

People with disabilities face barriers that limit their access to routine preventive care and are more likely to report anxiety, pain, sleepless-ness, and depression (Wilson, Armstrong, Furrie, & Walcot, 2009). Health professionals may need to make additional efforts to reach out to this population group, as people with disabilities are more likely to have behavioral health risks such as obesity, smoking, and being physically inactive, all of which can lead to poorer health and premature death. Adults with any disability were more likely to die of any cause compared to adults without any disability. Women with disabilities and those who are minorities experience additional social and environmental barriers that make them more vulnerable to certain health conditions. For instance, disabled women are more likely to suffer from pain, fatigue, osteoporosis, obesity, and depression. Disabled minorities are often said to be in double jeopardy because they have two characteristics, being disabled and being from a minority group, that place them at greater risk for health disparities (Jones & Sinclair, 2008; Zawaiza, Walker, Ball & McQueen, 2003).

Geographic Location

The place where we are born, grow up, and live has a strong influence on our health status. For example, international studies have found that geography has an important and independent influence on infant mortality and child malnutrition rates. Even in the United States, differences in physical and social environments are apparent and may account for the variations in illness and death (Centers for Disease Control and Prevention, 2015). In comparison with White children, Hispanic and African American children are more likely to live in communities near toxic waste sites. Further, African Americans are more likely to live in communities that are less likely to have parks, green spaces, walking or biking trails, swimming pools, beaches, or commercial outlets for physical activity such as physical fitness facilities, sports clubs, dance facilities, and golf courses (Robert Wood Johnson Foundation, 2009). Furthermore, those living in very poor neighborhoods often lack supermarkets with fresh produce. The differences in poverty rates by counties across the United States are displayed in Figure 2.2.

Health care access and quality of health care differ by neighborhoods. Figure 2.3 displays the results of the first-ever scorecard on local health system performance in the United States comparing 43 indicators spanning four dimensions of the health care system performance: access, prevention costs, treatment costs, and health outcomes. Comparing all 306 local hospital referral regions across the United States, the report found that access, quality, costs, and health outcomes all vary significantly from one local community to another, often with a two- to threefold variation in key indicators between leading and lagging communities (Radley, How, Fryer, McCarthy, & Schoen, 2012).

Sexual Orientation

Gay, lesbian, bisexual, and transgender (GLBT) people constitute a segment of our population with particular health concerns, including the highest rates of tobacco, alcohol, and other substance abuse. GLTB youth are more

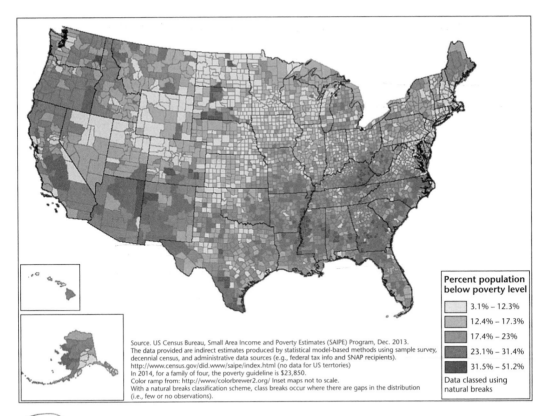

Percent population below poverty level

☐	3.1% – 12.3%
☐	12.4% – 17.3%
☐	17.4% – 23%
☐	23.1% – 31.4%
■	31.5% – 51.2%

Data classed using natural breaks

Source. US Census Bureau, Small Area Income and Poverty Estimates (SAIPE) Program, Dec. 2013.
The data provided are indirect estimates produced by statistical model-based methods using sample survey, decennial census, and administrative data sources (e.g., federal tax info and SNAP recipients).
http://www.census.gov/did.www/saipe/index.html (no data for US terrtories)
In 2014, for a family of four, the poverty guideline is $23,850.
Color ramp from: http://www.colorbrewer2.org/ Inset maps not to scale.
With a natural breaks classification scheme, class breaks occur where there are gaps in the distribution (i.e., few or no observations).

Figure 2.2 Poverty Rates by County, 2012
Source: Centers for Disease Control and Prevention, 2015.

likely to be homeless and 2 to 3 times more likely to attempt suicide. Lesbians are less likely to get preventive services for cancer and are more likely to be overweight or obese. Prejudice and lack of social acceptance contribute to violence and personal safety among GLBT people (U.S. Department of Health and Human Services, 2014).

Race and Ethnicity

Health disparities are well documented in U.S. minority populations for African Americans, Hispanics, American Indians, Alaska Natives, Asians, Native Hawaiians, and Pacific Islanders (Figure 2.4). It is important to keep in mind that the health disparities observed in these groups compared with the White majority population cannot be explained by biological and genetic characteristics or even by socioeconomic factors alone. Differences related to race and ethnicity have become a major focus of the national debate on health equity. The U.S. minority population in 2012 accounted for approximately 39% of the total population. By 2050, it is projected that

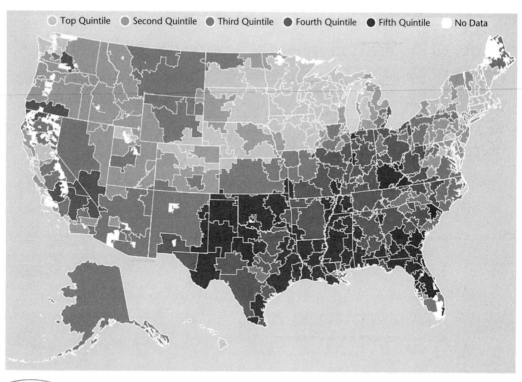

Figure 2.3 Performance of Local Health Care Systems by Quartiles
Source: Radley, How, Fryer, McCarthy, and Schoen, 2012.

they will account for more than half of the U.S. population (Haub, 2008).
✻This projection is significant, given that compared with non-Hispanic
Whites, racial and ethnic minorities are, in general, more likely to be
poor or near poor, less likely to have a high school education, and often
experience poorer access to care and lower quality of preventive, primary,
and specialty care.

Since 2003, the Agency for Healthcare Research and Quality (AHRQ)
has produced an annual report entitled the *National Healthcare Disparities
Report* (NHDR) which examines disparities in health care received by racial
and ethnic minorities, low-income populations, and people with special
health care needs. These reports measure trends in effectiveness of care,
patient safety, timeliness of care, and efficiency of care, tracking more than
200 health care process, outcome, and access measures, covering a wide
variety of conditions and settings. Disparities in quality of care are common
among Blacks and Hispanics who received worse care than Whites for
about 40% of quality of care measures, while American Indians/Alaska
Natives received worse care than Whites for one-third of quality measures.

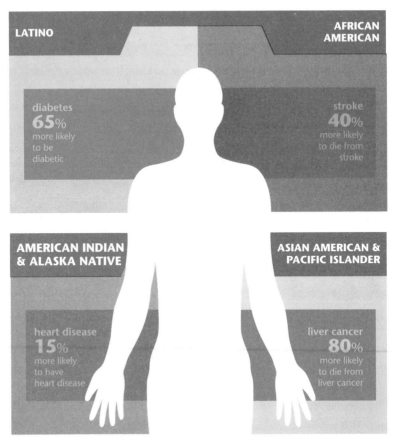

Figure 2.4   Illustrious Racial and Ethnic Health Disparities among Communities of Color Compared to Non-Hispanic Whites
Source: FamiliesUSA, 2014.

African Americans and American Indians/Alaska Natives also experience worse access to care than Whites for about 40% of access measurers, while Hispanics had worse access to care than Whites for about 60% of measures.

Understanding Racial and Ethnic Differences in Health

The Prevention Institute (2006) divided the causes for racial and ethnic disparities into four major categories: *societal factors*, which include poverty, racism, economics, health illiteracy, limited education, and educational inequality; *environmental factors*, including poor and unsafe physical and social environments, viral and microbial agents, exposure to toxins, inadequate access to nutritious food and exercise, and community norms that do not support protective behaviors; *individual and behavioral factors*, including sedentary lifestyles, poor eating habits, not wearing seat belts, and participating in high-risk behaviors such as smoking; and *medical care factors*, including lack of access to health care, lack of quality health care, and lack of *cultural competence* among providers.

Among the variety of causes of racial and ethnic disparities in health, racism is the one factor that needs some explanation. Race is a social construct, not a biological reality. Unlike age, neither race nor ethnicity have fixed, objective referents—that is, they have no scientific markers for anyone to verify but are terms that are self-adopted or imposed (Child Trends, 2015). In general, in the United States, one is assigned to a race based on the color of one's skin, which does not begin to capture the genetic and cultural differences among those residing in the United States who are assigned to the racial category of Black (Jones, 2001).

While we often characterize our American society as a great melting pot and while the relationships between individuals assigned to different racial categories have improved dramatically, race still governs the distribution of risks and opportunities in our society to a great degree. Jones (2001) describes three types of racism that affect health outcomes: institutionalized racism, personally mediated racism, and internalized racism. *Institutionalized racism* is described as differential access to goods, services, resources, and opportunities by race. For example, the majority of minority children attend high-poverty, underresourced schools, while the percentage of White children attending this type of school is much lower. *Personally mediated racism* is discrimination in which the majority racial group treats members of a minority group as inferior and views the minorities' abilities, motives, and intents through a lens of prejudice based on race. This type of racism is what most individuals think of when they hear the term *racism*. It manifests as lack of respect, suspicion, devaluation, scapegoating, and dehumanizing. *Internalized racism* is acceptance by members of the stigmatized race of negative messages about their own abilities and intrinsic worth. It manifests as self-devaluation, helplessness, and hopelessness, potentially leading to risky behaviors that can endanger a person's health.

Program Strategies to Achieve Health Equity and Eliminate Health Disparities Among Minorities

Health promotion programs that are designed with the goal of eliminating health disparities need to facilitate program participation. In order to do this, they first must establish rapport and cooperation by increasing participants' involvement in the designing of the program. Second, they must honor the program participants' autonomy, including people's right to retain their own cultural orientation in regard to their health.

Designing health promotion programs that address health disparities is important and fundamental work in changing people's health status and health care. In each phase of program planning, implementation, and evaluation, eliminating health disparities and achieving health equity needs to be a constant theme and consideration that permeates the process down to the smallest details and staff actions. To succeed, a health promotion program needs to be tailored to the people it serves. Successful customization of programs requires that program staff be aware of and sensitive to the culture of the program participants as well as incorporate and use *culturally appropriate* methods and interventions in the context of the culture.

To support the planning, implementation, and evaluation process, several strategies are available to health promotion program staff, stakeholders, and participants for reducing health disparities among racial and ethnic minorities. The strategies discussed in this section are overarching strategies to support program planning, implementation, and evaluation. These include (1) engaging minority groups and communities directly in addressing health issues, (2) creating culturally competent programs, (3) improving *cross-cultural staff training*, (4) recruiting and mentoring a diverse program staff, and (5) addressing *root causes of health disparities*.

As you move through the succeeding chapters of this text, think of these strategies as foundations on which to build and deliver health promotion programs.

The driving force for the strategies is the Office of Minority Health in the U.S. Department of Health and Human Services, which in 2011 published a strategic framework for achieving health equity (Table 2.2). While there is general acknowledgment that there needs to be equity in access to culturally and linguistically appropriate health care, there is a growing recognition that equitable health care in and by itself will not reduce health disparities. Attention must be directed to the economic, educational, and environmental inequities at the individual and the community level. ✳

Engage Minority Groups and Communities Directly in Addressing Health Promotion Issues

Talking with program participants and understanding their personal, cultural, social, and environmental realities provides the foundation for making sure that a program addresses the needs of the people it serves. Project *REACH* (Racial and Ethnic Approaches to Community Health) is one

Table 2.2   Regional and National Blueprint Strategies

Objective	Strategies
1. Awareness. Increase awareness of the significance of health disparities, their impact on the nation, and the actions necessary to improve health outcomes for racial and ethnic minority populations.	**1. Health Care Agenda.** Ensure that ending health disparities is a priority on local, state, regional, tribal, and federal health care agendas.
	2. Partnerships. Develop and support partnerships among public and private entities to provide a comprehensive infrastructure for awareness activities, drive action, and ensure accountability in efforts to end health disparities across the life span.
	3. Media. Leverage local, regional, and national media outlets, using traditional and new media approaches (for example, social marketing, media advocacy) as well as information technology to reach a multitier audience—including racial and ethnic minority communities, rural populations, youth, persons with disabilities, older persons, and geographically isolated individuals—to compel action and accountability.
	4. Communication. Create messages toward and appropriate for specific audiences across their life spans, and present varied views of the consequences of health disparities that will compel individuals and organizations to take action and to reinvest in public health.
2. Leadership. Strengthen and broaden leadership for addressing health disparities at all levels.	**5. Capacity Building.** Support capacity building as a means of promoting community solutions for ending health disparities.
	6. Funding and Research Priorities. Improve coordination, collaboration, and opportunities for soliciting community input on funding priorities and involvement in research.
	7. Youth. Invest in young Americans, to prepare them to be future health leaders and practitioners, by actively engaging and including them in the planning and execution of health initiatives.
3. Health and Health System Experience. Improve health and health care outcomes for racial and ethnic minorities and underserved populations and communities.	**8. Access to Care.** Ensure access to quality health care for all.
	9. Health Communication. Enhance and improve health service experiences through improved health literacy, communications, and interactions.
	10. Education. Substantially increase, with a goal of 100%, high school graduation rates by establishing a coalition of schools, community agencies, and public health organizations to promote the connection between educational attainment and long-term health benefits; and ensure health education and physical education for all children.
	11. At-Risk Children. Ensure the provision of needed services (for example, mental, oral, and physical health, and nutrition) for at-risk children.

(continued)

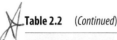

Table 2.2   *(Continued)*

Objective	Strategies
4. Cultural and Linguistic Competency. Improve cultural and linguistic competency.	**12. Workforce Training.** Develop and support broad availability of cultural and linguistic competency training for physicians, other health professionals, and administrative workforces that are sensitive to the cultural and language variations of racially and ethnically diverse communities.
	13. Diversity. Increase diversity of the health care and administrative workforces through recruitment and education of racial/ethnic minorities and through leadership action by health care organizations and systems.
	14. Standards. Require interpreters and bilingual staff providing services in languages other than English to adhere to the National Center on Interpreting for Health Care Code of Ethics and Standards of Practice.
	15. Interpretation Services. Improve financing and reimbursement for medical interpretation services.
5. Research and Evaluation. Improve coordination and utilization of research and evaluation outcomes.	**16. Data.** Ensure the availability of health data on all racial and ethnic minority populations.
	17. Authentic Community-Based Research. Invest in authentic community-based participatory research in order to enhance implementation and capacity development at the local level.
	18. Community-Originated Intervention Strategies. Fund the evaluation of community-originated intervention strategies for ending health disparities.
	19. Coordination of Research. Support and improve coordination of research that enhances understanding about and proposes methodology for reducing health and health care disparities.
	20. Knowledge Transfer. Expand and enhance knowledge transfer regarding successful programs that are addressing social determinants of health (for example, housing, education, poverty).

Source: National Partnership for Action to End Health Disparities, 2011.

example of how the federal government has encouraged a participatory approach to engage vulnerable populations who are experiencing racial disparities in addressing their own problems and reducing existing health disparities. Funded by the Centers for Disease Control and Prevention (CDC), Project REACH addresses a variety of priority health disparities concerns by (1) empowering and mobilizing community members to seek better health, (2) bridging gaps between the health care system and community members, (3) changing the social and physical environments of communities to overcome barriers to good health, (4) implementing evidenced-based strategies and public health programs, and (5) studying community systems changes. In turn, the funded communities have built and sustained effective long-term partnerships across community agencies, provided individuals with the tools to seek and demand better health care, shared lessons learned and best practices with other communities, and improved health care and reduced disparities in numerous communities, ✱proving that health care disparities are not inevitable and can be overcome (Centers for Disease Control and Prevention, 2010).

Create Culturally Competent Programs

Culturally competent programs facilitate all stakeholders—clients, patients, staff, families, community members—to access and engage with the goal of eliminating health disparities and promoting health equity. Actions and activities are required that honor the stakeholders, including their right to retain their own cultural orientation in regard to their health. At the same time, each organization has its values and ways of doing things, its own culture. Examples of organizational ideas that may get in the way of quality care include

- People who ask for help must be on time.
- Eye contact from the person seeking help is desirable.
- Paperwork is essential.
- Staff need to be distant and uninvolved with service recipients or applicants.
- All programs are suitable for all employees.
- Everyone needs be treated exactly the same.
- Employees seeking help need to follow our rules.
- The causes of problems are logical and rational.
- Experts know what is best for persons who ask for help.
- Drop-in care is impossible.
- Formal settings such as the workplace, hospitals, and clinics are the best places in which to provide care.
- Visiting hours in institutions need be limited.
- Medication is good.
- Mental health problems can be dealt with by strangers.
- People need to be responsible for paying for their health care.
- Technology is useful and not to be feared.

Table 2.3   Questions an Organization Needs to Ask When Assessing and Reflecting Upon Attempts to Be Culturally Competent

1.   How do staff, volunteers, and leadership represent the diverse population served by the organization?

2.   Do youth and families genuinely have a voice in program and service planning and implementation?

3.   Is there outreach to populations who are underserved or may not feel welcome or safe in approaching the organization?

4.   Are programs and services offered in neighborhoods and communities that are underserved or most greatly affected? If not possible, are connections made and networks built with local religious communities or businesses?

5.   Is the organization linguistically culturally competent?

6.   Does the organization aggressively advocate for the rights of all youth and families who are affected by the social problems (i.e., social determinants) of concern within the school community?

Culturally competent health promotion programs are not designed with the notion that "one size fits all"; rather, such programs offer a variety of alternatives and options to fit a variety of people. Individuals have access to as much choice as possible in a culturally competent organization. In addition, culturally competent programs realize and acknowledge that society has not always been fair to everyone and that oppression and discrimination are real. Culturally competent programs have as an underlying philosophy that each and every person deserves dignity and has value. An organization that wants to establish a culturally competent health promotion program needs to consider three critical points: (1) long before an individual becomes part of an organization, his or her health (physical and mental) has an established history; (2) organizations, neighborhoods, and homes shouldn't be hazardous to a person's health; (3) individuals need to have the opportunity to make the choices that allow them to live a long, healthy life, regardless of their income, education, or ethnic background (Robert Wood Johnson Foundation, 2009).

The list above (Table 2.3) includes six questions for organizations that want to assess their workplace health promotion programs and reflect upon the quality of their culturally competent practices (Fertman, 2015).

Improve Cross-Cultural Staff Training

Culture is the ways in which a group of people organize their beliefs and make sense of life, and is the glue that holds a community or group together. Cultural variations reflect what people hold to be worthwhile and help to determine what is believed about what is worth knowing and doing. The concept of culture is sometimes confused with concepts of race, color, or ethnicity.

A culturally competent system of care acknowledges and incorporates the dynamics of culture, an analysis of potential cross-cultural misunderstanding, a focus on interactions that can result from cultural differences and ethnocentric approaches, and the adaptation of services to meet specific cultural needs (National Alliance for Hispanic Health, 2011). A culturally competent person or organization validates similarities as well as celebrates differences. Some of the signs of a culturally competent person and organization include

- Being aware of personal assumptions, values, and biases

- Changing personal perceptions and behaviors as needed in order to respect the beliefs and values of others

- Respecting others' definitions of *family*

- Feeling and communicating empathy

- Being aware of barriers that the organization presents to persons from various cultures and addressing those barriers

- Seeking information about other cultures by reading, observing consultants from other cultures, and respectfully asking questions

- Using language that is deemed to be respectful by members of the group served

- Respectfully negotiating plans and approaches if there are differences of opinion

- Avoiding acting on stereotypes and unverified assumptions

- Striving to avoid offensive or hurtful language

- Approaching each person, family, culture, community, or group tentatively, seeking more information

Recruit and Mentor Diverse Staff

One of the strategies proposed for reducing health disparities is to boost the representation of minorities in the health care workforce (including health promotion programs). Having staff that look like the program participants is critical (staff selection is described later in this book, during the discussion of program implementation). The Institute of Medicine and the American Medical Association are actively seeking approaches to attract more minorities to medical schools to increase the pool and mentor minorities in a range of health professions. The National Institutes of Health and the Health Resources and Services Administration both support innovative, culturally competent approaches that encourage underrepresented minority and disadvantaged students to pursue a career in a health or allied health field.

At the other end of the health professional continuum of care the utilization of community health workers (CHWs) who are known by a variety of names—community health advocates, lay health educators, peer health promoters, outreach workers, and in Spanish, *promotores de salud*—has proven a useful strategy (U.S. Department of Health and Human Services, 2015). These community members often serve as the bridge between health care providers and the uninsured and underserved members of their community who often have lacked access to adequate health care. Because the CHWs live in the communities in which they work, they understand what is meaningful to community members, communicate in the language of the community members, and incorporate *cultural sensitivity* (e.g., cultural identity, traditional health practices), which help community members cope with their disease while promoting positive health outcomes.

Address Root Causes of Health Disparities

There are those who encourage health promotion program staff as they plan, implement, and evaluate their advocacy efforts to consider moving upstream and addressing the social determinants of health. A number of strategies are recommended.

1. *Increase high school graduation rates of poor and minority students.* Two major consequences for students living in a high poverty family include an achievement gap limiting students' success in school and a health disparities gap. These disparities are interrelated with students from families in the lowest quartile of income being about seven times more likely to drop out of high school than are their counterparts who come from families within the highest quartile of income. Children from poor families experience more chronic disease, infectious disease, childhood injury, social/emotional and behavioral problems, and violence compared to children who do not live in poverty. These health disparities increase absenteeism from school and affect learning. In addition, schooling for children in poverty is often substandard (SOPHE, 2012). Further, more teachers teaching minority students are not credentialed (U.S. Department of Education, 2014). Students of color also experience disproportionately higher suspension/expulsion rates, which increases the absenteeism rate of these students and which in turn contributes to failing classes and ultimately dropping out of school. To address educational inequities, the local health department and the local education agency could establish a community-wide school health council to

coordinate the health promotion activities of the community, linking the various health, social service, juvenile justice, and youth development agencies in the community to ensure that inequities in education are eliminated. Students who receive health interventions and other services have been linked with increasing academic success.

2. *Increase health literacy.* Health literacy requires that individuals have the capacity to obtain, process, and understand basic health information in order to make healthy choices and secure those interventions needed to prevent or treat disease. Low health literacy has been associated with poor self-reported health status in many diverse populations, including Latinos and Asian Americans, even when education and other well-established predictors of health status are controlled (Sentell & Braun, 2012). The problem is twofold. First, navigating the health care and health insurance systems with their jargon and terminology creates barriers to know where to go and what actions to take. Secondly, although there are many sources for health promotion information, individuals with low health literacy frequently have trouble taking the right medication and following prescribed health promotion assignments and programs (Koh & Rudd, 2015). In order to help individuals who have particular difficulty with health literacy, use jargon-free written materials, provide simple and understandable step-by-step instructions about health activities, and consider engaging English as a second language programs to address health literacy levels in their classes (Koh & Rudd, 2015; Soto Mas, Cordova, Murrietta, Jacobson, Ronquillo, & Helitzer, 2015).

3. *Improve air, water, and soil quality.* Environmental toxins that adversely affect health need to be reduced. For example, a healthier environment is achieved by reducing exposure to diesel particulates by prohibiting diesel trucks in residential neighborhoods, enforcing the no-idling law near schools, requiring the use of clean technology in new ships and trucks, reducing emissions in existing fleets, and implementing existing state and federal emissions regulations. Monitoring the impact of trucking and shipping activities needs to be expanded among low-income and vulnerable populations. Input from public health professionals on the impact of air pollution needs to also be incorporated in local land use and development decisions, using such tools as health impact assessments during planning phases (Health Trust, 2013).

4. *Improve housing options.* High-quality, affordable, stable housing located close to resources leads to reduced exposure to toxins and

stress, stronger relationships and willingness to act collectively among neighbors, greater economic security for families, and increased access to services (including health care) and resources (such as parks and supermarkets) that influence health. Policies need to be implemented that support transit-oriented development, along with incentives for mixed-use and mixed-income development. View one community's three-pronged plan to end homelessness at destinationhomesscc.org. (Health Trust, 2013).

5. *Improve transit options by providing incentives for use of mass transit and nonmotorized vehicle transportation.* Designing streets that are safe and accessible for all users (that is, *complete streets*) will encourage walking and bicycling. Enhancing the safety, accessibility, and affordability of mass transit is also essential. Increased use of these types of transit will decrease air pollution and increase physical activity, which will lead to healthier individuals and communities.

6. *Support healthy behaviors through increased opportunities to engage in physical activity and to access healthy foods.* Because physical activity is key to preventing disease and promoting health, policies are needed to encourage physical activity in school and facilitate after-hours use of school grounds and gyms to improve community access to physical activity facilities. Zoning laws and general plans need to be developed to improve the safety of parks, walking paths, and other recreational facilities in high-crime and low-income communities. In addition, provide support to ensure access to healthy foods in all communities through development of grocery stores in low-income communities; incentives for existing stores to offer more healthy food options, especially fresh produce; and incentives for alternative venues, such as farmers' markets and community or school-based produce stands.

Summary

Health disparities occur among various demographic groups in the United States, including groups delineated by gender, income, education, disability, geographic location, sexual orientation, and race or ethnicity. The federal government has led efforts to raise awareness of and identify potential solutions to reduce health disparities and achieve health equity. *Healthy People 2020* has identified reducing health disparities as one of the initiative's four main goals.

Effective health promotion programs address diversity with sensitive practice and awareness of program participants' cultural values and attitudes, resist stereotyping, and allow participants to communicate their views. Culturally competent programs are designed to eliminate health disparities and assess cultural practices that affect health status and health care while respecting cultural differences.

The five strategies for eliminating health disparities discussed in this chapter are overarching strategies that support program planning, implementation, and evaluation. These strategies are offered as foundations on which to build and deliver health promotion programs.

For Practice and Discussion

1. Compare and contrast disparities in health care among racial and ethnic minorities using the National Healthcare Quality and Disparities Reports as well as the 2014 infographic reports by FamiliesUSA (http://familiesusa.org/health-disparities) or the *National Healthcare Disparities Report, 2013* (http://www.ahrq.gov/research/findings/nhqrdr/nhdr13/index.html).

2. Discuss the consequences of being a member of two or more of the population groups who experience health disparities (for example, being a low-income African American with little education who has a disability). Begin using the *National Healthcare Disparities Report.*

3. Discuss the relative merits of implementing a health promotion program that addresses the major cause of death of a specific population or of implementing a health promotion program that addresses the root causes of that disease.

4. Culturally competent health promotion programs are not designed with the notion that one size fits all; rather, such programs offer a variety of alternatives and options to fit a variety of people. Culturally competent health promotion programs have an underlying philosophy that each and every person deserves dignity and has value. What are some ways that a health promotion program is culturally sensitive and respectful?

5. Using *About Health Literacy* (from http://www.hrsa.gov/publichealth/healthliteracy/index.html) discuss the impact on school health promotion programs (e.g. health education, physical activity and education, nutrition services, etc.,) when schools serve families and children who are not native English speakers.

6. How do health promotion program staff learn what is correct and respectful in building relationships with program participants?

KEY TERMS

Access	Income
Cross-cultural staff training	Individual and behavioral factors
Cultural competence	Institutionalized racism
Cultural sensitivity	Internalized racism
Culturally appropriate	Medical care factors
Disability	National Partnership for Action to End
Diversity	Health Disparities
Education	Office of Minority Health
Environmental factors	Personally mediated racism
Equity	Race
Ethnicity	Racism
Gender	REACH
Geographic location	Root causes of health disparities
Health disparities	Sexual orientation
Health literacy	Societal factor

References

American Psychological Association. (2011). *Study finds sex differences in mental illness.* Retrieved from http://www.apa.org/news/press/releases/2011/08/mental-illness.aspx

Brault, M. (2012). *Americans with disabilities: 2010* (Current Population Reports No. 70-131). Washington, DC: U.S. Department of Commerce, Economics and Statistics Administration, U.S. Census Bureau.

Centers for Disease Control and Prevention. (2008). Racial/ethnic disparities in self-rated health status among adults with and without disabilities—United States, 2004–2006. *Morbidity and Mortality Weekly Report, 57*(39), 1069–1073.

Centers for Disease Control and Prevention. (2010). *REACH: Finding solutions to health disparities.* Atlanta, GA: U.S. Department of Health and Human Services, Centers for Disease Control and Prevention. Retrieved from http://www.cdc.gov/chronicdisease/resources/publications/aag/pdf/2010/reach-success-stories.pdf

Centers for Disease Control and Prevention. (2015). NCHHSTP Atlas, slide 1: Poverty rates by county, 2012. Retrieved from http://www.cdc.gov/nchhstp/atlas/SDH-Slide-1.html

Child Trends. (2015, May 14). Measuring race/ethnicity. *Child Trends Indicator.* Retrieved from http://www.childtrends.org/?e-news=child-trends-indicator-spring-2015#news1

FamiliesUSA. (2014). Racial and ethnic health disparities among communities of color compared to non-Hispanic Whites. Retrieved from http://familiesusa.org/health-disparities

Fertman, C. I. (2015). *Workplace Health Promotion Programs: Planning, Implementation, and Evaluation.* San Francisco, CA: Jossey-Bass.

Health Trust. (2013). Initiatives of the Health Trust. Destination: Home. Retrieved from http://healthtrust.org/about/

Haub, C. (2008). U.S. population could reach 438 million by 2050, and immigration is key. Population Reference Bureau. Retrieved from http://www.prb.org/Publications/Articles/2008/pewprojections.aspx

Jones, C. P. (2001). Race, racism, and the practice of epidemiology. *American Journal of Epidemiology, 154*(4), 299–304.

Jones, G. C., & Sinclair, L. B. (2008). Multiple health disparities among minority adults with mobility limitations: An application of the ICF framework and codes. *Disability and Rehabilitation, 30*(12–13), 901–915.

Koh, H. K., & Rudd, R. E. (2015). The arc of health literacy. *Journal of the American Medical Association, 14*(12), 1225–1226.

National Alliance for Hispanic Health. (2001). *Quality health services for Hispanics: The cultural competency component* (DHHS Publication No. 99-21). Washington, DC: U.S. Department of Health and Human Services.

National Partnership for Action to End Health Disparities. (2011). *National stakeholder strategy for achieving health equity.* Rockville, MD: U.S. Department of Health & Human Services, Office of Minority Health. Retrieved from http://www.minorityhealth.hhs.gov/npa/templates/content.aspx?lvl=1&lvlid=33&ID=286

Nutbeam, D. (2000). Health literacy as a public health goal: A challenge for contemporary health education and communication strategies into the 21st century. *Health Promotion International, 15*, 259–267.

Paasche-Orlow, M. K., & Wolf, M. S. (2010). Promoting health literacy research to reduce health disparities. *Journal of Health Communication, 15*(Suppl 2), S34–S41.

Prevention Institute. (2006). *The imperative of reducing health disparities through prevention: Challenges, implications and opportunities.* Retrieved from http://www.preventioninstitute.org/documents/DRA_ReducingHDthruPrx.pdf

Radley, D. C., How, S. K. H., Fryer, A. K., McCarthy, D., & Schoen, C. (2012). *Rising to the challenge: Results from a scorecard on local health system performance.* New York, NY: Commonwealth Fund. Retrieved from http://www.commonwealthfund.org/Publications/Fund-Reports/2012/Mar/Local-Scorecard.aspx

Ratzan, S. C., & Parker, R. M. (2000). Introduction. In C. R. Selden, M. Zorn, S. C. Ratzan, & R. M. Parker (Eds.), *National library of medicine current bibliographies in medicine: Health literacy.* Vol. NLM Pub. No. CBM 2000-1. Bethesda, MD: National Institutes of Health, U.S. Department of Health and Human Services.

Robert Wood Johnson Foundation. (2009). *Beyond health care: New directions to a healthier America.* Retrieved from http://www.rwjf.org/en/library/research/2009/04/beyond-health-care.html

Sentell, T., & Braun, K. (2012). Low health literacy, limited English proficiency, and health status in Asians, Latinos, and other racial/ethnic groups in California. *Journal of Health Communication, 17*(3), 82–99.

Society for Public Health Education (SOPHE). (2012). *Reducing youth health disparities requires cross agency collaboration.* Washington, DC: Society for Public Health Education. Retrieved from http://www.sophe.org/Cross-AgencyCollaborationYHD_final.pdf

Soto Mas, F., Cordova, C., Murrietta, A., Jacobson, H. E., Ronquillo, F., & Helitzer, D. A. (2015). Multisite community-based health literacy intervention for Spanish speakers. *Journal of Community Health, 40*(3), 431–438.

Stone, C., Trisi, D., Sherman, A., & Brandon, D. (2015). *A guide to statistics on historical trends in income inequality.* Center on Budget & Policy Priorities. Retrieved from http://www.cbpp.org/research/poverty-and-inequality/a-guide-to-statistics-on-historical-trends-in-income-inequality

U.S. Census Bureau, Current Population Survey. (2012a). Available at https://www.census.gov/compendia/statab/2012/tables/12s0710.pdf

U.S. Census Bureau, Current Population Survey. (2012b). Table 229 Educational Attainment by Race and Hispanic Origin: 1970 to 2010. *Statistical Abstract.* Retrieved from https://www.census.gov/compendia/statab/cats/education/educational_attainment.html

U.S. Department of Education. (2006). *National Assessment of Adult Literacy (NAAL): A first look at the literacy of America's adults in the 21st century* (NCES Publication No. 2006-470). Washington, DC: Institute of Education Sciences.

U.S. Department of Education. (2014). Data snapshot: Teacher equity. *Issue Brief,* No. 4 (March 2014). Civil Rights Data Collection. Retrieved from http://ocrdata.ed.gov/Downloads/CRDC-Teacher-Equity-Snapshot.pdf

U.S. Department of Health and Human Services. (2015). *About health literacy.* Retrieved from http://www.hrsa.gov/publichealth/healthliteracy/healthlitabout.html

U.S. Department of Health and Human Services, Office of Disease Prevention and Health Promotion. (2010). *National action plan to improve health literacy.* Washington, DC: Author.

U.S. Department of Health and Human Services. (2014). Lesbian, gay, bisexual, and transgender health. *Healthy People 2020.* Retrieved from http://www.healthypeople.gov/2020/topics-objectives/topic/lesbian-gay-bisexual-and-transgender-health

U.S. Department of Health and Human Services. (2015). *Promotores de Salud Initiative.* Retrieved from http://minorityhealth.hhs.gov/omh/content.aspx?ID=8929

Wilson, A. M., Armstrong, C. D., Furrie, A., & Walcot, E. (2009). The mental health of Canadians with self-reported learning disabilities. *Journal of Learning Disabilities, 42*(1), 24–40.

Zawaiza, T., Walker, S., Ball, S., & McQueen, M. F. (2003). Diversity matters: Infusing issues of people with disabilities from underserved communities into a trans-disciplinary research agenda in the behavioral sciences. In F. E. Menz & D. F. Thomas (Eds.), *Bridging the gaps: Refining the disability research agenda for rehabilitation and the social sciences—Conference proceedings* (pp. 279–312). Menomonie: University of Wisconsin–Stout, Stout Vocational Rehabilitation Institute, Research and Training Centers.

CHAPTER 3

THEORY IN HEALTH PROMOTION PROGRAMS

Melissa Grim and Brian Hortz

Theory in Health Promotion Programs

Theories provide the conceptual basis on which health promotion programs are built, and guide the actual process of planning, implementing, and evaluating a program. The strongest programs focus on both purposes. Conversely, in the absence of theories it is difficult to identify how health promotion programs affect factors that influence health at individual, family setting, or societal levels. Theories used in the field of health education and promotion are derived from multiple disciplines, including education, sociology, psychology, anthropology, and public health. Health promotion theories are used to guide interventions that are delivered in multiple settings, including schools, communities, work sites, health care organizations, homes, and the consumer marketplace (Glanz, Rimer, & Viswanath, 2015). Understanding the history, purpose, constructs, and use of the prominent health theories provides the knowledge necessary to select the most appropriate theory to guide the development, implementation, and evaluation of health promotion programs (Goodson, 2010).

Kerlinger (1986) defines a *theory* as "a set of interrelated concepts, definitions and propositions that present a systematic view of events or situations by specifying relationships among variables in order to explain and predict the events or situations" (p. 25). Theories help us articulate assumptions and hypotheses regarding the strategies and focus of interventions. In health promotion we are primarily interested in predicting or explaining changes in *behaviors* or environments. Sometimes health promotion

LEARNING OBJECTIVES

- Define and explain the role of ideas, concepts, constructs, and variables in the development and support of a theory.

- Summarize the essential constructs of intrapersonal, interpersonal, and population-level theories and models.

- Apply theoretical constructs when developing health education or promotion activities or programs.

- Describe the leading models of contemporary health promotion program planning, implementation, and evaluation and suggest how they might be used in practice.

practitioners and researchers combine two or more theories to address a specific problem, event, or situation; when this occurs, health *models* are formed (Glanz, Rimer, & Viswanath, 2015; Hayden, 2014).

Theories are rooted in concepts or ideas that are abstract entities. They are not measurable or observable. *Concepts* are adopted and formed in theories and are considered the primary components of a theory (Glanz, Rimer, & Viswanath, 2015). Concepts that have been developed and tested over time and are components of theories are referred to as *constructs*. For example, in the theory of reasoned action and theory of planned behavior, behavioral intention is a construct. And when a construct is defined with specificity and can be measured, it becomes an indicator or *variable*. Converting a theory construct into a variable allows the construct to be refined through empirical testing. This empirical testing allows for relationships between constructs and a specific behavior to be explored. By exploring association with as well as mediation and moderation of these constructs and the behavior, health educators obtain a better knowledge of how the theory links to the specific behavior. Valuable constructs of theories must be able to explain phenomena, which for health promotion are behaviors and environmental conditions.

Theories in the early 1970s and 1980s focused primarily on the characteristics, risk factors, demographic characteristics, and life stages of individuals. Theories in the 1980s evolved to focus not only on characteristics of individuals but also on an increased recognition that behaviors take place in a social, physical, and environmental context. Prominent in the 1990s were models that identify steps in planning, implementing, and evaluating health promotion programs. The health theories and models presented in this chapter reflect this evolution of health promotion. Because health is dynamic, so too are theories. Likewise, these theories represent different paradigms. They were formed to address a range of health concerns, needs, and situations, and therefore they are used in different ways. Theories are an important tool for health practitioners and researchers as they address health concerns, problems, and situations.

This chapter first presents theories and models most used in health promotion programs. These foundational theories focus on one or more of the three levels of influence to consider in developing health promotion programs: intrapersonal (individual), interpersonal, and community or population (Hayden, 2014). When health promotion programs focus on multiple levels, they reflect the ecological perspective of health promotion that emphasizes the interaction between and interdependence of factors within and across all levels of a health problem. In other words, people are influenced at a number of levels and an individual's behavior both shapes and is shaped by the social environment.

Second, this chapter presents health models that focus on the process of developing a health promotion program. Such models guide planning, implementation, and evaluation of health promotion programs. The strongest health promotion programs use both foundational theories and models and planning models.

Foundational Theories/Models: Intrapersonal Level

The most basic level of health theory is the intrapersonal level. When we are designing or working in a program, it is critical to understand how the theory underlying or directing the program would work at an individual level. Ideally, individual health theories provide the framework for the approach (that is, methodology) in the classroom, in the group setting, and in the development of health promotion materials. In addition to structuring interventions, theories help us address intrapersonal factors such as knowledge, attitudes, beliefs, motivation, self-concept, and skills. The major intrapersonal health theories are highlighted in this section: the health belief model, the theory of reasoned action/planned behavior, and the integrative model, and the transtheoretical model and stages of change.

Health Belief Model

The *health belief model*, one of the more widely researched models, originated in the 1950s as a way to understand health-seeking behaviors (Rosenstock, 1974). In particular, it grew from work that sought to understand why very few people were participating in free and available disease detection programs. According to this model, a person's action to change his or her behavior (or lack of action) results from the person's evaluation of several constructs. First, a person decides if he or she is susceptible (*perceived susceptibility*) to a disease or condition, and weighs this against the severity of the disease or condition (*perceived severity*). For example, if a person believes that he or she is susceptible and the disease is severe enough to motivate him or her to change, he or she is more likely to take action to change. Alternatively, if a person does not believe he or she is susceptible, even though the disease might be severe, he or she will likely not act. A person also weighs the benefits of action to change (*perceived benefits*) versus the barriers to change (*perceived barriers*), and this analysis is the strongest predictive factor for behavior change (Sugg Skinner, Tiro, & Champion, 2015). If a person believes that the benefits outweigh the barriers, then he or she is more likely to take action to change. *Cues to action*, such as instructions or reminders, can also be used to facilitate change. The health belief model also takes other factors such as age, gender, and personality into account, with the assumption that these factors can influence a person's motivation to change behavior. *Self-efficacy*, a person's belief that he or she can engage in a behavior (Bandura, 1986), was added later as a factor in behavior maintenance (Rosenstock, Strecher, & Becker, 1988). The original health belief model was tested on short-term health-seeking behaviors and appears to have greater associations with these types of shorter-term behaviors. For more complex lifestyle health behavior such as regular physical activity, other theories allow for more complex understanding of the mechanisms involved in those behaviors. Recent research suggests a need to expand the health belief model (Orji, Vassileva, & Mandryk, 2012) to create a model that is more predictive of behavior.

Theory of Planned Behavior, Theory of Reasoned Action, and the Integrated Behavioral Model

The theory of planned behavior, a derivative of the theory of reasoned action, postulates that people are motivated to change based on their perceptions of norms, attitudes, and control over behaviors. Each of these factors can either increase or decrease a person's intent to change his or her behavior. Intention to change behavior, then, is thought to be directly related to behavior change.

Table 3.1 shows several important constructs that are involved in these value-expectancy theories: *attitude*, *subjective norm*, *perceived behavioral control*, *intention*, and *behavior* (Montano & Kasprzyk, 2015). Figure 3.1 shows the theory of planned behavior explanation of how behavioral intention determines behavior, and how attitude toward behavior, subjective norm, and perceived behavioral control influence behavioral intention.

Table 3.1   Constructs in the Theory of Planned Behavior, Theory of Reasoned Action, and the Integrated Behavior Model

External variables	Demographic variables, specific attitudes, personality, and other variables that can influence attitudes; subjective norm or perceived behavioral control
Attitude	Comprises a person's beliefs that the behavior will lead to certain outcomes as well as the value the individual places on those outcomes
Subjective norm	Comprises a person's perception of a social norm and his or her motivation to comply with that perceived norm
Perceived behavioral control	Comprises beliefs about facilitators or barriers and how easy or difficult it would be to change behavior in the face of those facilitators or barriers
Intention	The probability that a person will perform a behavior
Behavior	Single, observable action performed by an individual, or a category of actions with a specification of target, action, context, and time (TACT)

According to the theory, attitudes toward behavior are shaped by beliefs about what is required to perform the behavior and outcomes of the behavior. Beliefs about social standards and motivation to comply with those norms affect subjective norms. The presence or lack of things that will make it easier or harder to perform the behaviors affects perceived behavioral control. Thus a chain of beliefs, attitudes, and intentions drives behavior.

In a revision to the theory of reasoned action/planned behavior, Fishbein (2008) presents an integrated behavioral model, where distal factors such as demographic variables, attitudes, personality traits, and other individual variables are included to show their influence on beliefs. Proximal constructs are those that directly influence either intention or behavior (such as environment or skills). Additionally in the integrated behavioral model, perceived behavioral control is equated to self-efficacy, a more commonly known and widely used construct in health behavior research (Fishbein, 2008).

The strength of the relationship between the first three constructs in Table 3.1 and intention and behavior varies. A growing body of research has established what is being termed as the "planning-behavior gap" or the "intention-behavior gap" (Fernandez, Fleig, Godinho, Montenegro, Knoll, & Schwarzer 2015; Rhodes & Bruijn, 2013). Such research proposes the addition of action control variables to bridge this gap between planning and intention and actual behavior change (Fernandez et al., 2015).

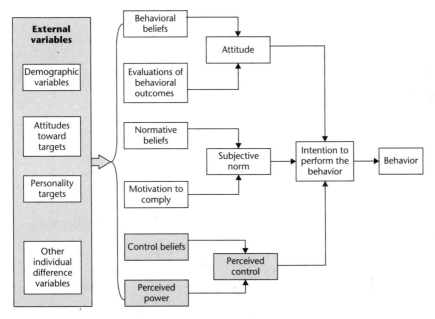

Figure 3.1 Theory of Planned Behavior and Theory of Reasoned Action, Integrated Behavioral Model
Source: Montano and Kasprzyk, 2015. Reprinted with permission of John Wiley & Sons, Inc.

Transtheoretical Model and Stages of Change

The *transtheoretical model* was developed in the early 1980s as a way to understand behavior change—in particular, change associated with addictive behavior (Prochaska, DiClemente, & Norcross, 1992). The transtheoretical model proposes that behavior change is a process that occurs in stages; a person moves through these stages in a very specific sequence using different strategies. The *stages of change* are one of the transtheoretical model constructs. The stages are precontemplation, contemplation, preparation, action, and maintenance. In the *precontemplation* stage, a person is not planning a behavior change within the next 6 months. In the *contemplation* stage, a person begins to consider behavior change and is intending to change within 6 months. In *preparation*, a person is planning a behavior change within the next month. In the *action* stage, a person has initiated a behavior change but has done so for 6 months or less. In *maintenance*, a person has maintained the behavior change for at least 6 months but less than 5 years. People move forward or backward (relapse) through the stages. The dimension of time—that is, each of the stages being associated with a specific time frame—is unique to the transtheoretical model.

This model postulates that *processes of change*, constructs that are used to facilitate behavior change during different stages of change (Prochaska, Redding, & Evers, 2015), help people move from one stage to the next. Table 3.2 lists the processes of change.

Throughout the entire process of changing behavior, people weigh the benefits and drawbacks of behavior change. This construct, called

Table 3.2 Transtheoretical Model Construct: Processes of Change

...ges	Process	Definition
Precontemplation to Contemplation	Consciousness raising	Increasing awareness of health factors
	Dramatic relief	No longer experiencing negative emotions
	Environmental reevaluation	Realizing the impact of a behavior on one's environment
Contemplation to preparation	Self-reevaluation	Understanding the personal impact of the behavior change
Preparation, action, maintenance	Self-liberation	Making a commitment to change
Maintenance	Counter-conditioning	Behavioral substitution
	Helping relationships	Social support
	Reinforcement management	Using and modifying reinforcement strategies
	Stimulus control	Manipulating cues for behavior change

decisional balance, is fluid throughout the process. For example, in the precontemplation stage, a person might associate more negatives than positives with a behavior change. A person moving through this stage to subsequent stages and to the action stage might find there are more positives than negatives associated with behavior change. When the perceived benefits outweigh the perceived barriers, action occurs.

Other transtheoretical model constructs appear to be linked to behavior progression across many stages. Two such constructs are *self-efficacy* (Bandura, 1986) and *temptation*. Temptation refers to the urge to engage in unhealthy behavior when confronted with a difficult situation (Prochaska, Redding, & Evers, 2015). Temptation is represented by three factors that denote the most common types of tempting situations: negative affect or emotional distress, positive social situations, and craving.

Foundational Theories/Models: Interpersonal Level

The second level of health theories and models focuses on individuals within their social environment. Our social environment includes the people with whom we interact and live in our daily lives (for example, family members, coworkers, friends, peers, teachers, clergy, health professionals). These theories and models recognize that we are influenced and influence others through personal opinions, beliefs, behavior, advice, and support, which in turn influence our health and that of others. This section discusses two theories that explore these reciprocal effects of relationships on our health behavior: *social cognitive theory* and *social network and social support theory*.

Social Cognitive Theory

Social cognitive theory (SCT; Bandura, 1986) evolved from social learning theory, which was created by Albert Bandura in the early 1960s (Bandura & Walters, 1963). SCT (Bandura, 1986) defines human behavior as an interaction of personal factors, behavior, and the environment. SCT theory is the most frequently used paradigm in health promotion. This theory is based on the reciprocal determinism between behavior, environment, and person; their constant interactions constitute the basis for human action. Bandura posits that individuals learn from their interactions and observations (Bandura, 1986). According to this theory, an individual's behavior is uniquely determined by each of these three factors (Bandura, 1986):

Personal factors: A person's expectations, beliefs, self-perceptions, goals, and intentions shape and direct behavior.

Environmental factors: Human expectations, beliefs, and cognitive competencies are developed and modified by social influences and physical structures within the environment.

Behavioral factors: A person's behavior will determine the aspects of the person's environment to which the person is exposed, and behavior is, in turn, modified by that environment.

Bandura has identified several important constructs in SCT, including the *environment, situations, behavioral capacity, outcome expectations, outcome expectancies, self-control, observational learning, self-efficacy,* and *emotional coping.* Each of these constructs is defined in Table 3.3.

APPLICATION ACTIVITY: SOCIAL COGNITIVE THEORY

Locate a peer-reviewed journal article focusing on the use of SCT in explaining, predicting, or attempting to increase physical activity levels.

1. What type of study is being conducted? What evidence did you use to make your decision?

2. How are the constructs defined?

3. How are the constructs measured?

4. Describe the purpose and methodology.

5. Describe the findings with respect to the limitations of the study.

In small groups, discuss the strengths and weaknesses of the study, specifically in regard to methodology and measurement. What areas of future study do you identify as needed after your discussion?

According to Bandura (1986), these constructs are important in understanding health behaviors and planning interventions to change them. The construct of self-efficacy is among the most analyzed psychosocial constructs in research. Bandura (1995) defines self-efficacy as the confidence a person has in his or her ability to pursue a specific behavior. Self-efficacy is a central construct, in that it can influence behavior both directly and indirectly (Bandura, 2004). It is a guide for and motivator of health behaviors and is rooted in the core belief that one has the power to produce desired effects through one's actions. Unless people believe that they can produce the desired changes by their own effort, there will be very little incentive to put in that effort (Bandura, 2004).

Table 3.3 Constructs of Social Cognitive Theory

Construct	Definition
Environment	Social or physical circumstances or conditions that surround a person
Situations	A person's perception of his or her environment
Behavioral capability	The knowledge and skill needed to perform a given behavior
Outcome expectations	Anticipation of the probable outcomes that would ensue as a result of engaging in the behavior under discussion
Outcome expectancies	The values that a person places on the probable outcomes that result from performing a behavior
Self-control	Personal regulation of goal-directed behavior or performance
Observational learning	Behavioral acquisition that occurs through watching the actions of others and the outcomes of their behaviors
Self-efficacy	A person's confidence in performing a particular behavior
Emotional coping	Personal techniques employed to control the emotional and physiological states associated with acquisition of a new behavior

Social Network, Social Support, and Social Capital Theory

It is widely recognized that social networks and the social relationships that are derived from them have powerful effects on important aspects of both physical and mental health. *Social network* refers to the existence of social ties that could be supportive (Valente, 2015). Social networks involve the network environment (influence and selection), the position of the individual in the network, and the network properties (Valente, 2015). Social networks can also be described by type (i.e., dyadic relationships, affective communities, etc.) (Vassilev et al., 2011).

Most obviously, the structure of network ties influences health via the provision of social support. *Social support* has been defined as the physical and emotional comfort given to us by our family, friends, co-workers, and others (House, 1981). Social support is structural or functional (Holt-Lunstad & Uchino, 2015). Structural support refers to the level of integration into social networks or how connected people are within their community. Functional support refers to the mechanisms of support, or the types of support that a person may perceive to have or receive. Common types of functional support are listed in Table 3.4. *Social capital* refers to resources individuals and groups have within their network (Villalonga-Olives & Kawachi, 2015). Relationships and social networks are central to social capital (Hayden, 2014). When relationships are solid at the community level, individuals feel strong bonds and attachment to places

Table 3.4   Subtypes of Functional Social Support

Subtypes	Definition
Emotional	Conveying that a person is being thought about, appreciated, or valued enough to be cared for in ways that are health promoting
Instrumental support	Provision of tangible aid and services such as gifts of money, moving furniture, food, assistance with cooking, or child care
Belonging	Sense of feeling connected to a social group
Informational support	Provision of advice, suggestions, or information that a person can use to address a particular situation

(for example, a neighborhood) and organizations (for example, voluntary or religious organizations)—bonds that may lead to improvements in psychological and physical health. For instance, scholars have recently focused on the role of social capital in chronic illness (Hu et al., 2014; Vassilev et al., 2011). Additionally, newer research attempts to integrate social capital into other behavioral theories based upon a review of behavioral literature (Samuel, Commodore-Mensah, & Himmelfarb, 2014).

Foundational Theories/Models: Population Level

Health promotion programs for diverse settings and populations, not just a specific group of individuals, are at the heart of the health promotion field. Theories at the population level explore how social systems function and change and how to mobilize individuals in the different settings. Because health is complex and not always modifiable solely on a behavioral level, ecological approaches can address broader influences, such as social economic issues (Fielding, 2013). For this reason, multicomponent interventions are often necessary to tackle overarching issues such as health disparities (Fielding, 2013). Ecological frameworks typically use multiple levels of influence, including the intrapersonal, interpersonal, institutional, community, and societal levels (Hayden, 2014). More recently, researchers suggest modifying the model to make the policy/societal level the core, moving outward toward individual, rather than the traditional model that begins with the individual moving outward toward the societal/policy level (Golden, McLeroy, Green, Earp, & Lieberman, 2015).

The conceptual frameworks in this section offer strategies for intervening at the population level. This section discusses how communication theory, diffusion of innovations, and community mobilization are used to affect health behavior.

Communication Theories

Though there are many *communication theories,* they typically are grouped into micro-level or macro-level theories (Viswanath, Finnegan & Gollust, 2015). Micro-level theories (such as information processing theories and message effects theories) investigate the impact of communication on individuals. Messages are directed toward a priority population based upon a shared characteristic (such as gender) or tailored toward a specific, measured characteristic (such as sedentary working mothers) (Kreuter & Wray, 2003). Macro-level models (e.g., knowledge gap, risk communication) investigate how the larger social structure and function impacts the process of creating messages through evaluating the impact of messages (Viswanath, Finnegan & Gollust, 2015). For example, knowledge gap research looks to decrease disparities in health knowledge by carefully selecting the message channel in order to reach those most in need of the message, while risk communication research involves investigating the delicate balance between communicating risk and promoting behavior change. Much of the research on health communication theory is limited to investigations of message type and level of interest in specific populations; how people sense and react to messages is still not well understood (Ruben, 2014). Edgar and Volkman (2012) provide examples about use of common communication theories and models (Activation Model, Extended Parallel Process Model, and Fisher's Narrative Theory) in health promotion efforts.

Diffusion of Innovations Model

Though there are many diffusion models, the *diffusion of innovations model* is one of the most widely known (Brownson, Tabak, Stamatakis & Glanz, 2015). This model focuses both on the adopter and on innovative characteristics of the intervention to tailor messages to adopter groups over time (Rogers, 2003). People are grouped into adopter groups based on when they buy in to an innovation (such as a new product, program, or service): innovators, early adopters, early majority, late majority, and laggards. The innovators are the first group to adopt an innovation, and adopt because they want to be on the cutting edge. Early adopters, the next group, typically adopt an innovation after seeing how it works for the innovators. The early majority and late majority are the next two groups to adopt; they usually wait to see the longer-term benefits and drawbacks of an innovation before adopting it. The last group to adopt an innovation, if they do adopt it, is the laggards. Table 3.5 shows key concepts in the diffusion of innovations model, along with questions that illustrate their application (Brownson, Tabak, Stamatakis & Glanz, 2015).

Table 3.5   Concepts in the Diffusion of Innovations Model

Concept	Questions Used to Make Decisions About Adoption
Relative advantage	Is the innovation easier or more cost-effective to use than other options?
Compatibility	Is the innovation compatible with the adopter's lifestyle?
Complexity	Is the innovation relatively simple to adopt and use?
Trialability	Can adopters try the innovation out before adopting?
Observability	Can the innovation's benefits be easily observed?
Impact on social relations	Will the innovation have a positive impact on the adopter's social structure?
Reversibility	Can an adopter discontinue the innovation easily?
Communicability	Is the innovation understandable?
Time	How much time must be committed in order to adopt the innovation?
Risk and uncertainty level	How much risk is associated with adoption of the innovation?
Commitment	How much commitment is needed for adoption of the innovation?
Modifiability	Will there be opportunities for modifications after adoption has occurred?

The diffusion of innovation model also uses marketing strategies to target individuals in specific adopter groups to change a behavior. Groups adopt an innovation through five stages: awareness, persuasion, decision, implementation, and confirmation (Rogers, 2003).

The concepts of the diffusion of innovations model help to define and structure the communications related to an intervention. The concepts guide program staff in how to pitch a program to a potential group of participants. For example, using the concept of complexity, the staff promoting a walking program to encourage employees at a particular work site to engage in physical activity might frame the idea of fitting walking into a busy schedule as something that is relatively simple to do. A staff member might advocate for employees to hold meetings while walking, or she might promote quick, 10-minute walking breaks during the day. The message would change depending on the characteristics of the adopter group (for example, innovators, early adopters). Recent research suggests a need to focus on implementation, specifically evaluating adoption and diffusion of messages and interventions in populations (Breslau, Weiss, Williams, Burness, & Kepka, 2015).

Community Mobilization

Community mobilization is broadly defined as individuals or groups taking action that is organized around specific community issues. Community mobilization focuses on community-based strategies to improve health outcomes. Grounded and guided by the seminal works of Cloward and Ohlin (1961), Alinsky (1971), Arnstein (1969), and Freire (1972), early community mobilization efforts attempted to view the individual in relationship to the community (for example, the individual's family or neighborhood) in order to better understand the interplay of individual characteristics, health conditions, and environmental factors. Though recent research is mixed regarding the efficacy of efforts of community mobilization, some point to the broad and sometimes varying definitions, as well as numerous measurements and evaluations of such efforts (Cornish, Priego-Hernandez, Campbell, Mburu, & McLean, 2014). Concepts associated with community mobilization include community empowerment, community participation, capacity building, community coalitions, and community organization and development.

As originally developed, community mobilization focuses on communities as defined in Chapter 1—that is, both as physical locations (for example, neighborhoods, towns, or villages) and as groups of people with common interests (for example, cultural, racial, faith, or hunger action groups). The community mobilization phases discussed in this section are now widely used in all types of settings (for example workplaces, schools, health care organizations, and communities).

Community mobilization attempts to engage all sectors of a community or setting in a community-wide (or setting-wide) effort to address a health, social, or environmental issue. Desired results of mobilizing stakeholders may include promoting collaboration between individuals and organizations; creating a public awareness; promoting shared ownership between individuals and organizations; expanding the base of support for an issue; promoting networking, training, and education; increasing opportunities for training and education; and increasing access to funding opportunities to support community (or setting) programming (Centers for Disease Control and Prevention, n.d.).

According to the CDC's model there are four phases in mobilizing a community: (1) planning for mobilization, (2) raising awareness, (3) building a coalition, and (4) taking action (Centers for Disease Control and Prevention, n.d.).

In the first phase, *planning for mobilization*, organizers initiate a planning process to determine the many factors that may affect the overall mobilization process. The second phase, *raising awareness*, focuses on the key individuals and organizations to contact in order to stimulate interest, participation, and collaboration. The third phase, *building a coalition*, emphasizes the need to build a coalition that includes key organizations and individuals like health care providers, clergy members, community-based organization leaders, housing authorities, members of the local media, school and university administrators, local police forces, local businesses, and, most important, citizens of the community.

Once an active, participatory coalition, along with formal goals and objectives, is put in place, the final phase, *taking action*, is critical to actualizing results. This phase involves the development and implementation of an action plan. The action plan is based on the results of a needs assessment of the community or setting (see Chapter 4) and the effective use of coalition members' strengths and talents. The action plan would address, for example, efforts to educate members of the community or people in the setting about important health issues that affect the community or setting and ways to reduce or eliminate health problems. Lippman and colleagues (2016) suggest six domains in measuring community mobilization: shared concern, critical consciousness, organizational structures and networks, leadership, collective actions, and social cohesion.

Foundational Theories/Models Applied Across the Levels

Health theories and models provide guidance and support for planning, implementing, and evaluating a health promotion program. Programs drawn from health theories use a body of knowledge and experience that allows health promotion staff, stakeholders, and participants to be confident that a program is based on current research and best practices. Theories are the foundation for evidence-based health promotion programs. All theories have the potential to contribute to the process of planning, implementing, and evaluating a health promotion program. To aid in the process, Table 3.6 lists examples of theory-based strategies that are used at different levels of influence.

By becoming familiar with theories and models, program staff, stakeholders, and participants gain access to tools that will allow them to generate creative solutions to unique situations. They are able to go beyond acting on instinct or repeating earlier ineffective interventions to adopt a systematic, scientific approach to their work. Theories and models help staff, stakeholders, and participants to understand the dynamics that underlie real situations and to think about solutions in new ways.

Table 3.6   Using Foundational Theories to Plan Multilevel Interventions

Change Strategies	Examples of Strategies	Ecological Level	Useful Theories

Change people's behavior	Educational sessions
	Interactive technologies
	Printed literature
	Social marketing
	  campaigns
		Individual
		  (intrapersonal)
			Health belief model
			Theory of planned
			  behavior
			Transtheoretical model

	Mentoring programs
	Lay health advising
	Goal setting
	Enhancing social
	  networks or
	  improving social
	  support
	Creating new
	  organizational policy
	  and procedures
		Interpersonal	Social cognitive theory
			Social network and
			  social support theory

Change the environment	Media advocacy
	  campaigns
	Advocating changes to
	  public policy
		Population	Communication theories
			Diffusion of innovations
			  model
			Community mobilization

Health Promotion Program Planning Models

The health promotion planning models discussed in this section have common elements, although the elements may have different labels. In fact, all the approaches involve three basic steps:

1. Planning the program, including conducting a needs assessment of a health problem and its related factors and influences, prioritizing actions, selecting interventions, and making decisions to create and develop the program

2. Implementation of the program interventions and activities that are based on health theory, eliminate disparities, and are rooted in a needs assessment

3. Evaluation of the program to determine whether it has been implemented as planned and whether it has actually affected the health problem or related factors (identified in assessment) that it was intended to affect

This general three-part process makes sense; the three parts work together to give continual feedback and opportunities to adjust the program. Sussman and colleagues (2000) outline how to use these processes iteratively to provide one with an empirical program development process. Sussman and colleagues (2000) state that health behavior programs are planned and evaluated on an ongoing basis to make sure they are theoretically sound and will achieve stated goals. This cyclical process allows for continuous quality improvement.

The remainder of this section presents several prominent models that are used by health promotion professionals: the *PRECEDE-PROCEED model*, *intervention mapping*, the *community readiness model*, and *social marketing*. These represent a wide range of models that share the three basic elements of planning, implementation, and evaluation.

PRECEDE-PROCEED Model

One of the most well-known approaches to planning, implementing, and evaluating health promotion programs is the PRECEDE-PROCEED model (Green & Kreuter, 2005). The PRECEDE portion of the model (phases 1–4) focuses on program planning, and the PROCEED portion (phases 5–8) focuses on implementation and evaluation. The eight phases of the model guide planners in creating health promotion programs, beginning with more general outcomes and moving to more specific outcomes. Gradually, the process leads to creation of a program, delivery of the program, and evaluation of the program. (Figure 3.2 presents the PRECEDE-PROCEED model for health program planning and evaluation; the direction of the arrows shows the main lines of progression from program inputs and determinants of health to outcomes.)

Phase 1: Social Assessment

In the first phase, the program staff are looking for quality of life outcomes—specifically, the main social indicators of health in a specific population (for example, poverty level, crime rates, absenteeism, or low education levels) that affect health outcomes and quality of life. For example, at a worksite where there is a high rate of smoking among employees, absenteeism might be high due to illness.

Phase 2: Epidemiological Assessment

In this second phase, after specifying the social problems related to poor quality of life in the first phase, the program staff need to identify which

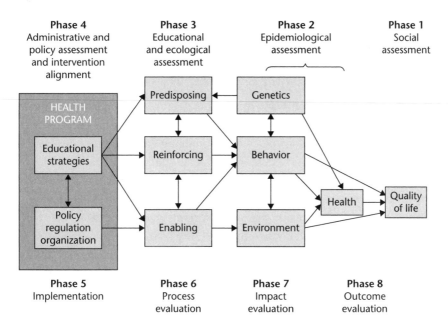

Phase 4	Phase 3	Phase 2	Phase 1
Administrative and policy assessment and intervention alignment	Educational and ecological assessment	Epidemiological assessment	Social assessment

Phase 5	Phase 6	Phase 7	Phase 8
Implementation	Process evaluation	Impact evaluation	Outcome evaluation

Figure 3.2 PRECEDE-PROCEED Model

Source: Green and Kreuter, 2005, p. 10. Reproduced with permission.

health problems or other factors play a role in impaired quality of life. The health problems are analyzed according to two factors: importance in terms of how related the health problems are to the social indicator identified in the social assessment and how amenable to change the health problems are. After a first-priority health problem is established, identification of the determinants that can lead to that health problem occurs. Specifically, which environmental factors, behavioral factors, and genetic indicators lead to a specific health problem? The same importance and changeability analysis would be performed to identify which factors to focus on a health promotion program. For example, the program staff would gather data on health problems in the population that might lead to absenteeism, such as obesity, heart disease, cancer, and communicable disease. After ranking the diseases according to importance and amenability to change, the planner might select one health problem. The next step in this assessment would be to investigate the underlying causes of these diseases, such as environmental factors (for example, toxins, stressful working conditions, or no control over working conditions), behavioral factors (for example, lack of physical activity, poor diet, smoking, or alcohol use), and genetic factors (for example, family history). Data on importance and changeability would be analyzed, and then one or several of these risk factors might be selected. To complete this phase, a measurable health status objective (or objectives), behavioral objective (or objectives), and environmental objective (or objectives) would be constructed.

Phase 3: Educational and Ecological Assessment

The focus of phase 3 shifts to mediating factors that help or hinder a positive environment or positive behaviors. These factors are grouped into three categories: predisposing factors, enabling factors, and reinforcing factors (Green & Kreuter, 2005). Predisposing factors are those that can either promote or detract from *motivation* to change, such as attitude or knowledge. Enabling factors are those that can promote or detract from change, such as resources or skills. Reinforcing factors are those that help continue motivation and change by providing feedback or rewards. These factors are analyzed according to importance, changeability, and feasibility (that is, how many factors is it feasible to include in a program). Factors are then selected to serve as a basis for program development, and educational objectives are composed.

Phase 4: Administrative and Policy Assessment and Intervention Alignment

The main focus of the administrative and policy assessment and the intervention alignment in the fourth phase is a reality check, to be sure that at the setting (the school, workplace, health care organization, or community) all of the necessary support, funding, personnel, facilities, policies, and other resources are present to develop and implement the program. For example, site policies and procedures are reviewed, revised, created, and implemented. Likewise at this point, there is an assessment at the site to clarify exactly what staff are needed to implement the program as well as to determine funding levels, space requirements (e.g. classroom, a gym, changing rooms, or showers might be needed), required materials. Finally as part of this phase examined is how best to recruit, retain, and recognize program participants.

Phase 5: Implementation

Delivery of the program occurs during phase 5. Also, the process evaluation (phase 6), which is the first evaluation phase, occurs simultaneously with implementation of the program.

Phase 6: Process Evaluation

The process evaluation is a formative evaluation, one that occurs during implementation of the program. The goals of this type of evaluation are to collect both quantitative and qualitative data to assess the feasibility of the program as well as to ensure quality delivery of the program. For example, participant attendance and attitudes toward the program might be recorded, as well as an assessment of how well the written lesson plans (describing what content is to be delivered, how it will be delivered, and how much time is allotted) align with actual delivery of the lesson (what content actually was delivered, how it was delivered, and how much time it took to deliver it). Achievement of educational objectives can also be measured in this phase.

Phase 7: Impact Evaluation

The focus of phase 7's summative evaluation, which occurs after the program ends, is to determine the intervention's impact on behaviors or environment. Timing may vary from immediately after the completion of all the intervention activities to several years later, depending on the objective and/or the sensitivity to change of the variable being assessed.

Phase 8: Outcome Evaluation

The focus of the last evaluative phase is the same as the focus when the entire process began—evaluation of indicators of quality of life and health status.

APPLICATION ACTIVITY: LEVELS OF EVALUATION

Locate one article for each level of evaluation—process, impact, and outcome. Read and prepare a summary, including how you have identified which level of evaluation is reported in the article. In small groups, discuss:

- Common activities/methodology in a process evaluation.
- Common activities/methodology in an impact evaluation.
- Common activities/methodology in an outcome evaluation.
- What is the value of each level of evaluation? What does it tell you? What does it not tell you? How do the levels of evaluation interact?

Intervention Mapping

Intervention mapping is another approach to planning health promotion programs. According to Bartholomew, Parcel, Kok, and Gottlieb (2011), the purpose of intervention mapping is to provide health promotion program planners with a framework for effective decision making at each stage of intervention planning, implementation, and evaluation. Interventions using this model have addressed health issues such as nutrition and physical activity, sexually transmitted infections, and mental health (Wisenthal & Krupa, 2014; Belansky et al., 2013; Wolfers, van den Hoek, Brug, & de Zwart, 2007). The intervention mapping process consists of six steps: (1) needs assessment, (2) matrices, (3) theory-based methods and practical strategies, (4) program, (5) adoption and implementation plan, and (6) evaluation plan. Although the model is presented in steps, program planners often go back and forth between steps as needed (Bartholomew, Markham, Mullen, & Fernandez, 2015).

Step 1 is a needs assessment of the priority population is conducted. Based on the needs assessment of the health issues, quality of life, and behavioral and environmental concerns of the priority population, the desired program outcomes are established. Step 2 involves creating a logic model and stating who and what will change at each ecological level as a result of the intervention. This step also involves crossing performance objectives for each ecolog-ical level with personal and external determinants in matrices in order to help write the change objectives (Bartholomew, Markham, Mullen, & Fernandez, 2015).

In Step 3, theory-based methods for bringing about changes at each ecological level are identified. In addition, practical strategies for realizing the change objectives are selected or designed. Step 4 involves consulting the intended program participants and implementers for their input, delineating the program's scope and sequence, compiling a list of needed materials, and developing and pretesting program materials with the priority population (Bartholomew, Markham, Mullen, & Fernandez, 2015).

Step 5 focuses on developing a program implementation plan. Matrices are created, similar to those in Step 2, by crossing adoption and implementation performance objectives with personal and external determinants. Last, Step 6 is to finalize the evaluation plan for the program. This step involves describing the program and its intended outcomes, writing questions for the process evaluation based on the matrices from Step 2, developing indicators and measures, and specifying the evaluation design (Bartholomew, Markham, Mullen, & Fernandez, 2015).

Community Readiness Model

The community readiness model is designed both to assess and to build a community's capacity to take action on social issues (Donnermeyer, Plested, Edwards, Oetting, & Littlethunder, 1997). It can and is applied in any setting (for example, school, workplace, healthcare organization, or

Table 3.7 Community Readiness Model

Stage	Description
1. Community tolerance	Issue is not generally recognized by the individuals at the site or leaders as a problem (or it may truly not be an issue).
2. Denial, resistance	There is recognition by individuals at the site that there is a local problem, but little concern is occurring locally.
3. Vague awareness	There is recognition by individuals at the site that there is a local problem but little or no specific knowledge of its extent. Leadership to do something about the problem is minimal.
4. Preplanning	There is clear recognition that there is a local problem; however, efforts to address it are not focused and detailed.
5. Preparation	Individuals at the site are actively engaged in developing a plan of action to address an issue.
6. Initiation	Enough information is available to justify efforts to address an issue.
7. Institutionalization	A program to address a social issue is up and running. Staff either are in training or have recently been trained to lead the effort.
8. Confirmation, expansion	Program continues to receive support and is perceived by individuals and leaders as useful. Data on the extent of the problem locally are collected regularly.
9. Professionalism	Data on prevalence rates and risk factors are collected periodically and used by staff to adjust program goals and target high-risk groups.

community). It provides a framework for assessing the social contexts in which individual behavior takes place by measuring changes in readiness related to community-wide efforts. The model integrates a community's culture, resources, and level of readiness to more effectively address an issue. The model consists of nine stages that are used as a guide to assess readiness and to determine the best intervention (or interventions) that align with a particular stage (see Table 3.7). Using the community readiness model will help increase community (as well as other settings) partnership, participation, and investment in the delivery of interventions at a site.

Social Marketing

Social marketing is not a theory but an approach to promoting health behavior that is used in conjunction with existing theoretic approaches (Luca & Suggs, 2013). Social marketing uses commercial marketing techniques to influence the voluntary behavior of specific audience members for a health benefit. Social marketing promotes a behavior change to a targeted group of individuals in several ways. It encourages persons to accept a new behavior, reject a potential behavior, modify a current behavior, or abandon an old behavior. Helping individuals to increasing walking (accept a new behavior) can aid in weight loss (Coulon et al., 2012). Discouraging the use of toxic fertilizers (rejection of a potential behavior) would enhance water supply and quality. Encouraging regular dental hygiene to including flossing regularly (modification of a current behavior) can reduce cavities (Brocklehurst, Morris, & Tickle, 2012). Encouraging smokers to quit smoking (abandon an old behavior) would reduce the incidence of lung illnesses (Green & Kreuter, 2005).

It is important to differentiate social marketing from commercial marketing. Marketing, in general, focuses on the process in which goods or services are exchanged for a profit, which is financial or for other goods and services. Social marketing, however, focuses on behavior rather than goods and services. Both conduct market research, which is research on a specific audience to understand their behaviors—for example, to understand how they perceive their needs, benefits to change, barriers, and opportunities (Green & Kreuter, 2005). Additionally, both require voluntary exchange, the idea that people will accept, reject, maintain, or modify a new behavior if the benefits exceed the cost of the behavior (Storey, Hess & Saffitz, 2015). Social marketing is similar to commercial marketing in that both have a customer-centered approach (Storey, Hess & Saffitz, 2015). Audience segmentation is the process of dividing larger markets of dissimilar individuals into a smaller market of more similar individuals for which an appropriate intervention is designed (Rogers, 2003). After an audience is segmented, then marketing principles are used to create a message tailored to each specific audience.

Table 3.8 outlines the differences between commercial and social marketing (Storey, Hess & Saffitz, 2015).

There are four basic marketing principles: product, price, place, and promotion. These elements are known as the *four P's of marketing*.

Table 3.8   Differentiating Social Marketing from Commercial Marketing

	Social Marketing	**Commercial Marketing**
Goal	Resolve certain social problems	Financial profit
Focus	Behaviors	Selling goods and services
Product	Often intangible (ideas)	Tangible (physical goods)
Funding	Taxes, donations (often limited)	Investments
Accountability	Public	Private
Performance	Hard to measure	Measured by financial profits

Product: the good, service, or idea being marketed in order to change behavior (for example, hand washing, safe sex, wearing a seat belt)

Price: the costs of and barriers to behavior change (for example, money, time, discomfort)

Place: the physical location and time in which the behavior change will take place (for example, at home, at school, in the car)

Promotion: the tactics used to communicate the message of behavior change (for example, media, brochures, billboards)

Using Health Theories and Planning Models

Developing health promotion programs can be an overwhelming task. Health theories and planning models have been developed and tested to guide professionals in the development of health promotion programs. Program staff members, stakeholders, and participants need to consider the setting, population, behavior, their desired level of influence, and practical issues such as resources when planning health promotion programs.

The planning models for developing health programs focus on the big picture. By becoming familiar with the theories and models, program staff, stakeholders, and participants gain access to tools that will allow them to generate creative solutions to unique situations. They are able to go beyond acting on instinct or repeating earlier ineffective interventions to adopt a systematic, scientific approach to their work. Theories and models help staff, stakeholders, and participants to ask the right questions and zero in on factors that contribute to a problem. The theories help everyone to understand the dynamics that underlie real situations and to think about solutions in new ways.

Summary

Health theories and planning models provide guidance and support throughout the planning, implementing, and evaluating of health promotion programs. No theory or model is perfect, and not all theories and their concepts are appropriate for all settings and behaviors. Each was designed to address a particular need or with a specific conceptualization of how best to address a health problem. Practitioners typically combine elements from different theories and models in their work. The theories and models are critical to effective health promotion programs and provide the foundation for evidence-based programs based on science, research, and practice across settings.

Health theories and models are dynamic, and the range of theories and models available for application in health promotion programs is rapidly expanding. Health theories describe, explain, and predict behavior at the intrapersonal, interpersonal, and population levels. Health theories reflect the ecological perspective of health promotion, which emphasizes the interaction between and interdependence of factors within and across all levels of a health problem. Health planning models can guide the creation and delivery of health promotion programs through planning, implementing, and evaluating. The strongest health promotion programs will use both health theories and planning models.

For Practice and Discussion

1. As a health educator in a community agency, you have been asked to develop a program to reduce bullying in the local schools. Use the social cognitive theory concept of reciprocal determinism and the constructs of environment, situation perceptions, outcome expectations and expectancies, self-control, observational learning, self-efficacy, and emotional coping to discuss potential intervention points for the program activities.

2. Adolescents engaging in sexual behaviors often do not feel susceptible to infection with a sexually transmitted infection. How might you use the health belief model to address this issue, and to motivate adolescents to abstain from sexual behavior or practice safer sex?

3. A local manufacturing company asks you to serve as a consultant to provide a healthy nutrition program for its 250 employees. The plan is to offer nutrition education activities (for example, cooking classes and home gardening workshops), personal nutrition counseling, a group weight management program, and improved employee food services (for example, low-calorie vending machine options) to employees at varied times. Several months pass, and only 50 employees have participated. The manager is concerned. She wants you to explain why 200 employees are not participating. She also wants you to change or revise the nutrition education program to make sure it is helping employees maintain and improve their nutritional health. Using the stages of change model, propose questions to assess employees' stages of change in regard to nutritional health in order to answer the manager's questions.

4. A group of stakeholders want to plan an innovative diabetes prevention program focused on elementary school students and uses a range of

activities and strategies. Using the PRECEDE-PROCEED model, discuss what would be involved with each phase of planning the program. In addition, discuss key concepts from the other planning models and how they might clarify for the stakeholders what to expect as they plan, implement, and evaluate their program.

5. Using the same innovative diabetes prevention program discussed in Question 4, apply the concepts from the diffusion of innovations model to discuss strategies the program developers can use to ensure that the program will be adopted and will change elementary school practices.

6. A hospital that serves a large farming population wants to increase childhood vaccinations among the families it serves. Using the four P's of marketing (product, price, place, promotion), design a social marketing mix for the hospital to use in order to increase childhood vaccinations among children living in rural farming communities.

KEY TERMS

Behavior	Model
Communication theory	PRECEDE-PROCEED model
Community mobilization	Social capital
Community readiness model	Social cognitive theory
Concept	Social marketing
Construct	Social network and social support theory
Diffusion of innovations model	Stages of change
Health belief model	Theory
Integrated behavioral model	Transtheoretical model
Intervention mapping	Variable

References

Alinsky, S. (1971). *Rules for radicals*. New York, NY: Random House.

Arnstein, S. (1969). A ladder of citizen participation. *Journal of Institutional Planning, 35*, 216–224.

Bandura, A. (1986). *Social foundations of thought and action: A social cognitive theory*. Englewood Cliffs, NJ: Prentice Hall.

Bandura, A. (1995). Exercise of personal and collective efficacy in changing societies. In A. Bandura (Ed.), *Self-efficacy in changing societies* (pp. 1–45). New York, NY: Cambridge University Press.

Bandura, A. (2004). Health promotion by social cognitive means. *Health Education and Behavior, 31*(2), 143–164.

Bandura, A., & Walters, R. H. (1963). *Social learning and personality development.* New York, NY: Holt, Rinehart & Winston.

Bartholomew, L. K., Markham, C., Mullen, P. & Fernandez, M. E. (2015). Planning models for theory-based health promotion interventions. In K. Glanz, B. K. Rimer & K. Viswanath (Eds.). *Health behavior: Theory, research, and practice* (5th ed., pp. 359–387). San Francisco, CA: Jossey-Bass.

Bartholomew, L. K., Parcel, G. S., Kok, G., & Gottlieb, N. H. (2011). *Planning health promotion programs: An intervention mapping approach.* San Francisco, CA: Jossey-Bass.

Belansky, E. S., Cutforth, N., Chavez, R., Crane, L. A., Waters, E., & Marshall, J. A. (2013). Adapted intervention mapping: A strategic planning process for increasing physical activity and healthy eating opportunities in schools via environment and policy change. *Journal of School Health, 83*(3), 194–205.

Breslau, E. S., Weiss, E. S., Williams, A., Burness, A., & Kepka, D. (2015). The implementation road: engaging community partnerships in evidence-based cancer control interventions. *Health Promotion Practice, 16*(1), 46–54.

Brocklehurst, P. R., Morris, P., & Tickle, M. (2012). Social marketing: An appropriate strategy to reduce oral health inequalities. *International Journal of Health Promotion & Education, 50*(2), 81–91.

Brownson, R. C., Tabak, R. G., Stamatakis, K. A. & Glanz, K. (2015). Implementation, dissemination, and diffusion of public health interventions. In K. Glanz, B. K. Rimer & K. Viswanath (Eds.). *Health behavior: Theory, research, and practice* (5th ed., pp. 301–325). San Francisco, CA: Jossey-Bass.

Centers for Disease Control and Prevention. (n.d.). *Community mobilization guide: A community-based effort to eliminate syphilis in the United States.* Retrieved April 22, 2016, from http://www.cdc.gov/stopsyphilis/toolkit/Community/CommunityGuide.pdf

Cloward R., & Ohlin, L. (1961). *Delinquency and opportunity: A theory of delinquent gangs.* New York, NY: Free Press.

Cornish, F., Priego-Hernandez, J., Campbell, C., Mburu, G., & McLean, S. (2014). The impact of community mobilization on HIV prevention in middle and low income countries: A systematic review and critique. *AIDS Behavior, 18,* 2110–2134. doi:10.1007/s10461-014-0748-5

Coulon, S. M., Wilson, D. K., Griffin, S., St. George, S. M., Alia, K. A., Trumpeter, N. N., . . . Gadson, B. (2012). Formative process evaluation for implementing a social marketing intervention to increase walking among African Americans in the Positive Action for Today's Health trial. *American Journal of Public Health, 102*(12), 2315–2321.

Donnermeyer, J. F., Plested, B. A., Edwards, R. W., Oetting, E. R., & Littlethunder, L. (1997). Community readiness and prevention programs. *Journal of the Community Development Society, 28*(1), 65–83.

Edgar, T., & Volkman, J. E. (2012). Using communication theory for health promotion: Practical guidance on message design and strategy. *Health Promotion Practice, 13*(5), 587–590.

Fernandez, B. R., Fleig, L., Godinho, C. A., Montenegro, E. M., Knoll, N., & Schwarzer, R. (2015). Action control bridges the planning-behavior gap: A longitudinal study on physical exercise in young adults. *Psychology and Health, 30*(8), 911–923. doi:10.1080/08870446.2015.1006222.

Fishbein, M. (2008). A reasoned action approach to health promotion. *Medical Decision Making, 28*, 834–844.

Freire, P. (1972). *Pedagogy of the oppressed.* London: Sheed & Ward.

Fielding, J. E. (2013). Health education 2.0: The next generation of health education practice. *Health Education and Behavior, 40*(5), 513–519.

Glanz, K., Rimer, B. K., & Viswanath, K. (2015). *Health behavior and health education: Theory, research, and practice* (5th ed.). San Francisco, CA: Jossey-Bass.

Goodson, P. (2010). *Theory in health promotion research and practice.* Sudbury, MA: Jones & Bartlett.

Green, L. W., & Kreuter, M. W. (2005). *Health program planning: An educational and ecological approach* (4th ed.). New York, NY: McGraw-Hill.

Golden, S., McLeroy, K., Green, L., Earp, J. A., & Lieberman, L. (2015). Upending the social ecological model to guide health promotion efforts toward policy and environmental change. *Health Education and Behavior, 42*(1S), 8S–14S.

Haider, M., & Kreps, G. L. (2004). Forty years of diffusion of innovations: Utility and value in public health. *Journal of Health Communication, 9*(Supp. 1), 3–11.

Hayden, J. (2014). *Introduction to health behavior theory.* Burlington, MA: Jones & Bartlett.

Holt-Lunstad & Uchino. (2015). Social support and health. In K. Glanz, B. K. Rimer, & K. Viswanath (Eds.), *Health behavior and health education: Theory, research, and practice* (5th ed., pp. 183–204). San Francisco, CA: Jossey-Bass.

House, J. S. (1981). *Work stress and social support.* Reading, MA: Addison-Wesley.

Hu, F., Hu, B., Chen, R., Ma, Y., Niu, L, Qin, X., & Hu, Z. (2014). A systematic review of social capital and chronic non-communicable diseases. *Bioscience Trends, 8*(6), 290–296.

Kerlinger, F. N. (1986). *Foundations of behavioral research* (3rd ed.). New York, NY: Holt, Rinehart & Winston.

Kreuter, M. W., & Wray, R. J. (2003). Tailored and targeted health communication: Strategies for enhancing information relevance. *American Journal of Health Behavior, 27*(Suppl 3), S227–S232.

Lippman, S. A., Neilands, T. B., Leslie, H. H., Maman, S., MacPhail, C., Twine, R., Kahn, K. & Pettifor, A. (2016). Development, validation, and performance of a scale to measure community mobilization. *Social Science in Medicine, 157,* 127–137.

Luca, N. R., & Suggs, L. S. (2013). Theory and model use in social marketing health interventions. *Journal of Health Communication, 18*(1), 20–40.

Montano, D., & Kasprzyk, D. (2015). Theory of reasoned action, theory of planned behavior, and the integrated behavioral model. In K. Glanz, B. K. Rimer, & K. Viswanath (Eds.), *Health behavior and health education: Theory, research, and practice* (5th ed., pp. 95–124). San Francisco, CA: Jossey-Bass.

Orji, R., Vassileva, J., & Mandryk, R. (2012). Towards an effective health interventions design: An extension of the Health Belief Model. *Online Journal of Public Health Informatics, 4*(3), e9.

Prochaska, J. O., DiClemente, C. C., & Norcross, J. C. (1992). In search of how people change: Applications to addictive behaviors. *American Psychologist, 47*(9), 1102–1114.

Prochaska, J. O., Redding, C. A., & Evers, K. E. (2015). The transtheoretical model and stages of change. In K. Glanz, B. K. Rimer, & F. M. Lewis (Eds.), *Health behavior and health education: Theory, research, and practice* (5th ed., pp. 125–148). San Francisco, CA: Jossey-Bass.

Rhodes, R. E., & Bruijn, G.J. (2013). How big is the physical activity intention-behaviour gap? A meta-analysis using the action control framework. *British Journal of Health Psychology, 18*, 296–309.

Rogers, E. (2003). *Diffusion of innovations* (5th ed.). New York, NY: Free Press.

Rosenstock, I. (1974). Historical origins of the health belief model. *Health Education Monographs, 2*, 328–335.

Rosenstock, I., Strecher, V., & Becker, M. (1988). Social learning theory and the health belief model. *Health Education Quarterly, 15*(2), 175–183.

Ruben, B. D. (2014). Communication theory and health education practice: The more things change, the more they stay the same. *Health Communication, 31*(1), 1–11. doi:10.1080/10410236.2014.923086

Samuel, L. J., Commodore-Mensah, Y. & Himmelfarb, C. R. (2014). Developing behavioral theory with the systematic integration of community social capital concepts. *Health Education & Behavior, 41*(4), 359–375.

Storey, J. D., Hess, R., & Saffitz, G. B. (2015). Social marketing. In K. Glanz, B. K. Rimer, & F. M. Lewis (Eds.), *Health behavior and health education: Theory, research, and practice* (5th ed., pp. 411–438). San Francisco, CA: Jossey-Bass.

Sugg Skinner, C., Tiro, J. & Champion, V.L. (2015). The health belief model. In K. Glanz, B. K. Rimer, & F. M. Lewis (Eds.), *Health behavior and health education: Theory, research, and practice* (5th ed., pp. 75–94). San Francisco, CA: Jossey-Bass.

Sussman, S. (Ed.). (2000). *Handbook of program development for health behavior research and practice*. Thousand Oaks, CA: Sage.

Valente, T. W. (2015). Social networks and health behaviors. In K. Glanz, B. K. Rimer, & F. M. Lewis (Eds.), *Health behavior and health education: Theory, research, and practice* (5th ed., pp. 205–222). San Francisco, CA: Jossey-Bass.

Vassilev, I., Rogers, A., Sanders, C., Kennedy, A., Blickem, C., Protheroe, . . . Morris, R. (2011). Social networks, social capital and chronic illness self-management: A realist review. *Chronic Illness, 9,* 60–86.

Villaloonga-Olives, E. & Kawachi, I. (2015). The measurement of bridging social capital in population health research. *Health & Place, 36,* 47–56.

Viswanath, K., Finnegan, J. R. & Gollust, S. (2015). Communication and health behaviors in a changing media environment. In K. Glanz, B. K. Rimer, & F. M. Lewis (Eds.), *Health behavior and health education: Theory, research, and practice* (5th ed., pp. 327–348). San Francisco, CA: Jossey-Bass.

Wisenthal, A., & Krupa, T. (2014). Using intervention mapping to deconstruct cognitive work hardening: A return-to-work intervention for people with depression. *BMC Health Services Research, 14*(1), 530.

Wolfers, M. E., van den Hoek, C., Brug, J., & de Zwart, O. (2007). Using intervention mapping to develop a programme to prevent sexually transmittable infections, including HIV, among heterosexual migrant men. *BMC Public Health Services Research, 7,* 141.

PART TWO

PLANNING HEALTH PROMOTION PROGRAMS

CHAPTER 4

ASSESSING THE NEEDS
OF PROGRAM PARTICIPANTS

James H. Price, Joseph A. Dake, and Britney Ward

Defining a Needs Assessment

To fully answer the question, "What is a needs assessment?" we need to answer the question, "What is a need?" A *need* is usually conceptualized as the difference between "what is" (the current status or state) and "what should be" (the desired status or state) (Altschuld & Kumar, 2010). A *needs assessment* is a formalized approach to collecting data in order to identify the needs of a group of individuals.

Understanding how the health of a group of individuals at a site might be improved requires information on both their current health status and their ideal health status. Traditionally, needs assessments have been associated with individuals living in a specific geographic area such as a city, county, state, or nation (commonly known as a community needs assessment, a reflection of health promotion's roots in health education). In 2010, the Affordable Care Act enacted new requirements that nonprofit hospitals must comply with to maintain their status as a 501(c)(3). One of these was the requirement for a hospital to conduct a community health needs assessment at least once every 3 years. While the structure and style of this assessment was not defined, it increased the use of this type of needs assessment across the country.

Needs assessments are also conducted in settings besides larger geographical communities. These include schools, universities, hospitals, worksites, and nonprofit organizations. While the settings may vary, the foundation

LEARNING OBJECTIVES

- Define *needs assessment*, and explain its relevance to health promotion programming.

- Evaluate sources of needs assessment data and information in terms of scope, timeliness, cost, and relevance to program recipients.

- Describe the four-step needs assessment process and the role of program stakeholders at each step.

- Describe how to report needs assessment findings in a way that meets stakeholders' requirements and uses for the data.

of a needs assessment remains the same. It is important to also consider the opportunity to assess needs beyond the intrapersonal level. Needs assessment can also assess the interpersonal, institutional, community, and policy factors that impact the health of a given group of people (Golden & Earp, 2012). This includes an assessment of a wide variety of *social determinants of health* such as unemployment, poverty, educational attainment, insurance status, access to health care, and many more (Niggel & Brandon, 2014). Understanding all of these issues helps to reduce the gap between "what is" and "what should be."

One common area in which gaps persist is between different racial/ethnic and socioeconomic groups. This is why there is such a focus on eliminating health disparities. In a needs assessment, the need to be culturally appropriate and culturally relevant is one of the guiding principles. Health theories and models also influence the questions asked and the information sought during the needs assessment.

The results of a needs assessment provide a foundation for the work of planning a health promotion program that addresses identified health problems and concerns. Furthermore, the results can be used to help allocate health resources and to establish a baseline against which to gauge the effectiveness of the program (through evaluation of interventions).

What Is Measured in Assessing Health? Focus on the Individuals

The first dimension of health that most agree is a component is physical health. Factors commonly included in the definition of *physical health* include being free from pain, physical disability, chronic and infectious diseases, and bodily discomforts that require the attention of a physician. Additionally, some include increased longevity. Table 4.1 identifies multiple examples of indicators commonly used in needs assessments.

Mental health is characterized by an ability to deal constructively with reality, adapt to change, and cope with adversity. In contrast, *mental illness* is characterized by alterations in thinking, mood, or behaviors that impair a person's relationships with others in their environment. Mental health and mental illness are not polar opposites but exist along a continuum of impairment. Mental illness typically affects about 18.5 percent of the adult population at any point in time (Substance Abuse and Mental Health Services Administration, 2014). Mental health insurance coverage is far less comprehensive than traditional health insurance coverage (Herrera, Hargraves, & Stanton, 2013). Assessments based on the volume of mental health care use are likely to underestimate the actual need for such services in a community, and even though more people are now receiving mental health care, significant gaps still exist (Mechanic, 2014).

Table 4.1   Dimensions of Health

Indicators of Physical Health

    Morbidity and mortality rates

    Life span

    Number of prescriptions

    Nutritional status

    Health care expenditures

    Environmental quality

    Level of physical disability

    Self-assessed health status

    Prevalence of health risk factors

    Number and types of health procedures

    Rate of premature births

    Prevalence of health insurance

    Health promotion or disease prevention programs

    Number and types of health professionals

    Number and types of health institutions

Indicators of Mental Health

    Mortality and mortality rates

    Number of psychotropic prescriptions

    Mental health care expenditures

    Number and types of mental health services

    Prevalence of insurance coverage for mental illness

    Self-assessed mental health status

    Hospitalization rates for mental illness

    Number and types of mental health professionals

    Number and types of mental health institutions

Indicators of Social Health

    Poverty levels

    Food insecurity rates

    Educational status

    Crime rates

    Divorce rates

    School dropout rates

    Out-of-wedlock pregnancies

    Social supports

(continued)

Table 4.1   *(Continued)*

Indicators of Social Health (*continued*)

Civic involvement

Community violence rates

Mortgage approval rates

Drug abuse

Unemployment rates

Number and type of social service agencies

Indicators of Environmental Health

Built environment

Environmental toxins

Pollutants (air, water, noise)

Population density

Transportation options

Recreational facilities

Housing facilities

Indicators of Spiritual Health

Level of sense of purpose in life

Number and types of religious institutions

Level of life satisfaction

Level of prejudice

A third dimension of health is termed *social health*. This area has been variously conceptualized by using variables such as educational status of a population, level of poverty and near poverty, crime rates, and a wide variety of other indicators (Table 4.1). This is commonly described as social determinants of health. A fourth dimension of health that can be measured is *environmental health*, which includes external conditions and influences that affect healthy growth and development.

The final dimension of health is *spiritual health* (Table 4.1). The spiritual dimension of health has not been explored or assessed in populations with the same intensity or depth as the other dimensions of health that we have discussed. People who conduct needs assessments have historically ignored this dimension of health because of the difficulty of assessing this concept and because of the limited research showing a direct connection to specific health problems.

What Is Measured in Assessing Health? Focus on the School, Workplace, Health Care Organization, and Community

Needs assessments focus on the health promotion program sites: school, workplace, health care organization, and community. This part of a needs assessment is known as a capacity assessment (Gilmore, 2012). A *capacity assessment* is a thorough and accurate assessment of the site to determine what resources are available in the setting to address the identified health concerns and problems—for example, health promotion materials, technology (computers, smartphones, software packages, Internet access, etc.), staffing, programs, funding, and services, as well as the gaps and needs in these areas. A key element of a capacity assessment is the empowerment of potential program participants, staff, and stakeholders to mobilize forces to address and solve the health problems or concerns identified in the needs assessment.

Tools for assessing capacity at each type of site are available. For example, for school sites, the *School Health Index: A Self-Assessment and Planning Guide* has been developed by the National Center for Chronic Disease Prevention and Health Promotion (2015) at the Centers for Disease Control and Prevention, in partnership with school administrators and staff, school health experts, parents, and national nongovernmental health and education agencies for the purpose of

- Enabling schools to identify strengths and weaknesses of health and safety policies and programs
- Enabling schools to develop an action plan for improving student health, which can be incorporated into the school improvement plan
- Engaging teachers, parents, students, and the community in promoting health-enhancing behaviors and better health

The *School Health Index* has two activities that are completed by teams from a school: the eight self-assessment modules and a planning for improvement process. The self-assessment process involves members of the school community coming together to discuss what the school is already doing to promote good health and to identify strengths and weaknesses. The *School Health Index* assesses the extent to which a school implements the types of policies and practices recommended by the Centers for Disease Control and Prevention's research-based guidelines for school health and safety policies and programs.

The areas covered by assessments in schools, workplaces, health care organizations, and communities can be quite broad. For example, they might include policies, procedures, health services and health promotion resources (for example, staff, space, materials, technology, and funding), service gaps and linkages, networks, health insurance and benefits, legal requirements and compliance, and accreditations.

Assessing the capacity of a site to operate and support a health promotion program provides early insight into the *culture* and *climate* of a setting. Culture is the beliefs, values, customs, experiences, and knowledge that gives meaning to what a particular group does and does not do. Culture refers to the basic assumptions about the world and the values that guide life in a given organization or community. Climate is the environment or mood of a particular group that emanates from their cultural background and the tenor of the group's official and unofficial leaders. Climate is also the meaning people attach to interrelated bundles of experiences at a site (Schneider, Herhart, & Macey, 2013). In addition to the items already discussed, examples of areas that are also explored as part of a capacity assessment include relationships that support health, opportunities to promote personal health for everyone at the site, and support systems for and barriers to implementation of the program.

Data Collection for Needs Assessments

Data collection plays a pivotal role in assessing the quality of life of the population of interest and in establishing *priorities* for health promotion programs. The needs assessment will use the principles of *epidemiology* and *demography*, which are essential in conducting a needs assessment. Much of this data can be obtained from federal and state sources (secondary data). There are two major categories of data: *primary data* and *secondary data*.

1. Primary data are new, original data that did not exist before, obtained directly from individuals at the site, usually by means of surveys, interviews, *focus groups*, or direct observation. Primary data constitute new information that will be used to answer specific questions.

2. Secondary data already exist because they were collected by someone for another purpose. The data may or may not be directly from the individual or population that is being assessed. Secondary data sources include *Healthy People* information, vital records, census data, and peer-reviewed journals. When large amounts and varying types of secondary data exist that can be analyzed for additional purposes, this can be referred to in the field of health promotion as "big data."

Primary data are more expensive and time consuming to collect than secondary data. Collection of quality primary data requires technical expertise in order to identify representative samples, design instruments, and complete data analysis. The problems with secondary data are that some information may not exist for some settings, the data is old, or the data may not have been correctly collected.

Information to be collected can be divided into two broad categories: quantitative and qualitative. *Quantitative data* are statistical information (for example, percentages, means, or correlations) such as one would typically find in professional journals. However, numbers alone do not provide sufficient insights to allow program staff to completely understand health problems or decide how to intervene in order to reduce a health problem. *Qualitative data* are more narrative, with fewer numbers. They include the perceptions and misperceptions of community members in regard to quality-of-life issues in the community. Qualitative methods include one-on-one key informant interviews, focus groups, public hearings, and observational methods. The two forms of data (quantitative and qualitative) complement one another, each type informing the other as staff derive conclusions and establish goals for community interventions.

Specific data-gathering techniques to be used depend on what one wants to know, the resources available, and the constraints of the priority population (for example, lack of reading ability, absence of telephones, or mobility problems). For initial phases of primary data collection, interactive group processes are recommended (for example, focus groups) because they allow those conducting the needs assessment to clarify both their own questions and respondents' answers. Interactive methods also provide the opportunity to collect specific words that members of the population group use to describe health issues, which can later be used to form questions for a final questionnaire that can be used to survey even more individuals. Later, these written questionnaires can be used to collect large amounts of data from many people over a wide geographic area. Such a large quantity of data will need to be aggregated and analyzed by the appropriate software package.

WEB RESOURCE: COMMUNITY TOOLBOX: ASSESSING COMMUNITY NEEDS AND RESOURCES

http://ctb.dept.ku.edu/en/table-of-contents/assessment/assessing-community-needs-and-resources

The Community Toolbox is a free online resource to provide a wide variety of information on building healthier communities. Chapter 3 of this resource has strategies and examples of the assessment of needs and assets within communities.

Conducting a Health Needs Assessment

Needs assessments consist of four basic steps: (1) determining the scope of the assessment, (2) gathering data, (3) analyzing the data, and (4) reporting the findings. Before you do anything, it is best to think about each of the steps and map out to the best of your ability what will happen in each step. This planning is important so that you can explain to stakeholders what they can expect from the process as well as how long it will take to complete the needs assessment.

1. *Determine the scope.* Work with the key informants and stakeholders (that is, an advisory committee) to determine the scope of the work and the purpose of the needs assessment. Ask who will be involved and what decisions will be based on the needs assessment. Who will use the results to make decisions about the intervention or prevention programs? Whenever possible, take an ecological approach to the needs assessment. Assess both the stakeholders and their environment. In the environmental assessment, include an analysis of organizational and community assets and capacity.

2. *Gather the data.* Gather only the needed data. Consider culturally appropriate data-gathering approaches tailored to the priority population and setting. Gather multiple types of data—both qualitative and quantitative. Table 4.1 provides an overview of types of data that could be secured in order to address the various dimensions of health.

3. *Analyze the data.* Use clear methods that people can understand.

4. *Report and share the findings.* Identify your options for sharing the findings of the needs assessment. Think about how best to communicate the findings. In sharing the information, identify any factors that are linked to the health problem. Validate the need for the program before continuing with the planning process. Tailor all communications to the program participants, stakeholders, and staff.

Many approaches can be used to conduct a needs assessment. Often, the methods that can be used will be limited by a lack of time, personnel, money or by political constraints.

Promoting a Needs Assessment

Conducting a needs assessment is an exciting event in the development of a health promotion program. It is often the first public acknowledgment that a school, workplace, health care organization, or community is working to address health problems at a site. Publicity to promote the needs assessment creates awareness of the needs assessment, enhances the chances that individuals and groups who have been asked to participate will respond, and increases the visibility of the organizations that form the advisory committee. Have a media kickoff for the needs assessment, and distribute press releases and information packets. Use social media to network with service clubs, community organizations, and their members. Numerous service clubs (for example, Rotary, Kiwanis, or chambers of commerce) may provide a forum in which to communicate the importance of the health needs assessment. Finally, be sure to obtain copies of newsletter articles and newspaper clippings to share with the advisory committee. This form of sharing can bolster support from the advisory committee.

Using Primary Data Methods and Tools

The sections that follow briefly describe a series of methods and tools that can be used to collect primary data for the needs assessment. Each method or tool has specific strengths and weaknesses.

Key Informant (One-on-One) Interviews

The idea underlying the qualitative technique of key informant interviews is that certain individuals possess unique and important information that can provide insights into the health issues at a site. These *key informants* are selected on the basis of their position or potential Influence (Barnett et al., 2007). For example, at schools, key informants might include teachers, principals, parents, school nurses, and students. Examples of key informants at work sites are human resource directors, company owners, supervisors, and union leaders. In communities, key informants might be local government officials, ministers, medical personnel, or agency directors. Another type of key informant is people who are chosen because of their reputation. Such individuals usually include opinion leaders, activists, or other socially prominent individuals. A needs assessment includes interviews with both types of individuals.

It is important that a specific set of questions be created ahead of time in order to create a uniform interview format. (See Table 4.2 for some questions that key informants in a community might be asked.) Pilot testing the interview questionnaire is essential. Again, remember that each person will share opinions (and biases) with the interviewer as if they were facts. Usually, not all key informants are interviewed, so the opinions collected will represent limited insights into the issues being assessed.

In-depth interviews with key informants typically take the form of conversation between the interviewer and the respondent. This type

Table 4.2   Interview or Focus Group Questions for a Community Assessment

1. What do you think the main health problems are in the community?
2. What do you think are the causes of these health problems?
3. How can these problems be reduced or eliminated in the community?
4. Are there any special health problems or issues affecting children and adolescents in the community?
5. Are there any special health problems or issues affecting the elderly in the community?
6. Is there a particular group of community residents that you would consider more unhealthy than the rest of the residents? If so, why are they less healthy?
7. Which one of the previously mentioned problems do you consider to be the most important one in the community?
8. If you were given $10 million to correct the health problems of the community, what would you spend it on?

of interaction gathers the views of the respondents in their own terms. Through probing questions, a well-trained interviewer can clarify statements made by an informant.

⁂ Focus Groups

A focus group is a qualitative data collection technique in which a small group of individuals meet to share their views and experiences on some topic. The ideal size of the group depends, in part, on the skills of the facilitator (Krueger & Casey, 2014). Usually the ideal group size is 6 to 12 participants who are similar in characteristics that may impact their perceptions (race/ethnicity, gender, educational status, socioeconomic status, etc.). This technique capitalizes on the interaction of the group members and reduces the chance that dialogue is inhibited (Krueger & Casey, 2014). The number of focus groups sufficient to study the perceptions of individuals at a site is impacted by the diversity of the population at the site. People of different age groups, sexes, and racial or ethnic groups may need their own focus groups.

Besides the group moderator, it is helpful to have an observer who serves as a recorder in order to capture the specific comments and unique words of the participants. The focus group leader does not take extensive notes because it might cause him or her to miss important elements of nonverbal communication. Respondents are usually provided with drinks and, sometimes, a snack and are paid for the time they spend to participate in a focus group. Results from focus groups are important in and of themselves but they can also be used to help develop surveys to further explore this issue among that population (Blair, Czaja, & Blair, 2014). Focus groups typically take 60 to 90 minutes (Krueger & Casey, 2014).

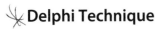 Delphi Technique

The *Delphi technique* is used to solicit information from individuals who cannot easily be brought together for, say, a focus group. This technique might be used with a group of health experts (for example, physicians or dentists) who cannot conveniently meet in person. First, a group of professionals are asked to respond to a few open-ended questions. Their responses are returned and are compiled into one list. Second, the experts are asked to respond to the combined list and add more items, eliminate items they do not support, and reword items that they think need to be clarified. The experts send their responses back, and again, the responses are compiled into one master list. The process can be stopped at this point, or the list of responses can be sent to the experts again in order for them to rate or rank the items. This process can be cumbersome if postal mail is used, or it can be simplified by using electronic or web-based communication.

Survey Questionnaires

Surveys, especially written questionnaires, are the most common form of gathering data for a needs assessment (public perceptions and behaviors in regard to issues). Questionnaires can be administered in four ways—as mail surveys, as telephone surveys, face to face (as discussed earlier), or as electronic/web–based surveys (Fowler, 2013; Dillman, Smyth, & Christian, 2014). Mail surveys allow a large quantity of data to be collected in a relatively short period of time. The main disadvantages are that special expertise is required to create valid and reliable mail surveys and to sample the population correctly. Techniques to increase the likelihood that one will obtain a satisfactory return rate can be employed (McCluskey, 2011); too low a return rate increases the likelihood of biased data (nonresponse error).

In contrast to mail surveys, telephone surveys are more time consuming, more expensive to conduct, and often result in a lower response rate (due to screening by telephone answering machines and the difficulty of interviewing people on cell phones). Recent research indicates that 44% of U.S. households did not have a landline phone and solely used cell phones (Blumberg & Luke, 2015). These homes are also more likely to be younger adults.

Some subjects may feel intimidated in a telephone interview and give socially desirable responses rather than authentic answers to some questions. However, the response rate for telephone surveys may be higher than that for mail surveys for groups of individuals who do not read well (for example, some elderly people, people of low socioeconomic status, and nonnative English language speakers). The longer the survey, the less likely it is that respondents will complete the questionnaire by phone.

Electronic surveys are increasing in their usage because of the relative cost and ease. These surveys are typically done through one of a wide variety of options such as Qualtrics, QuestionPro, SurveyMonkey, Zoomerang, or SurveyGizmo. These online services vary greatly in their price, interface, ease of use, customization, ability to conduct survey through mobile phones, and ability to download the collected data. These surveys require the potential respondent to click a link provided to them through a website, e-mail, or a text.

There still remains a significant difference in the economically disadvantaged to access surveys through electronic methods. While more now have access to the Internet at home though a computer or smartphone, the numbers are not high. A report from the American Community Survey from the U.S. Census reports that less than half (48%) of households with incomes less than $25,000 had Internet access at home (File & Ryan, 2014).

Another concern is that it is easier for people to decline an Internet survey, even with a promise of a mailed incentive, in contrast to mail surveys, which can contain a modest financial incentive. This incentive can be as simple as a one- or two-dollar bill (McClusky, 2011). Regardless of the survey method, it is essential to have a good survey instrument. Questionnaires have overall visual appeal; for example, they use large enough print and adequate white space, have directions at the beginning of the questionnaire, and present the most important questions first and the demographic questions at the end.

When developing a survey, a person with expertise in this area is included in order to appropriately ensure *validity* (*face validity*, *content validity*, construct validity, etc.) and *reliability* (test-retest reliability, internal reliability, etc.) (DeVon et al., 2007). Readability and acceptability are also important when using appropriate techniques (SMOG Dale-Chall, etc.).

CASE STUDY: RACIAL/ETHNIC HEALTH NEEDS ASSESSMENTS

Hispanics are the fastest growing ethnic minority population in the United States. Nationally, they are negatively impacted by higher rates of morbidity and premature mortality. A significant portion of Hispanics have low incomes, resulting in less access to health care because of high rates of being uninsured and underinsured. The National Alliance for Hispanic Health has identified *closing the gap in community services and medical practice* as a primary goal of their organization (http://www.hispanichealth.org/our-vision-and-mission.html).

Questions:

1. If you were assessing the community regarding access to care among the Hispanic population, what would you need to consider to ensure a quality outcome for your assessment?

2. How might segments of the Hispanic community are different from the rest of the community? How might they be different from each other? Why are these issues important to consider?

Selecting a Sample

Three techniques of survey research are key to obtaining results that represent the health-related perceptions, behaviors, and needs of the group being assessed at a site. First is correctly selecting the people who will receive the questionnaire. Second is selecting a large enough *sample* that the results will be representative of the entire population. Third is making sure the return rate is high enough (typically better than 50%) to help ensure that the results are valid when generalizing to the greater population.

Because limited resources prohibit surveying the entire population, obtaining a representative sample is an acceptable alternative. A representative sample can be accomplished through *random selection* of individuals to receive the questionnaire. In practice, true random selection for a needs assessment is unlikely to occur, but choosing methods that are as close as possible to random is ideal.

The second factor to consider is *power analysis* (Price, Dake, Murnan, Dimmig, & Akpanudo, 2005). Power analysis deals with having an adequate number of individuals to be able to generalize the findings from the sample to the population. To determine the necessary size of the random sample, one needs to know the following: how much sampling error (variation in how accurately the sample represents the entire population) one is willing to accept, the size (n) of the population, and how much variation (split) there is in the population with respect to the outcome variables (for example, health beliefs or behaviors) being surveyed (50/50 split is the most conservative estimate). Table 4.3 shows various population sizes and the number of sample responses needed in order to be able to generalize findings to that population.

The third factor is survey return rates. If a survey were sent to a random sample of 3,000 and 381 surveys were returned, the response rate is 13%

Table 4.3   Sample Sizes for Two Levels of Sampling Error at the 95 Percent Confidence Interval

Population Size	Sample Error +/−3% Variation in Responses		Sample Error +/−5% Variation in Responses	
	50/50 Split	80/20 Split	50/50 Split	80/20 Split
100	92	87	80	71
250	203	183	152	124
500	341	289	217	165
750	441	358	254	185
1,000	516	406	278	198
2,500	748	537	333	224
5,000	880	601	357	264
10,000	964	639	370	240
25,000	1,023	665	378	243
50,000	1,045	674	381	245
100,000	1,056	678	383	245
1,000,000	1,066	682	384	246
10,000,000	1,067	683	384	246

Note: Numbers in table refer to completed questionnaires returned.
Source: Price, Dake, Murnan, Dimmig, and Akpanudo, 2005.

(381/3,000). However, if the questionnaire were sent to a random sample of 700 and there were 381 returned, the response rate is 54% (381/700). Does it make a difference what the return rate is as long as the number of questionnaires returned meet the number needed for power? The answer depends on two issues: potential for *sampling bias* and potential for *response bias.*

Sampling bias occurs when the sample is selected in a manner (for example, a convenience sample) that results in people being left out who have unique characteristics (for example, race or ethnicity, health beliefs or behaviors, or socioeconomic status), which results in the final survey responses being uncharacteristic of the population. In contrast, response bias occurs when people who respond to the survey are different in their health beliefs or behaviors from those who do not respond to the survey. The more beliefs and behaviors reflected in the responses differ from the beliefs and behaviors of the nonrespondents, the greater the magnitude of the response bias. Another way of stating this is that a low return rate is a potential threat to external validity (being able to generalize the findings to the population from which the sample was drawn).

CASE STUDY: COLLEGE STUDENT MENTAL HEALTH NEEDS ASSESSMENT

College students are diverse groups of students. Their diversity includes racial/ethnic differences, intellectual ability, professional goals, socioeconomic status, and psychological traits and abilities that vary. Most students will for the first time operate in an environment with minimal personal guidance, requiring significant self-motivation in successfully progressing in their plans of study.

College students will deal with a variety of stresses, including academic pressures, interpersonal relationships, peer pressures, and financial stresses. These stresses often create thoughts for students of quitting their studies. In addition, this is a time when mental illnesses start to manifest themselves, resulting in the 18–25 age group having the highest rate of mental illness of any age group. Each year approximately 24,000 college students attempt suicide and another 1,100 of them end their lives by suicide.

This age group also has the highest rate of binge drinking. How would you go about conducting a college student mental health needs assessment at your university to answer the following questions?

1. What types of mental health problems do students report they have?

2. What are the students' self-reported needs for mental health services?

3. What mental health services are currently available for students?

4. How likely are students to use the existing mental health services?

5. What are the perceived barriers to using existing mental health services?

6. How knowledgeable are students regarding the mental health services currently available?

7. What additional mental health services would they like to have?

What behavioral theory could be used to structure a questionnaire to help answer the above questions?

Using Secondary Data Methods and Tools

Secondary data already exist because they were collected by someone for another purpose. From secondary sources, you can get the big picture as well as an overview of how to proceed to address a health problem. Working with secondary data, you can view a variety of approaches to defining and analyzing a problem. There are many other reasons for using secondary data:

 It is far cheaper to collect secondary data than to obtain primary data. In other words, you can get a lot of information for your money and time—usually, more than you would get using the same amount of money to collect primary data.

- National, state, and local health data are publicly available and accessible electronically. The time involved in searching these sources is much less than that needed to collect primary data. There are also online resources that combine large amounts of secondary data to help those working to improve the health of a particular community. This is often useful to help frame the local needs assessment.

- Local secondary data is important to understand details of the particular school, company, organization, or community. These include existing data such as attendance rates, grades, performance scores, number of sick days taken, production statistics, sales figures, clinical indicators, records, data from immunization programs, or insurance claims.

- Secondary sources of information usually yield more accurate data than those obtained through primary research. A government agency that has undertaken a large-scale survey or a census is likely to produce far more accurate results than custom-designed surveys that are based on relatively small sample sizes. However, not all secondary sources are more accurate.

- Secondary sources help define the population. Secondary data can be extremely useful both in defining the population and in structuring the sample to be taken. For instance, government statistics on a county's demographics will help decide how to stratify a sample, and, once sample estimates have been calculated, these can be used to project those estimates to the population.

- Sometimes sufficient secondary data is available that are entirely adequate for drawing conclusions and answering the questions, making primary data collection unnecessary.

WEB RESOURCE: COMMUNITY COMMONS

http://www.communitycommons.org/

Community Commons is an online resource that combines many secondary datasets to allow someone doing a needs assessment to generate reports and maps that can help frame the assessment or to communicate the importance of the needs assessment findings.

Problems with Secondary Information

The benefits of using secondary information are considerable; however, the quality of both the source of the data and the data themselves is evaluated. When deciding whether to use a particular source of secondary data, it is helpful to ask the following questions: How easy will it be to access and use the data source? Do the data help address the desired specific program area? Do the data apply to the priority population? Are the data relatively current? Are the data collection methods acceptable? Finally, are the data biased? Are the data trustworthy? If the answer to these questions is yes, the data source is good to use.

Whenever possible, use multiple sources of secondary data. In this way, different sources can be cross-checked and used to confirm one another. When differences occur, an explanation for the differences must be found or the data is set aside.

Reporting and Sharing the Findings

The last step in the process of needs assessment is to report and share the findings. What are your options for sharing the findings of a needs assessment? Think about how best to communicate. In sharing the information, identify any factors that are linked to the health problem. Identify the focus for the program, and validate the need for the program before continuing with the planning process. Tailor all communications to the program participants, staff, and stakeholders.

Analyzing Results

How the results of a needs assessment are analyzed largely depend on the purpose of the needs assessment. The data may be largely descriptive in order to provide a baseline assessment from which to do comparisons, write grants, plan programs, and so on. It is often useful when reporting descriptive statistics (percentages, means, standard deviations, and so on) to make comparisons with other appropriate data sources. For example, if the assessment of a site includes a question on the percentage of adults who are current smokers, it is useful to report the findings not only for that site but also for the state or nation, if the secondary data exist. This comparison is presented in tabular format or graphical format (Figure 4.1). The data also is separated by important characteristics such as gender, race, or socioeconomic indicators (Figure 4.2).

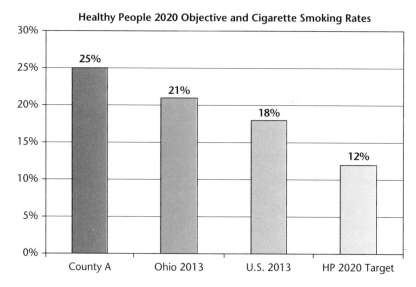

Figure 4.1 Comparisons to State and Federal Data

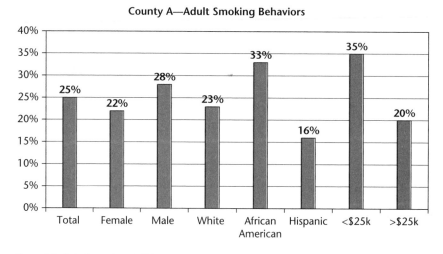

Figure 4.2 Data Comparisons to Subgroups

If data beyond descriptive statistics are desired, it is important to hire a statistician to determine what types of analyses are possible and appropriate based on the sample obtained for the needs assessment. If more in-depth analyses that compare subgroups are desired, increased sample sizes may be needed. It is sometimes inappropriate to calculate statistical comparisons on every subgroup that can be derived from needs assessment data. If an advisory committee wants to investigate a specific subgroup, it is important that this be decided prior to beginning the assessment so that oversampling of that subgroup is built into the assessment, ensuring adequate power in the subsample to calculate needed statistics.

One technique that can be used in reporting the results of needs assessments is through *geographic information system* (GIS) mapping. GIS technology has grown significantly in its ability and ease of use. In the field of public health, GIS can be used to visualize health data through mapping that presents the data in a spatial format, allowing interpretation and analysis that is different from what is possible through tabular or other graphical methods. Uses of GIS technology in health include determining the geographic distribution of various diseases, behaviors, resources, clinical sites, schools, or any other factor of importance and overlaying these maps to help understand possible spatial relationships among those data. This can help with identifying locations of greatest need and with planning the most effective interventions for those groups. This tool can help to make programming more efficient.

Such visual mapping of the data provides a unique perspective on the data and may lead to better policy making.

Establishing Priorities

Having an advisory board during the needs assessment is important to help establish program priorities. Most board members will come together (sometimes with program staff and other program stakeholders) to look at the needs assessment data (for example, numbers, summaries of interviews, and secondary data reports) and to discuss and decide on program priorities based on the data. Frequently the needs assessment produces a lot of information (such as numbers, tables, and charts), so the first task is to reduce the information to a manageable number of health concerns and topics. One way to group the data to facilitate ratings is to divide them into three areas: types of death or disability, behavioral risk factors, and nonbehavioral risk factors. (Social, physical, and environmental factors that affect health are considered nonbehavioral risk factors.)

Once the data are grouped, then the advisory board can prioritize what to address within each group and among groups. Identifying which problems to address will require that criteria (for example, importance, feasibility of change, magnitude of problem, and cost) be established by the advisory board. These priorities provide justification for starting new programs and continuing or terminating existing programs. The following issues might be factors to consider in establishing program priorities at a site.

- How large is the discrepancy between the incidence of the health problem locally and the incidence at state or national levels?

- How many individuals are affected by the health problem?

- Which problem has the greatest impact on disability or mortality?

- What are the leading perceived health problems of the stakeholders?

- What will be the consequences if the health problem is not corrected?

- Would not correcting the problem cause other health-related problems?

- Would other health-related problems be reduced if this health problem were reduced?

- What is the potential impact on others at the site if the health problem is reduced?

- How difficult would it be to correct the health problem?

- Which problems are already being addressed by other groups and organizations?

- How many resources would be required to solve the health-related problem?

- How effective are available interventions in preventing or reducing the health-related problem?

- Do you have the expertise to resolve the health-related problem?

- What are the barriers (obstacles) to correcting the health-related problem?

- Will the stakeholders want and accept the proposed solution to the health-related problem?

- Do current laws permit the proposed health-related program activities to be conducted?

These questions can guide the board's thinking when it is establishing priorities. Eventually, however, the criteria will probably need to be weighed numerically. One simple method of establishing priorities is to use only two categories to assess each health-related problem: *importance* and *feasibility* (Table 4.4). Importance factors include the number of people affected, mortality rate, and potential impact on the population. Feasibility factors include how difficult it will be to correct the problem, availability of resources, effectiveness of available interventions, and potential acceptance of solutions at the site. Each member of the advisory board rates the

Table 4.4   Process for Determining Health Priorities

		Feasibility		
		High (3)	Moderate (2)	Low (1)
	High (3)	6 points	5 points	4 points
Importance	Moderate (2)	5 points	4 points	3 points
	Low (1)	4 points	3 points	2 points

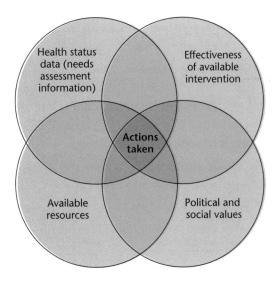

Figure 4.3   Factors in Decisions on Actions to Take After a Needs Assessment

health-related problems that have been identified in the priority population. The aggregated ratings of all board members are then used to determine the final priorities.

On the basis of the priorities it has set, the advisory board then establishes program goals. In other words, program goals are directed toward reducing a particular health problem. Which programs will actually be implemented is not based just on the results of an analysis but depends on a variety of issues. Figure 4.3 shows four factors that most often affect which actions are taken. Initially, it is the most serious health problems (based on data from the needs assessment) that you would think to address first. In reality, other factors—for example, insufficient resources, a lack of available effective interventions, or the political and social values of the school, workplace, health care organization, or community—may play significant roles in determining which needs are addressed.

A model that addresses the combination of these issues is the basic priority rating model 2.0 (BPR 2.0) (Neiger, Tackery, & Fagen, 2011). This model, which includes a detailed scoring system, has the following components:

Size: number of people with the problem (scored from 0 to 10 based on incidence or prevalence rates)

Seriousness: a combination of urgency, severity, economic loss, and impact on other people (scored from 0 to 5 each)

Effectiveness of intervention: strength of evidence to show that the intervention is effective (scored from 0 to 10)

PEARL score (Vilnius & Dandoy, 1990): Represents five feasibility factors that have a high degree of influence in determining how a particular problem can be addressed. Each of these five PEARL factors is scored as a 0 (if no) or 1 (if yes) and multiply together for a total score of either 0 or 1.

Propriety: Does the problem fall within the organization's overall mission?

Economic feasibility: Does it make economic sense to address the problem? Will there be economic consequences if the problem is not addressed?

Acceptability: Will the community or priority population accept an intervention to address the problem?

Resources: Are resources available to address the problem?

Legality: Do current laws allow the problem to be addressed?

The final priority score is calculated as follows:

$$((\text{Size score} + \text{seriousness score}) \times \text{effectiveness of intervention}/3)$$
$$\times \text{PEARL score})$$

As can be seen from the formula, if the answer on any of the five PEARL factors is scored as no, then the product will equal 0 and the health problem will not be addressed in the overall priority rating, regardless of the scores for the other factors.

Another approach to making program priority decisions, often used in combination with the two just mentioned, is *consensus building*. Essentially, consensus building (also called collaborative problem solving or collaboration) is bringing together advisory board members, program staff, program participants, and stakeholders to use the needs assessment results and data to express their ideas, clarify areas of agreement and disagreement, and develop shared program direction. Consensus can be difficult to reach. However, developing program priorities through consensus maximizes the opportunities to gain input and support from a wide range of individuals, groups, and organizations for the subsequent program planning decisions as well as program implementation and evaluation.

Writing the Final Report and Disseminating Findings

Once analysis of the data is complete and the ranking of priorities has been agreed on, then it is time to write the final report on the needs assessment. The final report contains an executive summary, acknowledgments, table of contents, demographics of the community, methods of data collection, main findings, established priorities, references, and appendices. The final report will be the face of the needs assessment for the next several years.

Before writing, think about the information that the audience needs and the format that is most appropriate. Both written and oral reports can be developed. Tailor presentations to program staff, participants, and stakeholders. Remember to plan ahead; don't wait until there are results to think about how to share them. *Needs assessment reports* do not need to be elaborate. It is most important that the information shared be clear, simple, and timely. Use brief sections and subsections, and make titles clear and informative. Whenever possible, depict findings pictorially in charts, graphs, figures, or maps, and combine these with explanations in the text. Mix didactic and data-rich information with supporting evidence and anecdotal descriptions. Varying the material in this way will make the report more interesting and readable and the findings more believable.

Consideration on dissemination is also important. Dissemination options include printing the entire report; preparing special reports or brochures for particular groups of individuals and stakeholders (such as funders or program participants); posting the report on the Internet; and informing people about the report through e-mail, public meetings, board and staff meetings, newspaper reports, radio and television interviews by advisory board members and staff, press releases, and news conferences.

Summary

Conducting a needs assessment provides an unbiased look at a priority population within a particular setting and provides a foundation for the work of putting together a program that is culturally appropriate and based on health theory in order to address identified health problems and concerns. When conducting a needs assessment, it is essential to use a variety of methods to collect and analyze data from both primary and secondary sources and to conduct a capacity assessment of the site: school, workplace, health care organization, or community. Then, working with the advisory board, program participants, staff, and stakeholders, establish program priorities using approaches such as BPR 2.0 and consensus building to maximize program support in the later program planning decisions as well as during the program implementation and evaluation.

Tailor the needs assessment report to the program participants, staff and stakeholders, and the setting. In the report, in plain language, identify the diverse factors that influence health behaviors as well as the behaviors and environmental conditions that promote or compromise health. Likewise, identify factors that influence learning and behavior, foster or hinder the health promotion process, and determine the extent of existing and available health promotion programs and services.

For Practice and Discussion

1. Identify several health theories and discuss how they might influence a needs assessment. Compare and contrast the theories. How do they help you to understand needs assessment for health promotion programs?

2. How would a needs assessment for a rural community of 5,000 people (including adults, children, and senior citizens) differ from a needs assessment for a large urban hospital with 1,500 employees working seven days a week, 24 hours a day, or for a school district with 4,000 students in kindergarten through 12th grade? How might the use of the primary data methods discussed in this chapter differ at the sites? What would be the pros and cons of the methods at the sites?

3. A manufacturing company is planning a program to promote physical activity among 1,000 employees at one of its sites. The company's directors have expressed interest in a particular physical activity program that is based on the Stages of Change model. How might this fact influence the needs assessment?

4. The first step toward eliminating health disparities is a culturally appropriate needs assessment. If you were assigned the task of preparing a needs assessment of incoming college freshmen at the University of Texas at El Paso, what steps would you take to implement and ensure a culturally appropriate needs assessment?

5. What important information is added to a needs assessment by conducting a capacity assessment at a workplace? Can you identify any resources that might help in completing the workplace capacity assessment?

6. You are working on a student health needs assessment for a school district. Your job is to conduct a survey by administering a health needs questionnaire to 1,500 students in grades 9–12. The school directors and the superintendent want you to identify how much it will cost. What are the costs?

7. Dissemination options for a needs assessment report include printing the entire report, preparing special reports or brochures for particular groups of individuals and stakeholders (such as funders or program participants), posting the report on the web, and informing people about the report through e-mail, public meetings, board and staff meetings, newspaper reports, radio and television interviews by advisory board members and staff, press releases, and news conferences. Which options do you think would work best, and why, at the different sites: schools, workplaces, health care organizations, and communities?

KEY TERMS

Capacity assessment

Climate

Consensus building

Content validity

Culture

Delphi technique

Demography

Epidemiology

Face validity

Focus group

Geographic information system (GIS)

Key informant interviews

Need

Needs assessment

Needs assessment report

PEARL score

Power analysis

Primary data

Priorities

Qualitative data

Quantitative data

Random selection

Reliability

Response bias

Sample

Sampling bias

School Health Index

Secondary data

Social determinants of health

Survey

Validity

References

Altschuld, J. W., & Kumar, D. D. (2010). *The needs assessment KIT—Book 1, needs assessment: An overview*. Thousand Oaks, CA: SAGE.

Barnett, E., Anderson, T., Blosnich, J., Menard, J., Halverson, J., & Casper. M. (2007). Key informant interviews. In *Heart healthy and stroke free: A social environment handbook* (pp. 61–66). Atlanta, GA: U.S. Department of Health and Human Services, Centers for Disease Control and Prevention.

Blair, J., Czaja, R. F., & Blair, E. A. (2014). *Designing surveys* (3rd ed.). Thousand Oaks, CA: Sage.

Blumberg, J. J., Luke, J. V. (2015). Wireless substitution: early release of estimates from the National Health Interview Survey, January–June 2015. National Center for Health Statistics. Available from: http://www.cdc.gov/nchs/data/nhis/earlyrelease/wireless201512.pdf

DeVon, H. A., Block, M. E., Moyle-Wright, P., Ernst, D. M., Hayden, S. J., Lazzara, D. J., et al. (2007). A psychometric toolbox for testing validity and reliability. *Journal of Nursing Scholarship, 39*, 155–164.

Dillman, D. A., Smyth, J. D., & Christian, L. M. (2014). *Internet, phone, mail, and mixed mode surveys: The tailored design method*. Hoboken, NJ: Wiley.

File, T., & Ryan, C. (2014). Computer and Internet use in the United States: 2013. American Community Survey Reports, ACS-28, U.S. Census Bureau, Washington, DC.

Fowler, F. J. (2013). *Survey research methods* (5th ed.). Thousand Oaks, CA: Sage.

Gilmore, G. (2012). *Needs and capacity assessment strategies for health education and health promotion*. Burlington, MA: Jones & Bartlett.

Golden, S. D., & Earp, J. L. (2012). Social ecological approaches to individuals and their contexts: Twenty years of health education & behavior health promotion interventions. *Health Education & Behavior, 39*, 364–372.

Herrera, C., Hargraves, J., & Stanton, G. (2013). The impact of the mental health parity and addiction equity act on inpatient admission. Health Care Cost Institute. Retrieved from http://www.healthcostinstitute.org/files/HCCI-Mental-Health-Parity-Issue-Brief.pdf

Krueger, R., & Casey, M. (2014). *Focus groups: A practical guide for applied research* (5th ed.). Thousand Oaks, CA: Sage.

McClusky, S. (2011). Increasing response rates to lifestyle surveys: a pragmatic evidence review. *Perspectives in Public Health, 131*, 89–94.

Mechanic, D. (2014). More people than ever before are receiving behavioral health care in the United States, but gaps and challenges remain. *Health Affairs, 33*(8), 1416–1424.

National Center for Chronic Disease Prevention and Health Promotion. (2015). *School health index*. Atlanta, GA: Author. Retrieved from http://www.cdc.gov/HealthyYouth/SHI/introduction.htm

Neiger, B. L., Tackery, R., & Fagen, M. C. (2011). Basic priority rating model 2.0: Current applications for priority setting in health promotion practice. *Health Promotion Practice, 12*(2), 166–171.

Niggel, S. J., & Brandon, W. P. (2014). Social determinants of health and community needs: Implications for health legacy foundations. *Health Affairs, 33*(11), 2072–2076.

Price, J. H., Dake, J. A., Murnan, J., Dimmig, J., & Akpanudo, S. (2005). Power analysis in survey research: Importance and use for health educators. *American Journal of Health Education, 36,* 202–207.

Schneider, B., Herhart, M. G., & Macey, W. H. (2013). Organizational climate and culture. *Annual Review of Psychology, 64,* 361–388.

Substance Abuse and Mental Health Services Administration. (2014). *Results from the 2013 National Survey on Drug Use and Health: Mental health findings* (NSDUH Series H-49, HHS Publication No. (SMA) 14-4887). Rockville, MD: Substance Abuse and Mental Health Services Administration.

Vilnius, D., & Dandoy, S. (1990). A priority rating system for public health programs. *Public Health Reports, 105*(5), 463–470.

CHAPTER 5

MAKING DECISIONS TO CREATE AND SUPPORT A PROGRAM

Jiunn-Jye Sheu, W. William Chen, and Huey-Shys Chen

Identifying a Mission Statement, Goals, and Objectives

One of the actions when creating a program is to decide what is the program *mission statement*. A mission statement is usually a short statement that describes the general focus or purpose of a program (McKenzie, Neiger, & Thackeray, 2013). The mission statement answers the question of why a health promotion program is being developed and established. As such, a mission statement reflects the program's overall purpose and values. A mission statement is sometimes referred to as the *philosophy* of a health promotion program.

The following are samples of mission statements:

- The Employee Wellness Program mission is to promote healthy and productive individuals and families.

- The Ohio Commission on Minority Health is dedicated to promoting health equity and high quality health care for minority populations through innovative strategies and financial opportunities, public health promotion, legislative action, public policy and systems change.

- The mission of the Brookfield Unified School District's Coordinated School Health Program is to prepare students to be healthy and productive individuals.

LEARNING OBJECTIVES

- Define *mission, goals,* and *objectives*; explain how they interact during program design and development.

- Write measurable process, action, and outcome objectives.

- Explain the link between measurable objectives and evidence-based practice approaches.

- Identify health promotion interventions designed to change knowledge, attitudes, and behavior.

- Create, write, and revise policies to support program implementation.

- Be able to make the transition to program implementation.

- Communities in Action for Peace promotes healthy communities by modeling peace and justice in action, as we strive to end violence and its causes in a nontraditional and culturally sensitive manner.

A *goal* sets a program's direction and intent (Gilbert, Sawyer, & McNeill, 2015). Goals clarify what is important in the health promotion program and state the end results of the program. A goal includes the program's priority population and, in general, uses action words such as *reduce, eliminate,* or *increase.* Some examples of program goals are listed here:

- A goal of the Employee Walking Program is to increase regular exercise among staff and their family members.

- A goal of the American Lung Association's Freedom from Smoking program is to decrease the number of smokers by helping people who already smoke to stop smoking.

- A goal of Brookfield Unified School District's Coordinated School Health Program is to increase the numbers of students in K to 12 who adopt healthy nutrition behaviors.

Program *objectives* are the specific steps (or subgoals) that need to be achieved in order to attain the goal. They are specific and measurable with a timeline that identifies by when the objective will be attained. An objective statement specifies who, what, when, and where and clarifies by how much, how many, or how often (U.S. Department of Health and Human Services, 1997). Each objective makes clear what is expected and is stated in such a way that the achievement can be measured. While achievement of objectives may not always be measured, the objectives must be measurable. If measurement is not possible, the objective is probably not clearly stated. Measurability is the major difference between goals and objectives. Goals provide an overview of the desired outcomes at the end of the program, while objectives provide specific and clear steps (tasks) that need to be achieved in order to attain the goal (or goals) of the program. Each goal may have several tasks (objectives) that need to be completed in order to achieve it. Different types of objective statements are used, depending on the needs of the program.

Process (or *administrative*) *objectives* are used to identify the needed changes or tasks in the administration of the program itself (for example, hiring staff, providing professional development for staff, seeking additional funding). These types of objectives are used to evaluate progress in the implementation of the program. Here are examples of process (administrative) objectives:

- By month 3 of the initiative, two qualified instructors will have been hired and received orientation in effectively delivering the curriculum of the initiative.
- By the end of the year, smoking cessation programs for college students will have been initiated in 70 of the 106 historically Black colleges and universities in the United States.

Action (or *behavioral*) *objectives* are used to identify needed changes in the actions or behaviors of the priority population. These types of objectives are used to evaluate the impact of a program on participants. Here are examples of action (behavioral) objectives:

- The percentage of binge drinkers among college students will decrease from 60% to less than 50% after completion of the social marketing program at the end of the year.
- By the end of the program, 50% of the participants will increase their exercise activities to at least 30 minutes a day, three times a week.

Outcome objectives are used to identify the long-term accomplishments of a health promotion program. Following are some examples of outcome objectives:

- The number of alcohol-related deaths and injuries will decrease by 25% within the city during the next 2 years.
- New cases of HIV among Hispanic women ages 18 to 25 will be reduced by 25% by the year 2020.

Writing Program Objectives

Writing a good objective takes skill and judgment. As we have discussed, objectives are the steps or tasks needed to achieve a goal. The objectives connect goals to the *interventions* that will facilitate achievement of the goals. The *Healthy People 2020* objectives are a good resource and model when writing objectives (http://www.healthypeople.gov/). When you begin to draft objectives, you ask questions like these:

- What does the priority population need to know or do in order to achieve this goal?
- What changes in knowledge, attitudes, or skills need to occur?

- What social support is needed to facilitate behavioral changes?
- What policy or environmental changes are needed to achieve the goal?
- Specifically, who is expected to change, by how much, and by when?

Reviewing data from the needs assessment will help in establishing target numbers. Being very clear by specifying numbers and percentages facilitates monitoring progress. For example, program planners shall review the infant mortality statistics and the prevalence of low birth weight babies in the county by key demographics such as age, race/ethnicity, income, education, marital status, and/or neighborhoods prior to writing up the objectives to provide prenatal care and nutritional supplements.

When writing objectives, make sure that the objectives (1) are measurable, relevant, and achievable; (2) drive action and suggest a set of steps that will help to achieve the goals within a specific time frame; (3) include a range of measures directed toward achieving program goals; (4) are established at the outset of the program in order to make evaluation possible; (5) support short-term as well as long-term plans; and (6) are based on sound scientific evidence (U.S. Department of Health and Human Services, 1997).

One approach to writing program objectives uses the mnemonic *SMART*, which indicates objectives that are specific, measurable, achievable, realistic, and time-phased (Evaluation Research Team, 2009). SMART objectives allow you to proceed with your program, knowing that you have a strong foundation on which implementation and evaluation plans can be developed. The SMART mnemonic is described in more detail in the following sections.

Specific

When you write an objective, clearly state exactly what you plan to achieve by providing the appropriate type and amount of detail and one specific action verb. The details can be summarized with the following "four W's" rule:

1. Who or what is expected to change or happen?
2. What or how much change is expected? (amount or degree of change)
3. Where will the change occur?
4. When will the change occur? (often indicated by a date)

For example, an objective of a program to prevent obesity among African American girls might state, "By May 30, 2020, 50% of the African American girls in grades 6 to 8 in the Riverside County Schools will engage in 40 minutes of moderate to vigorous physical activity each day as determined by an annual youth behavior risk survey (Baseline: 30% of African American girls work out 20 minutes of moderate to vigorous physical activity in 2015)."

- Who or what is expected to change or happen? African American sixth- to eighth- grade girls will increase daily physical activity from 20 to 40 minutes
- What or how much change is expected? Change from 30% to 80% of African American girls
- Where will the change occur? Riverside County Schools
- When will the change occur? May 30, 2020 (The change will occur over time beginning in 2017)

Some objectives do not have a quantifiable outcome and will not involve many numbers. However, this type of objective is still required to be specific, and the four W's rule still applies. Here is an example of this type of objective: "By June 30, 2018, Allegheny County commissioners will adopt and disseminate a policy to restrict the sale of sodas and other sugary drinks that are larger than 16 fluid ounces in food establishments such as restaurants, movie theaters, sports arenas, delis, food trucks, and street carts."

- What is expected to change or happen? Adoption of a policy to restrict the sale of sodas and other sugary drinks
- What or how much change is expected? Restrict the sale of sodas and other sugary drinks that are larger than 16 fluid ounces in food establishments such as restaurants, movie theaters, sports arenas, delis, food trucks, and street carts
- Where will the change occur? Allegheny County
- When will the change occur? By June 30, 2018

The action verb of an objective indicates a clear action. Verbs such as "understand" or "know" can be replaced by more specific ones such as "list" or "write." A list of frequently used action verbs can be found from http://www.cdc.gov/healthyyouth/tutorials/writinggoal/docs/wgg_verb-list.pdf.

Measurable (or Observable)

In the first example in the preceding section, the measurable outcome is whether the African American girls have increased their physical activity to 40 minutes per day. To measure the change that has occurred, you would compare the percentage of African American girls engaging in 40 minutes of daily physical activity as shown in the youth risk behavior survey that the school administers in 2017 to the percentage that were exercising in 2015 (30%).

In the second example, the achievement of the objective is a one-time event—the adoption of the policy—that does not involve measuring a quantity. However, one can observe whether the policy has been adopted and whether the policy has been disseminated. The observable outcome is whether the policy has been adopted. To verify that the policy has indeed been adopted, you could obtain official documents. Verification of dissemination could occur after the policy has been enacted and publicized as part of the public health department's periodic sanitary inspection of food establishments such as restaurants, movie theaters, sports arenas, delis, food trucks, and street carts.

Achievable (Reachable)

For objectives that have a quantifiable outcome, a baseline measure will assist in estimating the level of success that one might expect to achieve. Decide whether your objective is reachable by considering baseline measurements as well as by using your knowledge and experience in this area. For example, if at the start of the program, 30% of students engage in 20 minutes of physical activity per day, it may be too ambitious to aim to increase the proportion of students who exercise an hour daily to 80% by 2017. An increase to 50% might be more achievable.

In practice, your estimation would depend on the strategies that you were planning to implement as part of the health promotion program. In the first example in the preceding section, if the intervention strategies focused only on instruction about the value of exercise, one would choose a smaller number. But if the intervention included a program in which all K–6 teachers provide exercise breaks for students at their desk for 5 to 10 minutes several times a day, the number of students who achieve the goal would increase more than if the intervention were just instruction.

In the second example the objective is a step toward a healthy food environment. However, achieving a healthy food environment represents a large goal that will take time. The objective to adopt and disseminate a policy to prohibit the sale of large sugary drinks in all restaurants and public eating establishments is one of the items that needs to be accomplished. Objectives related to public education about the new policy and enforcement might be subsequent steps (objectives) once this objective is achieved.

Realistic, Meaningful, and Important

Objectives need to address concerns that are absolute priorities. Programs are expensive in terms of money and people's time and energy. Often, there is a limited window of opportunity in which to address a concern. A limited budget may force you to trim the scope of a program's activities. A program's objectives will determine its interventions and its advocacy agenda. For these reasons, from the beginning, you need to ask whether an objective is realistic and whether it is the most important and meaningful way to address a health concern.

Time-Phased

Effective objectives are time-phased. By what date do you want the outcome to be achieved? A time frame is important to establish because the type and intensity of your interventions, activities, and evaluation will depend on how much time you think it will take to achieve your goal.

Deciding on Program Interventions

Once the goals and objectives of a program have been written, the health promotion program staff, stakeholders, and participants need to identify the interventions or strategies that will facilitate attainment of each objective and all goals. The most effective interventions are culturally appropriate and based on health theories and models. An intervention is any set of methods, techniques, or processes designed to effect changes in behaviors or the environment. Identifying the interventions explains how you intend to achieve the objectives.

In planning program interventions, first consider the range of interventions available to be used in health promotion programs:

- Instruction: teacher-based lessons (for example, lecture, discussion, group work) and individual-based instruction (for example, web-based, wearable personal health devices, written or audiovisual materials, smart phones)

- Counseling: individual or group sessions, behavioral modification, behavioral contracting, skill building, or social support (texting)

- Regulatory strategies: policy mandates, legislation, ordinances, rules, regulations

- Environmental change: changes in the physical, social, or economic environment that provide incentives or disincentives for behavior change

- Social support: support buddy, support group, social networks

- Direct interventions: screening, referral, treatment, and follow-up to stimulate needed changes

• Communication or media outreach: mass media, such as radio, TV, newspapers; personal media, such as social media, personal health devices, and texting; printed media, such as pamphlets, billboards, posters, direct mail, and church bulletins

• Advocacy: organizing at the site, coalition building, community development, social action, meeting with legislative representative

In planning which interventions a health promotion program will use, it is important to match the intervention to the specific needs of the priority population as well as to choose interventions that represent a broad range of approaches in order to affect the priority population in different ways, depending on whether individuals need knowledge, practice in specific skills, change of attitudes, change in behaviors, support by significant others, or broad environmental change. For example, drug abuse prevention programs for school-age adolescents can achieve significant reductions in the rates of social, behavioral, and academic problems when interventions are designed for youths who are at risk to experiment with drug use. However, this instructional program designed to prevent alcohol and drug use in adolescents would not be effective for adolescents who already have an addiction problem; the interventions that they would need would be quite different. The selection of the intervention strategies is guided by health behavior theories. For example, the social cognitive theory, diffusion of innovation, and transtheoretical model are among the widely used theories.

The Institute of Medicine (1994) identified preventive interventions for different priority populations and different health problems and concerns. The model uses the range of identifiable risk to categorize preventive interventions. The three levels are:

1. **Universal preventive interventions:** The priority population is the general public or a population that has not been identified on the basis of individual risk. In other words, these interventions are designed for everyone. Universal preventive interventions are found to have mild to strong influences on different health concerns among different populations. Examples of this type of intervention include mass media campaigns via public service announcements on TV and social skills instruction provided to all K–12 students.

2. **Selective preventive interventions:** The priority population is individuals or a subgroup of the population whose risk of developing illness or disorders is significantly higher than average. Examples include an education program to encourage construction workers to wear earplugs or protective devices when operating noisy machinery and

grief counseling sessions provided to students who are experiencing a traumatic loss.

3. **Indicated preventive interventions:** The priority population is high-risk individuals who have detectable signs or symptoms but have not reached the diagnostic criteria of a particular health problem. Indicated preventive interventions are found to have better effects on identified health issues. An example would be a smoking cessation program for heavy smokers.

Weisz, Sandler, Durlak, and Anton (2005) expanded the Institute of Medicine's model of preventive intervention to five levels of strategies; health promotion and positive development strategies, and treatment strategies are added to the components of the Institute of Medicine's model.

1. **Health promotion and positive development strategies** address an entire population with the goal of enhancing strengths in order to reduce the risk of later problem outcomes or to increase prospects for positive development. Examples include programs that focus on building personal and social skills through teacher, parent, and youth training and development of individualized action plans to improve fitness levels after receiving the results of a fitness screening test.

2. **Universal preventive strategies** are approaches designed to address risk factors in an entire population without attempting to distinguish who is at elevated risk. Examples include programs that address risk factors in broadly defined population groups (for instance, a program in which all children in a particular grade or age range receive anti-bullying instruction and improved recess supervision in which teachers intervene with guided discovery when there is bullying on the playground).

3. **Selective preventive strategies** are approaches in which specific groups that share a significant risk factor, and interventions are designed to reduce that risk. An example of a selective preventive strategy is providing visits by a public health nurse to a young, unmarried, and economically disadvantaged pregnant woman to promote behaviors during and after pregnancy that will be healthy for both the woman and her child.

4. **Indicated preventive strategies** are approaches designed for individuals who have significant symptoms of a disorder but do not meet diagnostic criteria. An example of an indicated preventive strategy is a home-based and school-based intervention that focuses on disruptive boys in kindergarten.

Table 5.1   Typology of Health Promotion Interventions

Level	Strategies
Health promotion interventions for individuals	Focus on information, modeling, education, and training in order to promote change in knowledge, attitudes, beliefs, and behavior in regard to health risks such as smoking, eating, and physical activity.
Policy and practices of organizations	Focus on organizational change and consultancy in order to change organizational policies (rules, roles, sanctions, and incentives) and practices in order to produce changes in individuals' risky behavior and greater access to social, educational, and health resources that promote health.
Environmental actions and social change at sites	Focus on social action and social planning at existing sites and on creating new sites (for example, organizations, networks, or partnerships) in order to produce change in organizations and redistribute resources that affect health.
Public advocacy	Focus on social advocacy in order to change legislative, budgetary, and institutional settings that affect community, organizational, and individual levels.

Source: Adapted from Swerissen and Crisp, 2004.

5. **Treatment interventions** are approaches designed for individuals who have high symptom levels or a diagnosable illness or disorder. These interventions apply to those individuals' diagnosed illnesses and disorders. The interventions (treatment) usually take place in clinical settings.

Table 5.1 presents different types of interventions along with corresponding methods, techniques, or processes designed to effect changes in behaviors or the environment. The four types of interventions focus on health promotion interventions for individuals, policy of organizations, environmental actions and social change at sites and beyond, and public advocacy. While the types are nested within one another, they involve different processes (Swerissen & Crisp, 2004).

Health promotion interventions are often created (designed) for a priority population. Interventions that have already been developed can also be selected (or sometimes purchased) and used. Program staff can now select from an increasing number of evidence-based health promotion interventions that have been researched and reviewed for their effectiveness; evidence-based interventions will be discussed later in this chapter.

Selecting Health Promotion Materials

Many health promotion intervention materials are developed by government or commercial developers. Existing materials can be obtained from the catalogues published by government agencies or companies, but they need to be reviewed before use. Even if the materials are considered acceptable, they still need to be pilot-tested by a sample group of the priority population. The following questions in regard to the program objectives, theoretical foundation, interventions, and strategies can be examined:

- Do the program materials enable the objectives to be met?
- Do they deliver the intended theoretical methods and practical strategies?
- Do the materials fit with the priority population?
- Are the materials attractive, appealing, and culturally appropriate?
- Are the messages delivered by the materials consistent with the program objectives?
- Will the materials be properly used in the planned intervention?

After the materials are determined to be appropriate, the following criteria can be considered:

Availability. The availability of the material, in terms of quantity and time frame, can be considered in the planning stage. Reproduction may be possible if permission is granted. Companies that produce intervention materials may charge for them on the basis of quantity or frequency of use. Many materials are placed on the web in formats such as web pages, PDF documents, PowerPoint presentations, Word documents, videos, audio files, or graphics files. Increasingly personal health devices and smartphone and tablet apps are used to deliver programs. Attention is required to assure that participants have access to and know how to use the technologies. If modification is needed, permission is to be obtained from the developer in advance and proper acknowledgment can be included in the materials.

Reading level. The reading level of a piece of writing indicates how easy it is to read by assigning it a school grade level. The reading level often determines whether the intervention material is acceptable for the intended participants. Low reading literacy in the American general population has become a challenge in developing health promotion materials. Using graphics and short sentences helps to make materials accessible to populations with low levels of literacy.

Production quality and suitability. To address the overall suitability of materials (including reading level), Doak, Doak, and Root (1996) developed the suitability assessment of materials (SAM). Although SAM was developed for use with print materials, it has also been used to assess videotaped and audio instructions.

SAM scores materials in six categories: content, literacy demand, graphics, layout and typography, learning stimulation, and cultural appropriateness. SAM yields a final percentage score, which falls into one of three categories: superior, adequate, or not suitable. SAM can be used to identify specific shortcomings that reduce the suitability of materials either in the developmental stage or in final form. (A full description of SAM and a scoring sheet are available in Doak, Doak, & Root, 1996.)

Using Evidence-Based Interventions

Evidence-based health promotion interventions are conceptualized as the delivery of optimal care through integration of current best scientific evidence, clinical expertise and experience, and preferences of individuals, families, organizations, and communities. They provide to practitioners interventions that are critically appraised and that incorporate scientific evidence into practice. Evidence-based health promotion interventions identify the priority populations that would benefit from the intervention and the conditions under which the intervention works and may indicate the change mechanisms that account for intervention effects. The interventions include various tested strategies for different diseases or behaviors. A defining characteristic of *evidence-based interventions* is their use of health theory in both developing the intervention content (activities, curriculum, tasks) and evaluation (measures, outcomes).

Numerous health promotion interventions are initiated, evaluated, and found to be effective. Examples can be found in the published literature by using the free PubMed database (http://www.pubmed.gov) created by the National Library of Medicine and the National Institutes of Health. Use key words related to the health behavior that is of interest to you.

Three key sources of evidence-based health promotion interventions are operated by the federal government. The first is the *National Registry of Evidence-Based Programs and Practices* (NREPP), which was developed and is maintained by the Substance Abuse and Mental Health Services Administration (SAMHSA) in the U.S. Department of Health and Human Services. NREPP (http://www.nrepp.samhsa.gov) is a searchable database of interventions for the prevention and treatment of mental and substance use disorders (Figure 5.1). NREPP uses a voluntary, self-nominating system in which intervention developers elect to participate. There will always be some interventions that are not submitted to NREPP, and not all that are submitted are reviewed. Nevertheless, new intervention summaries are continually being added to the site. The registry is expected to grow to a larger number of interventions over time.

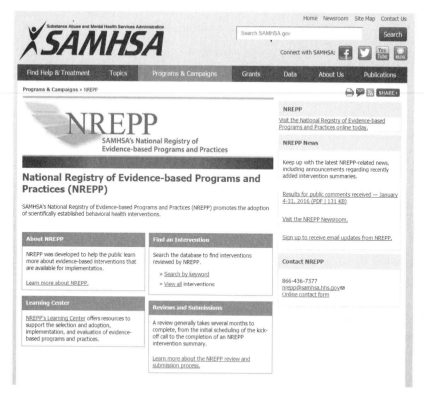

Figure 5.1 Search Page on the Website of the National Registry of Evidence-Based Programs and Practices

The second federal source of evidence-based health promotion interventions, *Guide to Community Preventive Services* (http://www.the communityguide.org), is a resource from the Centers for Disease Control and Prevention that evaluates the effectiveness of broad intervention categories through systematic research reviews. The Guide takes a broader approach looking at evidence-based policy and the community initiatives. Figure 5.2 shows an example of a summary of evidence from the Guide. The example is for tobacco cessation.

The third resource is *Research-tested Intervention Programs* (RTIPs) developed and maintained by the National Cancer Institute (http://rtips .cancer.gov/rtips/index.do). RTIPs is a database of programs as well as products that individuals, groups, and organizations can access and use (Figure 5.3). RTIPs is linked to the Guide to Community Preventive Services.

Identifying Appropriate Evidence-Based Interventions

Using NREPP, Guide to Community Preventive Services, and RTIPs, you have choices about interventions that you can use in your program.

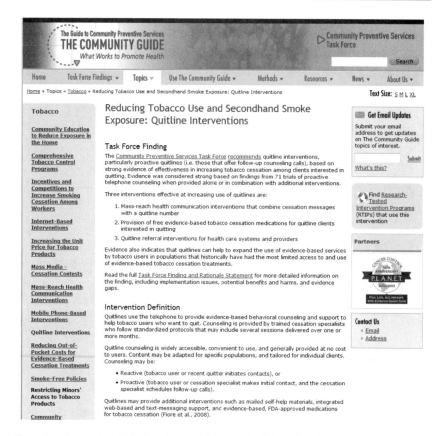

Figure 5.2 Community Guide Evidence Summary Example Using Tobacco Cessation

To identify evidence-based interventions that are appropriate for your health promotion program, consider the following:

Contexts for intervention. The array of settings in which the intervention might be based needs to be considered when deciding which evidence-based interventions would be most appropriate to address specific goals. Settings to consider include homes, schools, churches, primary care clinics, residential facilities, community centers, boys and girls clubs, after-school programs, teen social centers, sports team facilities, volunteer centers, and summer job settings. Preventive interventions can be sited in the places where the prioirty population lives or at the sites of other activities.

Coverage across the range of populations or settings involved in a health concern. Many of the most prevalent and significant risks and issues pertaining to specific health problems can now be identified through published empirical data, but significant gaps in

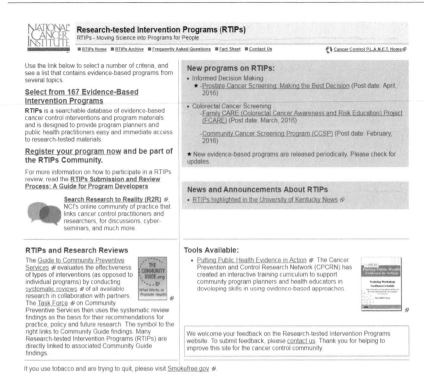

Figure 5.3 Home Page of the Research-Tested Intervention Programs (RTIPs) Website

coverage still remain, both in terms of information and appropriate interventions. For example, although anorexia interventions may have demonstrated effectiveness among the 15 to 24-year-old females who have the highest prevalence, the settings and program designs may not apply well to preadolescents. You would search extensively and find the most appropriate design for your audience.

Knowledge of what population interventions will be effective for— and under what conditions. For each intervention that works, you need to know as much as possible about the population within which benefits accrue. You need to know in what settings an intervention works. Even the best-supported interventions are apt to be beneficial for some groups (defined by age, gender, socioeconomic status, or other demographic characteristics) but not for others and in some settings but not in others. Understanding factors (in terms of population groups and conditions) that moderate intervention effects is essential to understanding how and to whom to apply various health promotion interventions.

Impact of race, ethnicity, and culture. Factors of race, ethnicity, and culture—for example, norms, beliefs, and values derived from their respective cultures—influence the priority population and program site. An effective intervention must be compatible with relevant norms, beliefs, and values or must incorporate the ability to understand, respect, and work with differences. Responses to health promotion interventions may differ on the basis of participants' ethnicity or culture.

Staff creativity, experience, and clinical expertise. Evidence-based interventions have explicit protocols described in intervention manuals that may provide essential principles and guidelines but still allow considerable flexibility and use of staff's creativity, experience, and clinical expertise in the effort to achieve desired intervention outcomes. Specific elements of these interventions, combined in ways that fit the distinctive characteristics of the individuals, may produce genuine benefits. For example, an element such as a role-playing activity to strengthen self-efficacy in refusing a cigarette could be modified and used in another intervention program to model how to ask friends to wear seat belts when one is driving.

Balancing Fidelity and Adaptation

Evidence-based interventions have prescribed protocols to direct the implementation or use of the intervention, including a detailed set of instructions, materials, and staffing requirements. Furthermore, there is a prescribed implementation process as well as staff training and development. Developers of evidence-based health promotion interventions try to facilitate maximum *fidelity* to the essentials of intervention while still allowing maximal *adaptation* for the specific needs of a setting.

Fidelity defines the extent to which the delivery of a health intervention conforms to the curriculum, protocol, or guidelines for implementing that intervention. Intervention fidelity is rated from high to low. A high-fidelity intervention would be delivered exactly as intended by the people who created it. A low-fidelity program would be delivered quite differently than intended by the people who created it. Adaptation defines the degree to which an intervention undergoes change in its implementation to fit the needs of a particular delivery situation. The apparent antithesis of fidelity, adaptation could alter program integrity if an intervention is adapted so drastically that it is not delivered as originally intended. However, it is possible for an intervention to be rendered more responsive to a particular priority population through the adaptation process. For example, adaptation could increase an intervention's cultural sensitivity and its fit within a new setting.

Researchers suggest that modifying an intervention is acceptable up to a *zone of drastic mutation*; after that point, further modification will compromise the program's integrity and effectiveness (Hall & Loucks, 1978). In working with evidence-based interventions, it is necessary to have a balance between fidelity and adaptation in order to fine-tune the complex, dynamic interaction between a health promotion intervention and its priority population and environment. Schinke, Brounstein, and Gardner (2002) recommend guidelines to help balance fidelity and adaptation:

1. Identify and understand the theory behind an intervention. What are the intervention's theoretical underpinnings? Reading the published literature on the intervention and talking with the individuals who developed the intervention are two strategies for answering this question. Understanding the mission, goals, and objectives of a particular intervention can help program staff to persuade stakeholders of the current health promotion program of an intervention's utility to them in the given environment.

2. Assess fidelity and adaptation concerns for a particular site or setting. Determine what adaptation might be required to meet the needs of the priority population and the environment where the intervention is to be implemented.

3. Involve the individuals who developed the intervention. Talk with them about their thinking as they shaped the intervention. Consultations with other groups that have implemented the intervention in similar environments may also be helpful.

4. Talk with the stakeholders at the site where the intervention will be implemented. Discuss your thoughts on the balance of fidelity and adaptation in order to understand concerns, build support, and generate input on how to achieve successful implementation.

5. Employ an analysis of core components. A core component analysis is a listing of an intervention's core ingredients followed by discussion with program staff, participants, and stakeholders about which are essential for success and which are more amenable to modification in order to meet local conditions and needs. Table 5.2 shows a list of core components for an intervention to prevent substance abuse in elementary schools and areas to consider for adaptation. A core component analysis can be a bridge between intervention developers and practitioners.

Table 5.2   Core Component Analysis for an Intervention to Prevent Substance Abuse in an Elementary School

Core Component	Description of Areas to Consider for Adaptation
Content focus	Intervention focuses on generic life skills and specific skills for avoiding the use of alcohol and tobacco. Consider adding marijuana as a content area.
Modeling and behavioral rehearsal	Instructor demonstrates new skills using set scripts; participant then performs the skill within the session. Consider student-produced scripts and use of upper elementary and middle school students as peer leaders in sessions.
Homework assignments	Assignments (for example, journaling, practicing a skill at home with a parent or others) reinforce concepts.
Cueing	Instructor cues students to use new behavior in a specific situation. Consider having the upper elementary and middle school student peer leaders cue students during school activities (for example, during lunch or before and after school programs).
Self-monitoring	Participants log behavior in order to enhance awareness and enactment of desired behavior. Consider using web postings and discussion boards.

6. Develop an overall implementation plan based on these inputs. Include a strategy for achieving and measuring the balance between fidelity and adaptation as the intervention is implemented

These guidelines inform and facilitate an implementation process that maintains fidelity to the concept of the intervention and makes necessary adaptations to facilitate effective delivery.

Developing Effective Policies and Procedures

Health promotion programs do not operate in a vacuum. They operate within the structure of their setting. Each setting (school, workplace, hospital, community) has its *policies*—operating rules that specify people's rights and responsibilities as well as spelling out the rights and responsibilities of the organization in regards to its stakeholders (for example, students, employees, clients, or members). Policies are the backbone of health promotion programs. Effective policies clearly state the health values and priorities of the organization and are tailored to the unique requirements and needs of the setting and stakeholders. Drawn from the policies are *procedures*, which typically address program logistics and day-to-day operating details such as recruitment, retention, and recognition of program participants.

The model smoke-free workplace policy in Table 5.3 was promulgated and promoted by the New York City Health Department for use by businesses and organizations at their sites in order to clearly state that smoke-free workplaces are required by law and, furthermore, that each organization, by personalizing the policy through such action as adding its

Table 5.3   Sample Smoke-Free Workplace Policy for New York City

- Purpose. A smoke-free policy has been developed to comply with the New York City Smoke-Free Air Act (Title 17, Chapter 5 of the Administrative Code of the City of New York) and New York State Clean Indoor Air Act (Article 13-E of the New York State Public Health Law), and to protect all employees and visitors from secondhand smoke, an established cause of cancer and respiratory disease. The policy set forth below is effective March 30, 2003, for all [company name] locations.

- Smoke-Free Areas. All areas of the workplace are now smoke-free without exception. Smoking is not permitted anywhere in the workplace, including all indoor facilities and company vehicles with more than one person present. Smoking is not permitted in private enclosed offices, conference and meeting rooms, cafeterias, lunchrooms, or employee lounges.

- Sign Requirements. "No Smoking" signs must be clearly posted at all entrances and on bulletin boards, bathrooms, stairwells, and other prominent places. No ashtrays are permitted in any indoor area.

- Compliance. Compliance with the smoke-free workplace policy is mandatory for all employees and persons visiting the company, with no exceptions. Employees who violate this policy are subject to disciplinary action.

- Any disputes involving smoking needs to be handled through the company's procedure for resolving other work-related problems. If the problem persists, an employee can speak to [company department and phone number for complaints] or lodge an anonymous complaint by calling the New York City Department of Health and Mental Hygiene's complaint line, 1-877-NYC DOH7 (1-877-692-3647) or on the web at nyc.gov/health. DOHMH's enforcement staff will take appropriate action to resolve the problem.

- The law prohibits employers from retaliating against employees who invoke the law or who request management's assistance in implementing it in the workplace.

- Smoking Cessation Opportunities. [Company name] encourages all smoking employees to quit smoking. [The company medical department or worksite wellness program offers a number of services for employees who want to quit.] Smoking cessation information is available from the New York Smokers' Quit Line at 1-866 NY QUITS (1-866-697-8487).

- Questions. Any questions regarding the smoke-free workplace policy can be directed to [company department and phone number handling inquiries].

Source: City of New York, 2003.

name and placing the policy on the organization's stationery, agrees with the policy and supports smoke-free workplaces. What makes this a good policy is its clarity, nonjudgmental approach, grievance alternatives, and resources for support and for having questions answered about the policy.

There are many reasons to put health policies in writing:

- It creates a supportive health-promoting environment.
- A written policy is required by a law or by the organization's insurance carriers.
- It makes legal review possible.
- It provides a record of the organization's efforts and a reference if the policy is challenged. It may protect the employer from certain kinds of claims by stakeholders such as employees, families, or students.

- A written policy is easier to explain to stakeholders.

- Putting the policy in writing helps stakeholders concentrate on important policy information.

Developing a Health Promotion Policy

The policy development process guides the creation, writing, revision, and adoption of policies. It can also identify outdated policies for archiving health promotion goals and objectives, and it can identify gaps in policy. The process for developing and implementing a health promotion policy is as follows:

1. Generate support from organization leaders and stakeholders.

    Leaders. Provide leaders with a rationale for establishing a policy. Offer them data that emphasize cost-effectiveness and benefits. Ask for representatives to serve on the advisory committee.

    Stakeholders. Provide stakeholders with knowledge about health concerns (for example, passive smoking, cardiovascular disease, cancer, or personal hygiene). Select representatives from different stakeholder groups to serve on the advisory committee that will set policies. Stress individual, family, and community benefits.

2. Organize a cooperative process for policy development.

    Form an advisory committee to develop the policy. Designate one person as chair. Include representatives from all segments of the setting (for example, school, workplace, health care organization, or community).

    Review policy options.

    Disseminate reports on the process, including the results and findings of the needs assessment.

3. Develop policy content.

    Locate policy samples from other similar organizations or government agencies.

    Draft the policy that is the best fit for prevention of disease or for health promotion in the specific setting. Incorporate comments from the public and input from stakeholders.

4. Prepare for implementation.

    Send notification of the policy to those who will be affected well in advance of the date when it takes effect. Notify people individually.

Allow time for questions and adjustments during the transition period, and have a contingency plan.

5. Implement the policy.

Devise a comprehensive plan, including a process for dealing with grievances.

Make enforcement policy operational and consider any unanticipated consequences or problems as learning opportunities to improve the policy and its implementation.

6. Support stakeholders.

Support stakeholders—for example, by providing counseling, preventive health care, or social support.

Continue to enforce the policy.

7. Evaluate the policy.

Periodically review the policy and its effectiveness. Reviewing the policy will provide feedback on how to best implement the policy.

The most important task for every organization is to ensure that its policy meets the needs of its stakeholders and setting. Whether or not laws and regulations apply, the policy needs to address the key health topics of concern. Organizations can write (or adapt) and organize content on the key topics using whatever language and structure will best communicate the information to their stakeholders. Organizations do not need to start from scratch. They can borrow and adapt information from other organizations and settings. For example, since the Drug-Free Workplace Act was passed, many national, regional, and local programs have been set up to help employers create effective policies. The programs provide free or low-cost information, technical assistance, or model policies that organizations can customize to meet their particular needs. For more information, visit SAMHSA's Workplace website and Helpline information at http://www .samhsa.gov/workplace.

Basic Elements of an Effective Policy

The effective policy elements presented in this section are examples from workplace policies in city government and small businesses to promote drug-free workplaces. However, the elements can be adapted for schools, health care organizations, and community settings in order to develop *health promotion policies* across a range of health concerns, problems, and issues.

Statement of Purpose

Background

- How was the policy developed? (For example, was it developed in meetings with union representatives or employees representing different and diverse segments of the workforce, after consultation with other organizations in the same industry, or in collaboration with the organization's legal counsel?)

Goals

- What are the drug-free workplace laws and regulations (federal, state, or local) with which the organization must comply?

- What other goals does the organization expect to achieve? (For example, does the organization hope to reduce or eliminate drug-related accidents, illnesses, or absenteeism?)

- Does the organization want to address the issue of preventing and treating workplace drug use and abuse in the context of accomplishing a broader goal of promoting worker health, safety, and productivity?

Definitions, Expectations, and Prohibitions

- How does the organization define substance abuse?

- What employee behaviors are expected?

- Exactly what substances and behaviors are prohibited?

- Who is covered by the policy?

- When will the policy apply? (For example, will it apply during work hours only or during work hours and also during organization-sponsored events after hours?)

- Where will the policy apply? (For example, will it apply in the workplace while workers are on duty, outside the workplace while they are on duty, or in the workplace and in organization-owned vehicles while they are off duty?)

- Who is responsible for carrying out and enforcing the policy?

- Will the policy include any form of testing for alcohol or other drugs?

- Are any employees covered by the terms of a collective bargaining agreement, and if so, how do the terms affect the way the policy will be carried out and enforced for those employees?

Implementation Approaches

Dissemination Strategies

* How will the organization educate employees about the policy? (For example, the organization could train supervisors, discuss the policy during orientation sessions for new employees, or inform all employees about the policy through a variety of means—such as a section in the employee handbook, posters in gathering places at work sites, or information on the organization's intranet system.)

Benefits and Assurances

* How will the organization help employees comply with the policy?
* How will the organization protect employees' confidentiality?
* How will the organization help employees who seek help for drug-related problems?
* How will the organization help employees who are in treatment or recovery?
* How will the organization ensure that all aspects of the policy are implemented fairly and consistently for all employees?

Consequences and Appeals

* What are the consequences of violating the policy?
* What are the procedures for determining whether an employee has violated the policy?
* What are the procedures for appealing a determination that an employee has violated the policy?

Transitioning to Program Implementation

Once program staff, stakeholders, and participants decide on a program's mission, goals, objectives, interventions, outcomes, policies, and procedures, a transition to program implementation occurs. Program implementation is a process, not an event. It happens over time (maybe over a number of years). Implementation will not happen all at once and probably will not proceed smoothly, at least not at first. In the most effective health promotion programs, staff, stakeholders, and participants are aware of how the program changes and develops over time as it is implemented.

According to Fixsen, Naoom, Blase, Friedman, and Wallace (2005), there are six program implementation stages:

1. **Exploration and adoption** involves program planning, including needs assessments and programmatic decisions about mission, goals, objectives, interventions, outcomes, policies, and procedures. Achieving acceptance and support for the program in the setting is part of this stage.

2. **Program installation** focuses on the structural supports necessary to initiate a program. A capacity assessment (discussed in Chapter 4) is the basis of program installation. A capacity assessment includes ensuring the availability of funding streams, human resource strategies, and supportive policy as well as creating referral mechanisms, reporting frameworks, and outcome expectations. Additional resources may be needed to realign current staff, hire and train new staff members, secure appropriate space, or purchase needed technology (for example, smartphones or tablets). These activities and their associated start-up costs are necessary first steps in beginning a new program in any setting (for example, a school, workplace, health care organization, or community).

3. **Initial implementation** means operating a program for the first time with the priority population in the setting. No amount of planning and discussion can account for all the complexities involved when staff members run a program with the program participants; there are too many unknowns until a program has been operating for some period of time. During initial implementation, the compelling forces of fear of change, inertia, and investment in the status quo combine with the inherently difficult and complex work of implementing something new at a time when the program is struggling to begin and when confidence in the decision to do the program is being tested. Learning from this initial experience and in particular from unanticipated consequences (both good and bad) is important to meeting the priority population's needs. Surprises and challenges may change the trajectory of the program but hopefully will not derail its work to address peoples' health needs. The strength of many programs can be traced to what is learned during the initial implementation about program participants' needs, critical staff skills, program policies and procedures, and the match between the program interventions and participant needs.

4. **Full operation** occurs when a program is operating with full staffing and full client loads, and all of the realities of doing business are impinging on the newly implemented program. Once an implemented program is fully operational, referrals are flowing according to the

agreed-on inclusion or exclusion criteria, practitioners are carrying out the evidence-based practice or program with proficiency and skill, managers and administrators are supporting and facilitating the new practices, and the setting has adapted to the presence of the program. Over time, the program becomes accepted practice and a new operationalization of "business as usual" takes place in the setting (see, for example, Faggin, 1985). At this stage, the anticipated benefits are realized as the program staff members become skillful and the procedures and processes become routine.

5. **Innovation** happens over time as staff, stakeholders, and participants learn what works with a priority population in a particular setting. Changes in staff, feedback from evaluations, and new conditions present opportunities to refine and expand the program. Ensuring cultural competence of the program is an important part of program innovation.

6. **Sustainability** is about long-term program operation. Skilled practitioners and other well-trained staff leave and must be replaced with other skilled practitioners and well-trained staff. Leaders, funding streams, and program requirements change. New social problems arise; partners come and go. External systems change with some frequency; political alliances are only temporary; and champions move on to other causes. And in spite of all these changes, program staff, stakeholders, and participants adjust without losing the functional components of the program or letting the program die from a lack of essential financial and stakeholder support. The goal during this stage is the long-term survival and continued effectiveness of the implementation site in the context of a changing environment.

Summary

Planning a health promotion program requires that staff, stakeholders, and participants all know what a program seeks to accomplish and how it will go about trying to accomplish it. As part of planning, decisions are made about the program's mission statement, and goals and objectives are set. Questions about using existing interventions, creating new interventions, or adapting and modifying interventions to achieve program goals are all explored. Increasingly, health promotion programs use evidence-based interventions drawn from health theory, paying attention to the balance between fidelity to the core functions of an intervention and adaptation to meet specific needs in a particular setting, in order to maximize a program's success in achieving its goals and objectives. Cultural sensitivity and appropriateness of the interventions are critical considerations at this point in the planning process if the program is to eliminate health disparities among the priority population.

Another part of planning for a successful program is reviewing, creating, or refining policies in order to clearly state the health values and priorities of the organization or community in ways that are tailored to the unique requirements and needs of the setting, staff, stakeholders, and participants. Procedures support a program by addressing the health concerns within the context of the site as well as by serving as a foundation for the program's day-to-day operation and logistics.

With all of the decisions about mission, goals, objectives, interventions, policies, and procedures made, the staff can move forward with implementing the program.

For Practice and Discussion

1. Identify the main differences between mission statement, goals, and objectives in planning a health promotion program. How are these statements related to each other?

2. What is the SMART approach to writing program objectives? What does SMART stand for? Write clear objective statements using the SMART approach, including the four W's rule, for an intervention program to reduce childhood obesity in a low-income African American community.

3. In your opinion, what are the key factors in selecting different types of interventions to achieve program objectives? What are the differences between universal preventive interventions, selective preventive interventions, and indicated preventive interventions?

4. Explain the critical components in designing a health promotion intervention for HIV/AIDS prevention among college students. What theory, method, and materials would you select? What website might provide evidence-based programs? If the materials are from the Internet, how would you determine their appropriateness?

5. What would be the process for developing policies for a smoke-free campus? Who would be the leaders, stakeholders, and enforcer? Where can you find sample policies? What elements do you need to consider in developing the policy?

6. You have been hired by a business to plan, implement, and evaluate a program to promote physical activity among its 450 employees in Los Angeles, California. Fully one-third of the employees are Latino,

one-third third Asian, and one-quarter of the employees are African American. The plan is to offer various physical activities (for example, walking, aerobics, biking, and yoga) to employees at varied times and locations. Using the transtheoretical model stages of change and the health belief model, develop a set of questions to explain and help people understand potential issues pertaining to employees' participation, and propose questions to assess employees' health beliefs. Explain how the employees' responses can be used to recruit participants for the program.

KEY TERMS

Action objectives

Adaptation

Evidence-based interventions

Fidelity

Goal

Guide to Community Preventive Services

Health promotion policies

Implementation stages

Indicated preventive interventions

Intervention

Mission

National Registry of Evidence-Based
  Programs and Practices (NREPP)

Objectives

Outcome objectives

Policies

Process objectives

Procedures

Research-tested Intervention Programs
  (RTIPs)

Selective preventive interventions

SMART

Universal preventive interventions

Zone of drastic mutation

References

City of New York. (2003). *A sample smoke-free workplace policy.* Retrieved from http://www.nyc.gov/html/doh/downloads/pdf/smoke/tc9.pdf

Doak, C. C., Doak, L. G., & Root, J. H. (1996). *Teaching patients with low literacy skills* (2nd ed.). Philadelphia, PA: Lippincott.

Evaluation Research Team. (2009). *Writing SMART objectives.* Atlanta, GA: Centers for Disease Control and Prevention. Retrieved from http://www.cdc.gov/healthyyouth/evaluation/pdf/brief3b.pdf

Faggin, F. (1985). The challenge of bringing new ideas to market. *High Technology*, 2, 35–39.

Fixsen, D. L., Naoom, S. F., Blase, K. A., Friedman, R. M., & Wallace, F. (2005). *Implementation research: A synthesis of the literature* (FMHI Publication No. 231). Tampa: University of South Florida, Louis de la Parte Florida Mental Health Institute, National Implementation Research Network.

Gilbert, G. G., Sawyer, R. G., & McNeill, E. B. (2015). *Health education: Creating strategies for school and community health* (4th ed.). Burlington, MA: Jones & Bartlett.

Hall, G. E., & Loucks, S. F. (1978). Teacher concerns as a basis for facilitating staff development. *Teachers College Record, 80*(1), 36–53.

Institute of Medicine. (1994). *Reducing risks for mental disorders: Frontiers for preventive intervention research.* Washington, DC: National Academies Press.

McKenzie, J. F., Neiger, B. L., & Thackeray, R. (2013). *Planning, implementing, and evaluating health promotion programs: A primer* (6th ed.). San Francisco, CA: Pearson Education.

Schinke, S., Brounstein, P., & Gardner, S. (2002). *Science-based prevention programs and principles.* Rockville, MD: U.S. Department of Health and Human Services.

Swerissen, H., & Crisp, B. R. (2004). The sustainability of health promotion interventions for different levels of social organization. *Health Promotion International, 19*(1), 123–130.

U.S. Department of Health and Human Services. (1997). *Developing objectives for Healthy People 2010.* Washington, DC: U.S. Government Printing Office.

Weisz, J. R., Sandler, I. N., Durlak, J. A., & Anton, B. S. (2005). Promoting and protecting youth mental health through evidence-based prevention and treatment. *American Psychologist, 60*(6), 628–648.

PART THREE

IMPLEMENTING HEALTH PROMOTION PROGRAMS

CHAPTER 6

IMPLEMENTATION TOOLS, PROGRAM STAFF, AND BUDGETS

Jean M. Breny, Michael C. Fagen, and Kathleen M. Roe

From Program Planning to Action Planning

One of the most critical steps in the health promotion planning process is the creation of practical and specific *action plans*. These practical documents are based on the program's goals, objectives, and interventions. A good action plan provides a summary of how the program needs to progress. The plan links the specific activities that will be undertaken with the outcomes desired. Once developed, the action plan helps staff members track progress, adapt to changes, and document accountability as the program unfolds. Because the action plan shows what is planned, it can also serve as a key document in process evaluation—an ongoing review of the process by which the program is implemented and of the impact that the process has on the outcomes. Process evaluation, an important part of program evaluation, is discussed in detail in Chapter 10.

Table 6.1 provides an abbreviated example of how goals, objectives, interventions, and activities can be written into an action plan that ensures that all the steps needed to accomplish each intervention are identified and assigned to a staff member to be completed by a certain date. In the example in Table 6.1, one of the goals of the school is to maintain the number of children who are within their healthy weight zone as they progress through school.

LEARNING OBJECTIVES

- Compare action plans, logic models, and timelines and describe their application to program implementation.

- Discuss approaches to recruiting, hiring, training, and retaining program staff with the necessary skills, commitment, and ability to work effectively with a variety of stakeholders.

- Suggest methods of advertising program staff openings to attract highly qualified applicants.

- Describe the relationship between income and expenses as it pertains to the sound fiscal management of programs.

- Describe the role of program staff, their rights, and their responsibilities to program funders.

Table 6.1   Constructing an Action Plan That Documents Activities Needed to Execute Strategies

Goal: Decrease the number of students who are overweight and at risk of being overweight in Adams County Middle Schools while maintaining the number of students who are at their correct weight for their height and age.

Objective 1. Increase the number of students who are physically active for sixty minutes each day from 30 percent to 55 percent by the end of the school year.

Objective 2. Increase the number of students who can achieve the Healthy Fitness Zone on all components of the FITNESSGRAM from 15 percent to 30 percent by the end of the school year.

Objective 3. Increase the number of students who can identify and describe the components of fitness from 65 percent to 85 percent by the end of the school year.

Objective 4. Increase the number of students who choose to eat five fruits and vegetables each day from 15 percent to 35 percent by the end of the school year.

Objective 5. Decrease the number of students who daily eat high-fat, high-salt, low-nutrient foods from 80 percent to 65 percent by the end of the school year.

Interventions (What will facilitate achieving the specific objective?)	Activities (What are the - action steps to implement the intervention strategy?)	Personnel (Who will ensure that each action step is completed?)	Time Frame (By what date does the action step need to be completed?)
Interventions for Objective 1:			
1.1. Purchase evidence-based physical activity program that promotes physical activity breaks within the classroom as a means to improve academic achievement as well as increase daily physical activity.	1.1.1. Schedule professional development for elementary teachers.	1.1.1. Project director	1.1.1. January 30
	1.1.2. Identify and secure needed resources.	1.1.2. Project administrative assistant	1.1.2. January 30
	1.1.3. Provide professional development.	1.1.3. Project director	1.1.3. February 10
	1.1.4. Start sixth-grade program.	1.1.4. Sixth-grade team	1.1.4. March 1
1.2. Add program components to increase amount of time students engage in moderate to vigorous activity while in physical education classes.	1.1.5. Start seventh-grade program.	1.1.5. Seventh-grade team	1.1.5. March 15
	1.1.6. Implement coaching initiative to reinforce the implementation of classroom activities.	1.1.6. Project director	1.1.6. March 15
1.3. Implement fitness testing followed by development of individualized self-improvement fitness action plans by each student.	1.1.7. Evaluate the implementation of classroom activities.	1.1.7. Project evaluator	1.1.7. April 20

Another goal is to reduce the number of children who are overweight or at risk of being overweight. Five objectives are provided that address both goals. Objectives 2 and 3 both require a similar strategy: an improved or enhanced physical education program. Objective 1 will also benefit from an enhanced physical education program that increases the amount of time that students engage in vigorous physical activity during physical education classes. In addition, the plan for objective 1 includes an intervention of promoting physical activity as a way to take "brain breaks" within the classroom, an intervention that is facilitated by the regular teachers, thus increasing the number of minutes that students are actively involved in aerobics, strength building, or flexibility exercises. (Only the activities for the first intervention in objective 1 [scheduling classroom breaks] are identified in the abbreviated action plan.)

In the following sections, two additional useful tools for moving from planning to implementation—a logic model and a Gantt chart—will be introduced. A logic model helps communicate the relationships between program elements to stakeholders and potential partners as well as the priority population (Erwin et al., 2003; McKenzie, Neiger, & Thackeray, 2012). Gantt charts help put program elements into a specific timeline in an at-a-glance format that allows staff and stakeholders to better manage the program (Timmreck, 2003). While the action plan also identifies a time when each activity is accomplished, the Gantt chart displays this information in the most useful format. Both logic models and Gantt charts are dynamic tools that can be revised and updated at regular intervals to reflect program development and growth.

Preparing a Logic Model

As its name suggests, a logic model is a visual depiction of the underlying *logic* of a planned initiative. It shows the relationship between the program's resources (*inputs*), its planned activities (*outputs*), and the changes that are expected as a result (*outcomes*). Logic models can take many forms, but they all are designed to provide a simple graphic illustration of the relationships assumed between the actions that will be initiated and the anticipated results. Figure 6.1 shows how to set up a logic model. A logic model reads from left to right. Each column flows into the next, indicating that what is in each column depends on the column before it in order to be successful. The logic model thus shows what the planners are assuming will happen as the program progresses. It also allows the staff and stakeholders to track any changes from what was assumed and analyze the impact of those changes on program outcomes. Logic models are useful for program staff and stakeholders, helping them to succinctly communicate and agree on the overall plan (Gilmore, 2011; Keller & Bauerle, 2009; MacDonald et al., 2001). A clear and simple logic model will explain in a single page how what is planned will make a difference in the health behavior or health status of a population.

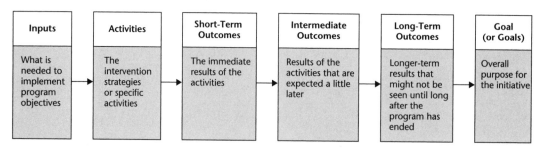

Inputs	Activities	Short-Term Outcomes	Intermediate Outcomes	Long-Term Outcomes	Goal (or Goals)
What is needed to implement program objectives	The intervention strategies or specific activities	The immediate results of the activities	Results of the activities that are expected a little later	Longer-term results that might not be seen until long after the program has ended	Overall purpose for the initiative

Figure 6.1 Schematic Logic Model

Source: Adapted from W. K. Kellogg Foundation, 2004.

Figure 6.2 is an example of a logic model for a program to prevent the initiation of tobacco use among young people (MacDonald et al., 2001). The program's long-term goals are to reduce tobacco-related morbidity and mortality and to decrease tobacco-related health disparities.

Program Inputs and Activities

The first two columns in the logic model in Figure 6.2 contain information generated during the program planning process when the planners developed the goals, objectives, and strategies. In the first column (*Inputs*), the major resources from the state public health department, along with its partners, are represented. These resources could include funding and staff from the health department's office of tobacco use prevention, the program staff of the health department's bureau of drug and alcohol education, and the staff and resources of various community agencies, as well as the staff and resources of the local education authorities (superintendent, principals, school health council or school health teams, school health coordinator). The shorthand notation of the logic model is used so that the entire plan can be reduced to one page that identifies all the critical elements that are needed to implement the program as well as their relationship to each other. Resources could be staff, locations to hold program events, organizational resources, appropriate supplies, equipment, technology, curricula, or instructional resources.

Moving to the right from *Inputs* to *Activities* brings into focus the specific strategies and interventions that were selected during the planning process on the basis of the staff and stakeholders' understanding of the underlying problem, its context, the program's theoretical framework, and the desired outcomes. In this second column, the key strategies

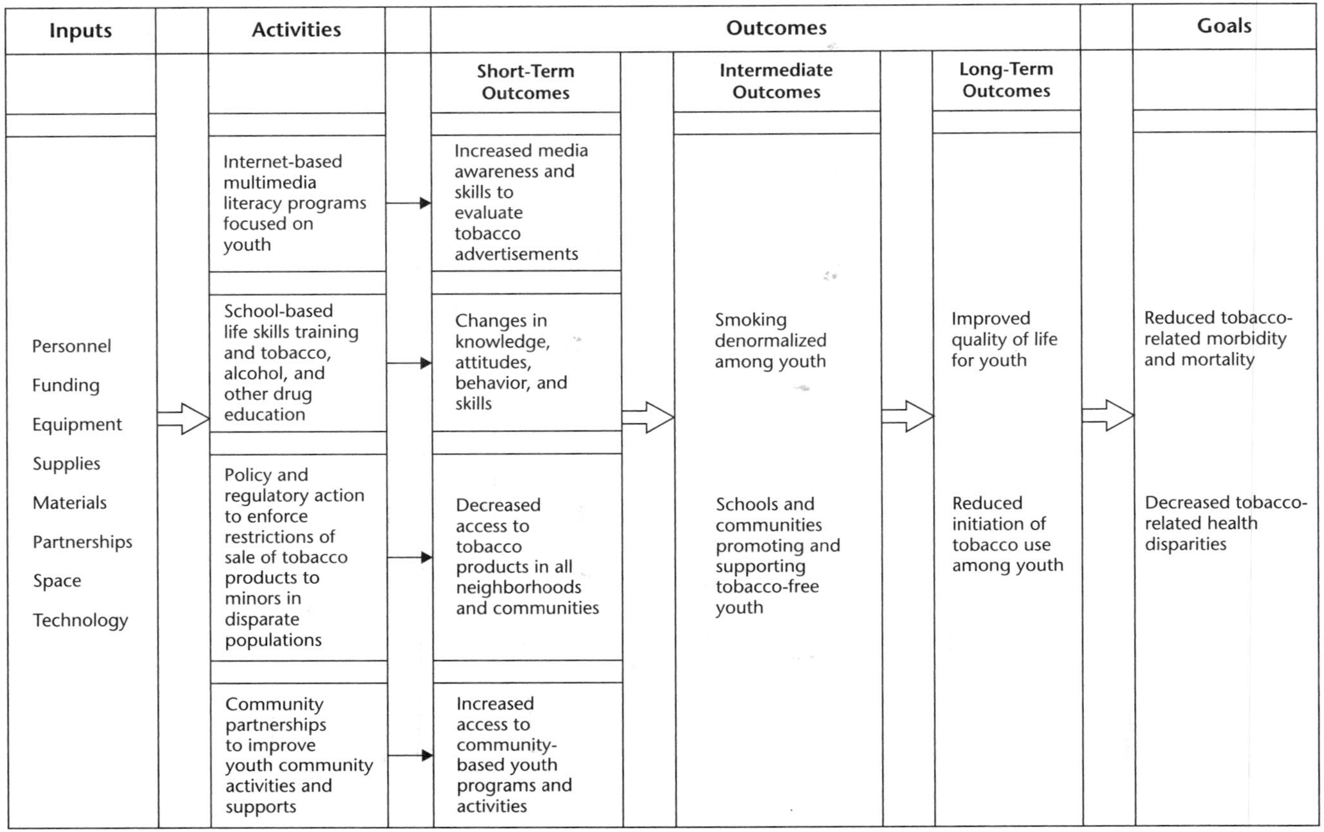

Inputs	Activities	Outcomes			Goals
		Short-Term Outcomes	**Intermediate Outcomes**	**Long-Term Outcomes**	
Personnel Funding Equipment Supplies Materials Partnerships Space Technology	Internet-based multimedia literacy programs focused on youth	Increased media awareness and skills to evaluate tobacco advertisements			
	School-based life skills training and tobacco, alcohol, and other drug education	Changes in knowledge, attitudes, behavior, and skills	Smoking denormalized among youth	Improved quality of life for youth	Reduced tobacco-related morbidity and mortality
	Policy and regulatory action to enforce restrictions of sale of tobacco products to minors in disparate populations	Decreased access to tobacco products in all neighborhoods and communities	Schools and communities promoting and supporting tobacco-free youth	Reduced initiation of tobacco use among youth	Decreased tobacco-related health disparities
	Community partnerships to improve youth community activities and supports	Increased access to community-based youth programs and activities			

Figure 6.2 Logic Model for Preventing the Initiation of Tobacco Use Among Young People

specified in this plan are Internet-based multimedia literacy programs focused on youth; school-based life skills and tobacco, alcohol, and other drug education; policy and regulatory action; and community partnerships focused on youth community activities and supports.

Outcomes

Moving from what is planned to what is hoped will happen, we arrive at the three *Outcomes* columns on the right side of the logic model. The *Short-Term Outcomes* column lists the things that we expect will happen as an immediate result of each of the planned activities. For example, the media literacy program, school-based prevention, policy initiatives, and the community activities and supports increases students' knowledge, awareness, and skills, as well as produce changes in students' attitudes. The key is making sure that there is a logical link between the items that are specified in the *Activities* column and what is assumed will happen if these are properly implemented (specified in the *Short-Term Outcomes* column).

The *Intermediate Outcomes* column is next; it refers to results that may not be seen after a single activity but can be measured or verified at some future point. In the example, the planners are hoping to denormalize tobacco use. This intermediate outcome could be assessed by doing student surveys at school or within the community after the instructional programs have been delivered for several years.

The column *Long-Term Outcomes* depicts the ultimate extension of the program's impact. If the activities are effective and the planners achieve both the short-term and the intermediate outcomes, the logic model specifies that the related long-term results that could be reasonably expected are reduced initiation of tobacco use among youths and improvement in youths' quality of life. In this case, the program manager might think that the program has been successful if measurements completed each year of the program and for three years after the program is terminated demonstrate a steady decline in youth tobacco use.

Most health promotion programs are designed to achieve a very long-term outcome that is health- or disease-related. The ultimate very long-term outcomes that are envisioned are the program's *goals*. In this case, as shown in the *Goals* column, a reasonable long-term outcome for the program to set as a goal might be a 20% reduction in tobacco-related morbidity and mortality 20 to 40 years later, when the youths who received the intervention are adults. Another very long-term result (goal) for the program to strive for is a decrease in tobacco-related health disparities.

Not all programs achieve their desired outcomes; others achieve the outcomes but not at the levels anticipated. If, in the example shown in Figure 6.2, participants gain the intended knowledge by the end of the exposure to the lessons but do not demonstrate any change in attitudes or behavioral intention, the project manager will be able to identify the point in the logical chain that needs reinforcement. Working backward and forward within a logic model throughout the action phase of a program provides valuable checks that can greatly enhance the program's effectiveness if the project manager is able to learn through analyzing what has happened and why.

Logic models can be created several ways. The process can be participatory and community building, such as when a community advisory group is facilitated through the design of a logic model on a white board or posted paper. This approach aims to build consensus around the program's key elements and expected outcomes among key players in a way that fosters inclusion and ownership. The key staff members responsible for moving from program proposal to implementation may elect to develop the logic model as an internal document, limiting input and review to a smaller group and using the resulting document as a staff roadmap. Logic models can even be developed by program evaluators through key informant interviews, designed to illuminate what different stakeholders assumed and noticed as the program got under way.

Logic models can be sketched by hand, developed in Word or Excel, or created through the many templates available online (for example: http://www.uwex.edu/ces/pdande/evaluation/evallogicmodelworksheets.html). Just type "logic model template" into your browser and you'll see the range of styles (Logic Model Templates, 2010). The online Community Toolbox offers several different logic model styles: http://ctb.ku.edu/en/table-of-contents/overview/models-for-community-health-and-development/logic-model-development/example (KU Work Group for Community Health and Development, 2015a). The most important thing is to go through the process, alone or in a group, and then get that logic into a chart that will help guide implementation.

Using a Gantt Chart to Guide Implementation

A logic model, as was just illustrated, provides a visual picture of the underlying logic of a program and how its key components rely on and build on each other. However, it does not provide one very important thing—a timeline. This is where a *Gantt chart* comes in handy.

A Gantt chart is a visual depiction of a schedule for completing a program's objectives. This particular method of charting project activities and phases over time was developed in the early 1900s by a mechanical engineer, Henry Gantt. Originally drawn by hand on graph paper, Gantt charts and other project management planning tools are now easily developed with software such as Microsoft Excel or Project. Ideally, a Gantt chart is no more than a single page, even for a complex project. The goal is to show in clean and simple lines the development of the project across time and on time. (Remember that the action plan has the details of who will do what by when in order to implement each strategy.) A Gantt chart will help program staff to organize all of those people and activities across the time that is available to complete the program (McKenzie, Neiger, & Thackeray, 2012). It will also help communicate this calendar to all of the program staff and stakeholders. A good Gantt chart can quickly become one of the most useful tools available to program staff.

While an action plan lists everything that must be accomplished by date and by the person responsible, the items are presented in order of the program's goals and objectives. The action plan does provide the staff with useful information, but completing a Gantt chart that puts all activities on a common calendar allows the staff to make sure that nothing is overlooked and to see at a glance what activities need to be accomplished—and by when. In order to move from an action plan to a program timeline (a Gantt chart), the following questions need to be answered:

Which activities need to be done before others?

What are the critical deadlines for each activity?

How much time will be needed for each activity?

Are there any scheduled holidays, vacations, or other predictable periods in which less work might get accomplished or activities won't be successful?

When are our evaluation and progress reports due?

In the example in Figure 6.3, the intervention is a set of educational activities: a workshop series, including a skill-building session, and a follow-up workshop.

The Gantt chart in Figure 6.3 identifies all of the things needed in order to complete one full cycle of the educational intervention. For example, if program funding begins January 1, staff need to be hired and trained immediately. If it is assumed that it will take 8 weeks to get the staff on board and ready, the first workshop series can begin in late March and conclude by late April, if the workshop is going to use instructional materials that

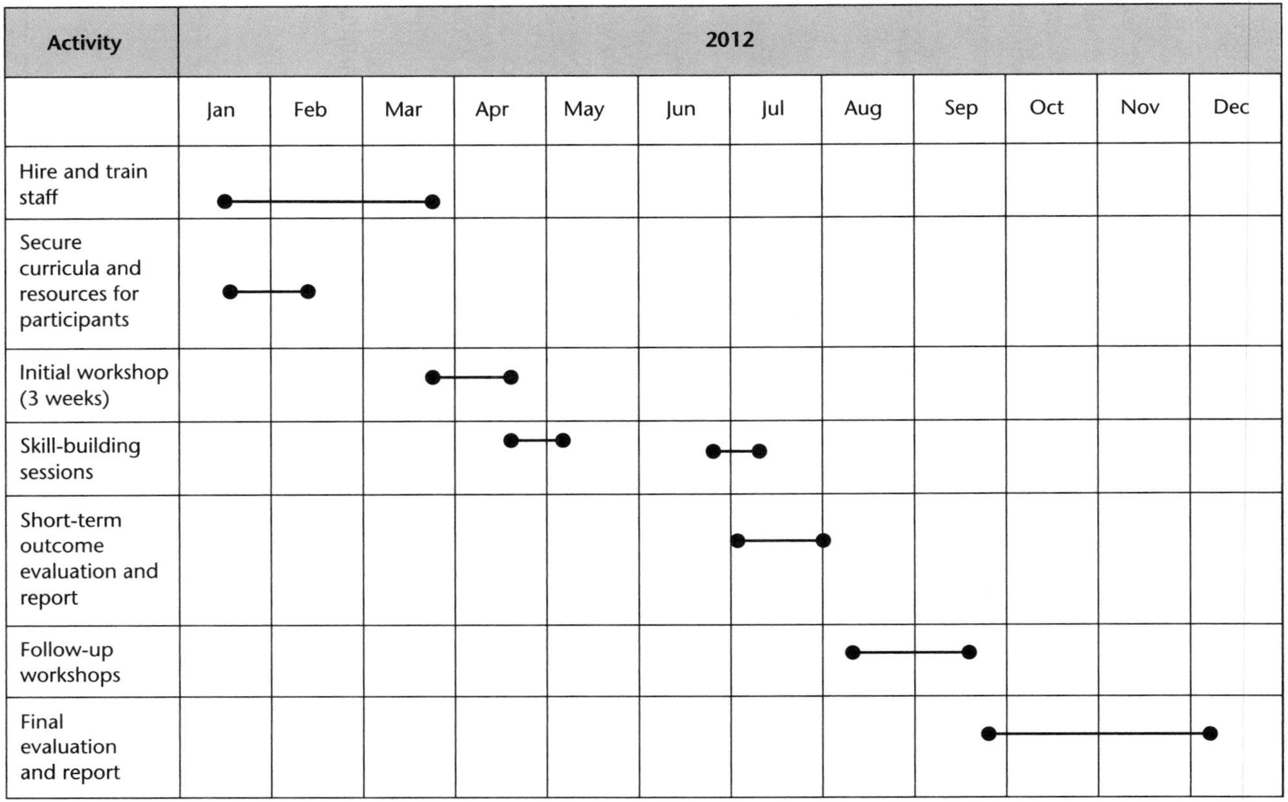

Activity	2012											
	Jan	Feb	Mar	Apr	May	Jun	Jul	Aug	Sep	Oct	Nov	Dec
Hire and train staff	●——————————●											
Secure curricula and resources for participants	●————●											
Initial workshop (3 weeks)			●————●									
Skill-building sessions				●————●		●————●						
Short-term outcome evaluation and report							●————●					
Follow-up workshops								●————●				
Final evaluation and report									●————————————————●			

Figure 6.3 Abbreviated Gantt Chart of Educational Activities

151

have already been developed. If the staff is to construct or adapt the lessons, additional time for curricula development would need to be built into the Gantt chart. Continuing to plot the activities across actual time, it becomes evident that the first full set of educational activities—and evaluation data collection and reporting—will be completed by the end of July. But what if the teaching staff assigned to the project typically take vacation in July? Or what if staff are ready to start the workshops in February but the weather is typically so harsh or unpredictable at that time of year that participants might have trouble attending? These kinds of considerations stemming from the organizational or community context are crucial when moving from planning to action. A carefully designed and updated Gantt chart helps the manager plan ahead, adjust, and stay on top of the program as the specifics of implementation unfold.

A good Gantt chart also includes critical evaluation and reporting deadlines. Figure 6.3 shows the evaluation data collection periods associated with each component of the educational intervention. Each period concludes with an evaluation report. However, the funder or stakeholders may require progress reports on a regular basis. If so, these need to be added to the Gantt chart. If the process evaluation plans call for ongoing monitoring of program activities for fidelity to the original design, that monitoring also needs to be added to the chart.

There are several online tools planners can use for designing and managing Gantt charts and project timelines. Among these are Smartsheet, Gantter, and Google's program, Ganttproject. All are easy to use, are interactive, and can be shared with program staff. The most popular online program management tool, however, is Microsoft Project, which comes with the Office software suite of programs. Project is a great tool to manage large or small projects. It creates timelines and Gantt charts, allows you to assign resources to tasks, and easily manage the timelines when implementation challenges occur. Tutorials for all of these programs are available for free on the Internet. Find one that works for you and helps you with the daily tasks of managing a program.

Additional Implementation Planning Tools

Logic models and Gantt charts are excellent implementation planning tools. As health promotion programs increasingly emphasize changes to the policies and environments ("structural changes") that influence health behaviors, additional planning tools are useful. One important resource for structural change planning is provided by the CDC's Healthy Communities Program's Action Guides (see Figure 6.4). Some of these guides provide a

Action Guides

Working with Schools to Increase Physical Activity Among Children and Adolescents in Physical Education Classes 🔖 [PDF–1.8M] ⮥

This action guide, developed by Partnership for Prevention, provides resources and key steps for working with schools to increase physical activity among children and adolescents in physical education classes. It translates a specific recommendation from *The Guide to Community Preventive Services* into "how to" guidance.

Facilitating Development of a Community Trail and Promoting Its Use to Increase Physical Activity Among Youth and Adults 🔖 [PDF–2M] ⮥

This action guide, developed by Partnership for Prevention, provides resources and key steps to facilitate the development of a community trail and promote its use among youth and adults. It translates a specific recommendation from *The Guide to Community Preventive Services* into "how to" guidance.

Working with Healthcare Delivery Systems to Improve the Delivery of Tobacco-Use Treatment to Patients 🔖 [PDF–1.6M] ⮥

This action guide, developed by Partnership for Prevention, provides resources and key steps for working with health care delivery systems to improve tobacco-use treatment for patients. It translates a specific recommendation from *The Guide to Community Preventive Services* into "how to" guidance. Tobacco-use screening and brief intervention is among the top clinical preventive services.

Promoting Health Equity: A Resource to Help Communities Address Social Determinants of Health 🔖 [PDF–1.5M]

This action guide is for public health practitioners and partners who want to improve health equity in their communities. The guide offers advice from experts in local community leadership, public health, medicine, social work, sociology, psychology, urban planning, community economic development, environmental sciences, and housing.

Media Access Guide: A Resource for Community Health Promotion 🔖 [PDF–1.5M]

This action guide helps communities to develop effective relationships with the media and gain valuable news coverage for health-related issues. It offers:

- Instructions, tips, and templates for writing press releases, media advisories, and other media-related materials.
- Methods for monitoring media coverage.
- Strategies for placing public service announcements and hosting press conferences.

^ Top of Page

Figure 6.4 CDC's Healthy Communities Action Guides

series of action steps for conducting specific initiatives, such as developing a community trail that promotes physical activity. Others provide case studies of initiatives designed to produce far-reaching structural change, such as promoting health equity. Additional guides focus on important skills necessary for effective health promotion programming, such as working with the media. All guides provide practical advice written in plain language, and are helpful implementation planning tools that supplement your use of logic models and Gantt charts.

Planning for Implementation Challenges

There are no right or wrong formats for an action plan, logic model, or Gantt chart. All need to be thoughtful, living documents that help the program staff and stakeholders accomplish the program objectives on time and in the way intended. They are tools that program staff and stakeholders (and even participants) can use to build and shape a program. Ideally, they also reflect the energy, passion, and excitement of the program stakeholders for addressing health problems by proactively promoting health and eliminating disparities.

Program staff prepare for changes and *challenges* during a program's implementation period; programs are planned on paper, but they take place in schools, workplaces, health care organizations, and communities, where change and challenge are to be expected. Talking about a program is very different from actually implementing it. Chapter 5 discusses the transition from planning to implementation and the six stages of implementation (Fixsen, Naoom, Blase, Friedman, & Wallace, 2005): exploration and adoption, program installation, initial implementation, full operation, innovation, and sustainability. In the remainder of this section, we discuss implementation challenges that are often encountered when moving through the stages, particularly program installation, initial implementation, and full operation.

Lack of attention to details is hampering execution of the program.
Attention to the details at the start of a program's operation is necessary and important. As the first day of program operation approaches, brainstorm a list of details to attend to, down to "open the doors and let people into the program." Anticipating how staff members will get to know participants' names and contact information, establishing how participants will arrive at the program (for example, taking a bus, being dropped off by parents, walking from their offices), having room door keys and equipment ready to use, and having computer access are small details that, if not attended to, will disrupt the flow and progress of a program. Tending to these details establishes staff and participant relationships that are trusting, supportive, and caring, which is important because good staff-participant relationships are fundamental to an effective health promotion program. It also has the wider effect throughout the organization or setting on the program's image and creditability as a competent and caring resource that is an asset to the organization.

The realities of actual program operations are more difficult than program planners anticipated. Rarely do programs function as planned, at least initially. There are too many unknowns and variables to permit program staff to plan for everything. Some typical problems are confusion on the part of participants about start and finish times (for example, date, day of the week, time) or location (for example, street address, building, room number), equipment problems, technology failures, program schedule conflicts caused by allotted times being either too long or too short, too few or too many participants, and erratic attendance (for example, some participants come late, others miss parts of the program, and some have to drop out). All of these initial problems have the potential to derail operations. These situations require staff members to troubleshoot by quickly assessing problem areas and what actions are needed to address them. When problems arise, it is essential to avoid blaming the participants or the organization. Focus on what is being learned, and incorporate it into the operation of the program.

Staff and stakeholders do not follow the action plan or Gantt chart. Staff and stakeholders often need to make decisions as the program is developing, particularly in response to participants' needs. Adherence to the plan and schedule may be viewed as no big deal by a staff member but have real consequences if future program segments depend on sequential completion of activities and tasks. Not everyone has to agree on every detail in the plan during program implementation; however, staff knowledge of what is actually occurring is critical to problem solving when programs struggle. Sharing the timeline and routinely referring back to it helps everyone see the way in which their responsibilities contribute to the integrity and ultimate success of the project. It also helps people realize in advance what the consequences will be for the entire program if they make independent decisions about the program without communicating them to the entire staff. Having frank and honest discussions of progress to date on a regular basis and adjusting the timeline as needed can help keep everyone on track. The Gantt chart will also help make expectations about timelines very clear for staff, which is helpful in both program process evaluation and staff performance evaluation.

Conflicts occur. Conflict and struggles are natural parts of program implementation. Each staff member and stakeholder will have his or her own work style, priorities, and level of commitment. For some, working with the health promotion program may be only one of their responsibilities. Complicating staff and stakeholders' concerns is the fact that participants will each have their own reasons and motivations for participating in the program. All of these personal concerns can lead to conflicts in the daily operations and delivery of a program. Agreed-on deadlines are missed. Conflicts are opportunities for program staff and stakeholders to learn how best to move from theory to practice, from plan to action. Most adults are shy about engaging in conflicts, yet conflicts and struggles are hard to avoid, given the nature of the work and of working with people and organizations who may have very different agendas and needs. It is best to talk about the struggles. Creative problem-solving and conflict resolution strategies can be used in these situations. It is difficult and awkward to deal with the conflicts and struggles, but there is a lot to be learned from them.

- **Unanticipated staff turnover leaves vacancies in positions that are critical to accomplishing the plan.** Hiring, training, and retaining staff is an integral part of program implementation, as we will discuss later in this chapter. The person who was hired to provide instruction in the planned workshops may leave for another position or is reassigned to another department, or the process evaluation may indicate that this staff member is not capable of delivering the instruction and must be assigned to other responsibilities. When such emergencies occur, the Gantt chart will help prioritize the next steps by identifying how much time is available before the vacancy seriously disrupts the program. If the disruption is for more than a very short time, updating the Gantt chart to reflect the time spent dealing with the situation and getting back on track will help guarantee that subsequent activities are completed on time. It will also document what really happened during implementation—a critical data element for the process evaluation.

- **Crisis occurs in the organization or community, and the program has to be put on hold.** Despite the best planning, events sometimes require staff or participants to focus their efforts in another area for short or long periods of time. Deadlines for new proposals, year-end reports, and emergencies can all interfere with health promotion programs. If a program needs to be placed on hold, the Gantt chart will be very helpful in getting back on track once the crisis is resolved.

- **The timeline is unrealistic.** This also happens. The process of moving from an action plan to a Gantt chart timeline helps identify whether this might be the case as all the necessary activities are placed on one calendar. If the timeline turns out to be unrealistic, the staff may need to "rightsize" the plan. Discussing the situation with a supervisor or funder is helpful; it may be possible to get an extension or additional support in order to bring the program to completion on time and as planned.

✳ **Staff members are unhappy with their jobs.** Unhappy staff members typically do not perform to their capabilities and contribute to turbulent work environments. The best way to promote staff satisfaction is through systematic hiring decisions followed by quality training, management, and evaluation. Despite managers' best efforts, however, some staff members may become dissatisfied with their jobs. In these instances, it is important to help the staff member find work in a different program or organization.

✳ **Staff members are challenged by working in teams.** Working in teams has become a common approach to implementing health promotion programs. While some staff members naturally work well in these types of small groups, others are challenged in a variety of ways, which may include not being able to compromise, share leadership, or make meaningful contributions. Effective leaders engage their staff in a variety of team-building activities that are designed to maximize overall team performance, ensure contributions from each team member, and minimize conflict. However, even effective leaders sometimes need to reorganize staff teams when teams are not performing near their capacity.

Planning is analytical, but implementation is an art. The more experience that a program's staff and stakeholders have with program implementation, the better they will be able to anticipate, deal with, and adjust to the many challenges that can happen once a program is under way. Each experience in implementing a health promotion program provides insight and information for the next time. Clear and current action plans, logic models, and Gantt charts can be critical tools that facilitate the open and proactive communication with the program's stakeholders, staff, and participants that keeps a program moving forward, even when change happens. Regularly updating and modifying the action plans, logic model, and Gantt chart can create a visual record of a program's growth and development. These tools can tell the story of how the planned program was implemented in real time with real people, reflecting the actual changes and challenges.

Hiring and Managing High-Quality Program Staff

Hiring staff is one of the most important program leadership functions. Quality hiring decisions contribute to effective programs and positive work environments. Conversely, hiring mistakes can lead to program implementation problems and turbulent work environments. Thus, investing time, energy, and resources in making effective hiring decisions is critical for producing successful programs (Hunt, 2007).

Hiring Considerations

A number of strategies can be used in order to make effective hiring decisions. In general, seek to hire staff who

- **Have skills and experience that are specifically matched to program goals.** If a youth development program is to be implemented, seek staff who have experience in working with young people.

- **Have interpersonal qualities that are desirable for the program.** If the program's work is highly collaborative, seek staff who value compromise and working in teams.

- **Are culturally competent.** Cultural competence is a requirement for program staff. Staff diversity and cultural competence contribute to supportive and caring relationships with stakeholders and participants as well as among the staff members. These relationships are critical to participants' participation in a program and their motivation to address a health concern.

- **Have an interest in the organizational mission.** If the organization's mission is to help eliminate health disparities, seek staff who are committed to this work.

In addition, use the following techniques to improve the hiring process:

- **Create high-quality job announcements.** An effective job announcement will describe the organization, program, minimum qualifications, and desired skills and experiences in an easy-to-understand and attractive format. Interested candidates will know how to apply, to whom, and by what deadline.

- **Distribute job announcements widely.** Circulate the job announcement in multiple formats and places, including Internet career sites, electronic mailing lists, professional journals, and local bulletin boards. The object is to generate the largest possible pool of qualified applicants.

- **Screen applicants systematically.** Identify leading candidates by using a grid that rates each applicant on qualifications, skills, and experience. Table 6.2 shows a sample grid in which applicants' attributes are rated on a scale of 1 (lowest) to 5 (highest). Such grids help clarify which traits are applicants' strengths and which are most important to the project. Augment this rating process with brief telephone interviews of 10 to 15 minutes as necessary. The object is to create a short list of three to five candidates who will be interviewed.

Table 6.2   Applicant Screening Grid

| | Desired Trait | | | |
Applicant	Suitable Educational Background	Ability to Design Program Materials	Ability to Work in Collaborative Teams	Experience with Similar Programs
Applicant 1	5	2	3	3
Applicant 2	4	4	4	4
Applicant 3	5	3	4	2
Applicant 4	3	4	2	5

Interview Leading Candidates

Conduct in-person interviews with the short list of candidates. Ask inter-view questions that will help clarify candidates' relevant skills, experiences, and potential fit with the rest of the program staff and your organization's mission (Camp, Vielhaber, & Simonetti, 2001). One way to identify the best candidates is by asking them to describe potential approaches to program-specific scenarios. Table 6.3 provides a list of sample interview questions. You might also ask applicants to perform some appropriate skill—for example, teaching an abbreviated sample lesson or constructing a letter to a specific group of program participants. If you keep your hiring considerations in mind as you interview the candidates, the chance that the staff member hired will be a good fit for your program and your organization increases.

Training, Coaching, Managing, and Evaluating Staff

After making good hiring decisions, effective leaders retain qualified staff by investing in staff development: training, coaching, management, and

Table 6.3   Sample Interview Questions

Describe your previous work experience that is relevant to this position.

Describe a needs assessment you performed as part of planning a health promotion program.

How have you applied health theories and planning models in your work?

How have you adapted an evidence-based health promotion intervention to fit a population in a setting different from the intervention's intended use while maintaining the intervention's fidelity?

Provide a logic model or Gantt chart you have prepared as part of a grant application.

How have you addressed challenges during a health promotion program implementation in a school, workplace, health care organization, or community setting?

How do you engage and support program participants and stakeholders?

Describe how you have used program evaluations to improve a health promotion program.

evaluation (Barbazette, 2007; Fixsen, Naoom, Blase, Friedman, & Wallace, 2005). Staff development focuses on supporting staff so that they can (1) perform their work effectively, (2) contribute meaningfully to the organization's mission, (3) achieve high levels of satisfaction with their job, and (4) continue to expand the depth and breadth of their knowledge of health promotion.

The best staff development programs are concrete, tailored to staff needs, and ongoing. Initial sessions cover the organization's mission, policies, and procedures. Orientation sessions often match new staff members with more experienced ones in a shadowing or mentoring relationship. The new staff member learns from the established staffer through a series of observations, initial implementation efforts, and debriefing sessions. Ideally, the relationship develops on a basis of trust, understanding, and mutual respect. If so, the new staffer then has a person to consult for discussion and support about implementation challenges as they are encountered. The initial sessions will be followed closely by training sessions on the program and its implementation.

Professional development does not stop once staff members are grounded in program implementation. Rather, training includes ongoing supervision. In most program structures, staff members report to a specific program director. The best programs provide time and space for these directors to meet regularly with their staff in supervisory meetings that focus on problem solving. The process of learning from a mentor continues with supervisors, who coach their staff members, using the same process (observations, debriefing, discussion). Supervisors may also demonstrate skills and work directly with staff members on tasks, helping to strengthen and refine staff skills. Furthermore, good supervisors will help their staff identify areas for additional training, which may include technical skills (such as techniques for designing program materials) or process skills (such as techniques for motivational interviewing). These training sessions might be provided by the organization or via external professional development opportunities.

Effectively trained staff is pleasant to manage because they understand their job responsibilities, have the skills to fulfill them, and are supported through mentoring and supervision. Strong leaders are effective managers who understand the importance of structuring programs so that staff members will be poised for success. Preparing staff members for success means matching staff skills and experience with job functions while providing opportunities for growth and learning. Staff members must feel comfortable approaching their managers with concerns and requests for additional professional development opportunities. In turn, managers must create work environments that allow these requests while ensuring that all staff members perform in ways that are beneficial to both the program and the organization.

The primary method that effective leaders use to manage for staff success is *performance evaluation*. Workplace performance evaluation is often thought to mean year-end reviews that determine raises, bonuses, or even job cuts. While annual reviews play a role in performance evaluation, the best leaders evaluate their staff on a continual basis. Such ongoing evaluation starts with staff goals that are formulated in partnership with supervisors and that meet staff, program, and organizational needs. These goals provide the blueprint for staff work, are discussed in regularly scheduled meetings with the primary supervisor, and are adjusted as necessary on the basis of changes at the staff, program, or organizational level. In this manner, the year-end review becomes a culminating event that synthesizes and summarizes staff performance instead of providing a single high-stakes, make-or-break performance rating (McDavid & Hawthorn, 2005).

Budgeting and Fiscal Management

The extent to which staff members of a health promotion program need specialized training in finance, accounting, and funding and resource development depends, to some degree, on the size and complexity of the health promotion program for which they work. Generally, the larger or more complex the organization, the greater the likelihood that the program will use specialized financial management expertise. For example, the norm for major health promotion organizations with large health promotion programs (for example, the American Heart Association or the Centers for Disease Control and Prevention) is to appoint senior staff members as the chief financial officer and business manager. These individuals assume primary responsibility for coordinating the organization's cash and credit, financial planning, accounting, budgeting, funding development, and management information services.

Despite the increased presence of trained financial specialists in organizations that operate health promotion programs, it is important to understand that almost all decisions made by program directors and program staff—no matter what their role in the organization—have financial implications. Even in organizations in which staff members take on specialized roles in direct services (for example, health educators, social workers, physical therapists, physicians, or nurses), it is critical for those individuals to understand how their decisions affect and are affected by available funds, cash flow considerations, project revenue streams, and budget constraints.

Therefore, it is extremely important for any person who is working or aspires to work in a health promotion program and organization to develop skills in basic accounting, financial analysis and planning, funding and resource development, and budgeting.

At the minimum, a well-prepared health promotion staff member has the ability to interpret three basic financial documents: *balance sheet, income statement,* and *cash flow statement.* A balance sheet shows what an organization owns and how it is financed. An income statement shows the financial performance of an organization over a specified time period—typically, a year. Finally, a cash flow statement shows how an organization's operations have affected its cash position. Effective interpretation of these three documents is crucial to making sound business decisions. These documents equip health educators with information that is essential to analyzing, controlling, and improving their organization's day-to-day operations and long-term prospects. In addition to acquiring basic skills in financial and managerial accounting, students who are contemplating senior executive roles in health promotion organizations gain knowledge of the fundamental concepts of corporate and public sector finance.

During the planning process, a budget needs to be developed for the program that is to be implemented. Effective program implementation requires careful adherence to the budget and timely reporting of any variation between what was planned and what actually happens. Effective leadership establishes a tone of honesty, problem solving, and transparency in every aspect of the program, but particularly in regard to budget and resources. An effective program leader is a good steward of the trust that comes with the position and the resources of the organization.

Budget Basics

A *budget* is simply a detailed statement of the resources available to a program (income) and what it costs to implement it (expenses). In the planning phase, the budget is a reasoned prediction; in the implementation phase, the budget is a living document, changing as resources come in and funds are spent. Budgets for small programs are simple and fairly straightforward; they often have a limited number of expense categories and a single funding source. More complex health promotion programs may have more complicated budgets, with multiple funding streams, varied expenses, and anticipated changes in both expenses and income at various program stages. Whether the budget is large or small, complex or simple, the principles of sound financial management are the same (http://ctb .ku.edu / en / table- of- contents / assessment / assessing- community- needs- and- resources / conduct - concerns - surveys / main; KU Work Group for Community Health and Development, 2015b).

Resources

Some health promotion programs have fixed incomes. They are funded at a certain level to implement a set of activities over a given period of time. In the case of multiple-year funding, annual reports that show how the resources for one year have been used may be required before funds are released for the next year. Careful spending of resources according to the approved categories and within the approved limits makes this kind of *fiscal management* relatively easy.

In contrast, some health promotion program budgets are based on variable factors, such as the number of people who enroll, the number of clients who complete a series of program activities, matching funds, revenue from services, fundraising, or in-kind contributions from other sources. Luckily, when a program has this many moving parts in its resource base, it is usually housed in an organization that has professionals who can help program staff and program leaders understand, manage, and utilize their resources to ensure their program's viability (Johnson & Breckon, 2007).

Expenses

Most program budgets have four primary expense categories:

Personnel: the compensation to the paid staff of the program. In most cases, the personnel category is actually divided into two categories: wages and benefits. Personnel who work more than 50% of full time on the program usually have associated benefit costs, including health insurance and retirement benefits. Benefits can add 15 to 30% to the amount allocated for wages.

Supplies: items that are needed to implement the program. Standard supply categories include printing and copying, postage, office supplies, telephone, and equipment. Depending on the program plan and the rules of the organization or funder, it may be possible also to include reasonable costs for entertainment or incentives in supply categories (for example, lunch for an advisory group, food and music for a volunteer thank-you reception, grocery store gift cards for participants).

Services: specific skills, talent, or expertise that must be hired—usually for a short period of time. Examples might include kitchen staff for two nights to supervise a school-based family health night, translators to adapt or create materials, or transportation for a youth group's field trip. These services are usually priced by the hour and do not include benefits. A funder or organization may place limits on the hourly rate or number of hours allowed.

Travel, training, and dissemination of results: the travel and professional development costs needed to train staff or participants and the costs of sharing what the program has done with others. This expense category may include modest compensation for local or regional travel required for site visits or program delivery in remote areas, usually calculated as cost per mile. Some funders who require grantees or staff to attend an annual meeting include the associated costs in the program's travel budget. Some funders even encourage program staff or leadership to present program findings at regional or national conferences in order to disseminate results in the field. If so, full or partial travel costs may be funded as a program expense.

It is very important that program staff understand in advance what can and cannot be claimed against the expense projections in the budget. For example, organizations may require proof of defensive driving instruction prior to authorizing travel reimbursement. Some funders will fund meal expenses, but most will not fund alcohol. Reviewing the expenses in the program budget and the rules and procedures of both the funder and the fiscal agent in their own organization will help program staff manage the budget, pay the bills, and keep their program running smoothly—at least on the financial end.

Monitoring the Budget

Program resources and expenses can be monitored with simple spreadsheet software such as Microsoft Excel or Apple's Numbers. It is very important to monitor the budget on a regular basis in order to make sure that expenses and income are within the projected range (Dropkin, Halpin, & La Touche, 2007). It is also important to make sure that program staff, stakeholders, and participants understand the rules and procedures for spending money and obtaining reimbursement for program-related expenses. Submitting requests for reimbursement without appropriate receipts, submitting requests too late, or expecting reimbursement for items that are not approved by the funder wastes time and resources and disappoints everyone.

The program director is responsible for making sure that the allocated funds are spent by the end of the time periods designated by the funder. For example, a three-year grant for $60,000 may require that $20,000 be spent each year. Underspending in year 1 will not benefit the program if the funder cannot allow funds for year 1 to be spent in year 2 (called *carryover* or *roll-forward*). The program director needs to make sure that everyone involved is aware of the key deadlines for each reporting period and does his or her part to make sure that the resources are used for the intended purpose within the designated time frame.

Budget Challenges

A budget lays out what is expected to happen with program resources and expenses and then tells the story of what actually happened. Ideally, the two scenarios are identical. However, even the best-planned program may deviate from its budget during the implementation phase (Johnson & Breckon, 2007). Two common budget challenges are presented here, along with strategies for overcoming them.

First, what if there's not enough money in the budget? Sometimes this happens despite careful planning. If a resource shortfall is identified during the planning phase, the program staff can search for funding or resources that will cover the additional expenses. For example, some federal grants cannot pay for food at program-related events. If this is known, yet the plan involves training or events at which the staff would like food to be served, donations (for example, from local stores) could be requested, a small grant (from a local organization or foundation) could be solicited, or resources from another source could be explored. Perhaps another resource stream within the agency that is running the program could be tapped to cover the expenses not included in the base funding.

If the staff are not successful in obtaining additional funds to cover providing lunch at the training event, the implementation plan will need to be adjusted so that program activities stay within budget. Overspending without prior approval from the funder might result in fewer resources for the next phase of the program. Even worse, overspending might jeopardize the program's continued or future funding, the project manager's position as a program leader, or the ability of the agency to successfully seek future support from this funder. These are serious consequences, but they can be avoided by carefully planning and monitoring the program budget.

Second, what if money is left over? This is a good problem to have, and it can happen for several reasons. Sometimes an expense item ends up costing less than anticipated or personnel costs are reduced through in-kind contributions of staff time from other sources. Careful monitoring of the budget on at least a monthly basis helps staff members to identify places where savings are occurring in plenty of time to make wise decisions about what to do with the extra money.

Minor changes within budget categories (for example, spending money saved on printing costs to upgrade the cover of a training manual) usually only need careful accounting in the next budget report. More significant changes within categories (for example, using money saved on printing volunteer manuals to print banners promoting program events) is raised with the funder or at least the grant or fund manager within the host agency prior to investing the resources. Changes across budget categories (for example, using the money saved on printing to fund travel for an additional staff person to the national conference where program results are being presented) must be cleared with the funder in advance. Remember that money left over at the end of a project year may not be allowed to roll forward into the next year. Similarly, unspent funds that were awarded to an agency in order to carry out a particular program may need to be repaid if they are not spent within the designated period. So watch the budget carefully, process expenses and reimbursements on time, and maintain open communication with the funder so that there are no surprises for anyone at year's end.

And when exactly does a project year end? That depends. The term *fiscal year* refers to the dates of the funding year. Some grants or contracts begin on January 1 and end on December 31, so the funding cycle follows the calendar year. Other funding, particularly that associated with schools or universities, begins on July 1 and ends on June 30. Still other funds may have a start date based on the day the award was made—March 1, October 1, or any other month in the year. It can be challenging for managers to handle grants with different fiscal years. However, it is manageable, given careful planning, organized files, and someone who can help with questions. Never be afraid to ask questions about managing a program's budget; both one's supervisor and the funder will appreciate proactive attention to the responsibilities of budget management. Good stewardship shows commitment to the program participants, the organization, and the funder. It also communicates to potential funders that the agency is a good investment for future funding.

Summary

Action plans, logic models, and Gantt charts are tools that program staff and stakeholders can use to implement a program and reach the desired program objectives and goals. All need to be thoughtful, living documents that help program staff and stakeholders accomplish the program's objectives on time and as intended.

Program staff and stakeholders need to be prepared for changes and challenges during a program's implementation period; programs take place in schools, workplaces, health care organizations, and communities, where change and challenge are to be expected. While it can be anticipated that challenges and struggles will arise, what they will be for any one specific program is unknown until the program is operating. It is difficult and awkward to deal with challenges and struggles, but there is a lot to be learned from them.

During implementation, staff and stakeholders manage the program's human and fiscal resources. Recruiting, selecting, developing, and supporting a skilled, motivated, diverse, and culturally competent staff contributes to caring and supportive relationships between and among program staff, stakeholders, and participants. A program's finances are a shared responsibility; everyone involved in the program needs to be made aware of his or her role in maintaining good fiscal practices that will contribute to long-term program growth and sustainability.

By using tools such as action plans, logic models, Gantt charts, budgets, and staff resources, the challenges of program implementation can be made manageable and often turned into learning opportunities.

For Practice and Discussion

1. A middle school is implementing a program to promote students' eating healthy lunches that include fresh vegetables and fruit, healthy beverages, whole grains, and low-fat choices. Program components include increasing healthy school lunch selections and providing classroom education and personal nutrition counseling for children, parents, and guardians. What challenges might be expected as the program moves from installation to initial implementation and full operation (stages discussed in Chapter 5)?

2. Have you ever had to plan anything big, like a wedding, a Thanksgiving dinner, or a graduation party? Did you use any kind of program management tool? Using a program like Microsoft Project and a budget of $2,000, develop a project plan for your college graduation party. Develop a Gantt chart and budget to see what you need to create a successful party.

3. What have your experiences been with on-the-job training? Has any job you have worked at provided training for you? Describe how the training was helpful, how it could have been improved, and what it entailed. Next, design a training program for a health promotion staff working in a school-based health clinic. What do they need to know in order to do their job? In what areas do you thinking coaching by program supervisors will be effective?

4. What tools do you use for your personal financial record keeping and financial planning? Do you use computer programs like Quicken or Excel? Or do you use paper-based products? How might any of these tools help you implement your program's budget? Complete a tutorial for Microsoft Excel. What makes this a useful budgeting tool for health promotion professionals?

5. Draw a logic model based on the academic program in which you are enrolled. Start with the program's resources, then its objectives, and finally its long-term goals. Discuss whether you see the program activities being able to reach the program goals.

KEY TERMS

Action plan	Implementation challenges
Balance sheet	Income statement
Budget	Intermediate outcomes
Cash flow statement	Logic model
Fiscal management	Long-term outcomes
Fiscal year	Performance evaluation
Gantt chart	Short-term outcomes

References

Barbazette, J. (2007). *Managing the training function for bottom line results: Tools, models and best practices.* San Francisco, CA: Pfeiffer.

Camp, R., Vielhaber, M., & Simonetti, J. L. (2001). *Strategic interviewing: How to hire good people.* Hoboken, NJ: Wiley.

Dropkin, M., Halpin, J., & La Touche, B. (2007). *The budget-building book for non-profits: A step-by-step guide for managers and boards* (2nd ed.). San Francisco, CA: Jossey-Bass.

Erwin, D. O., Ivory, J., Stayton, C., Willis, M., Jandorf, L., Thompson, H. . . . Hurd, T. C. (2003). Replication and dissemination of a cancer education model for African American women. *Cancer Control, 10,* 13–21.

Fixsen, D. L., Naoom, S. F., Blase, K. A., Friedman, R. M., & Wallace, F. (2005). *Implementation research: A synthesis of the literature* (FMHI Publication No. 231). Tampa: University of South Florida, Louis de la Parte Florida Mental Health Institute, National Implementation Research Network.

Gilmore, G. D. (2011). *Needs and capacity assessment strategies for health education and health promotion* (4th ed.). Boston, MA: Jones & Bartlett.

Hunt, S. (2007). *Hiring success: The art and science of staffing assessment and employee selection.* Alexandria, VA: Society for Human Resource Management.

Johnson, J. A., & Breckon, D. J. (2007). *Managing health education and health promotion programs: Leadership skills for the 21st century* (2nd ed.). Sudbury, MA: Jones & Bartlett.

Keller, A. & Bauerle, J. A. (2009). Using a logic model to relate the strategic to the tactical in program planning and evaluation; An illustration based on social norms interventions. *American Journal of Health Promotion, 24,* 89–92.

KU Work Group for Community Health and Development. (2015a). *Chapter 2, Section 1: Developing a Logic Model or Theory of Change.* Lawrence, KS: University of Kansas. Retrieved April 29, 2016, from the Community Tool Box: http://ctb.ku.edu/en/table-of-contents/overview/models-for-community-health-and-development/logic-model-development/example

KU Work Group for Community Health and Development. (2015b). *Chapter 43, Section 1: Planning and Writing an Annual Budget.* Lawrence, KS: University of Kansas. Retrieved April 29, 2016, from the Community Tool Box: http://ctb.ku.edu/en/table-of-contents/finances/managing-finances/annual-budget/main

Logic Model Templates (October, 2010). Retrieved from http://www.uwex.edu/ces/pdande/evaluation/evallogicmodelworksheets.html

MacDonald, G., Starr, G., Schooley, M., Yee, S., Klimowski, K., & Turner, K. (2001). *Introduction to program evaluation for comprehensive tobacco control programs.* Atlanta, GA: Centers for Disease Control and Prevention, Office on Smoking and Health.

McDavid, J. C., & Hawthorn, L. R. L. (2005). *Program evaluation and performance measurement: An introduction to practice.* Thousand Oaks, CA: Sage.

McKenzie, J. F., Neiger, B. L., & Thackeray, R. (2012). *Planning, implementing, and evaluating health promotion programs: A primer* (6th ed.). San Francisco, CA: Pearson Benjamin Cummings.

Timmreck, T. C. (2003). *Planning, program development, and evaluation* (2nd ed.). Boston, MA: Jones & Bartlett.

W. K. Kellogg Foundation. (2004). *WK Kellogg Foundation Logic Model Development Guide.* Retrieved from http://www.wkkf.org/resource-directory/resource/2006/02/wk-kellogg-foundation-logic-model-development-guide

CHAPTER 7

ADVOCACY

Regina A. Galer-Unti, Kelly Bishop, and Regina McCoy Pulliam

Creating an Advocacy Agenda for a Program

Advocacy is action in support of a cause or proposal. It is political, as in lobbying for specific legislation, or social, as in speaking out on behalf of those without a voice. Broadly, advocacy is part of being a professional in a health field. At the same time, from the narrow perspective of a staff member, stakeholder, or participant in a health promotion program, advocacy is championing the program, fighting for funding, and engaging others in order to sustain the program, address a specific health problem, and eliminate health disparities. Health promotion programs live with the tension that on any given day, changes may happen: funding is cut for political reasons, regardless of program performance; legislation may divert funding to new, higher-priority initiatives; changes in program participants' eligibility criteria may affect the priority population's access to a program; economic factors such as a recession might make money tight; or a new national (or state, local, school, business, hospital, or community) health priority might usurp a program's place in funders' and people's consciousness, leaving the program and its staff, stakeholders, and participants vulnerable to program closure.

Clearly, if there were unlimited resources, all health needs would be met, but given limited resources of time, materials, knowledge of what works best, and people's energy, advocacy is one tool that health promotion programs staff, stakeholders, and participants need.

LEARNING OBJECTIVES

- Compare and contrast the perspectives of health educators and health promoters on the role of advocacy in health programs.

- Describe the essential elements of a successful health advocacy effort and the relative importance of each element.

- Define the roles played by advocacy, media advocacy, community engagement, and mobilization in moving a health agenda forward.

- Describe the key methods of gaining support from elected officials for a health promotion agenda.

- Identify the ways that 501(c)(3) status affects agency efforts.

For without advocacy, programs disappear and public policy that protects and promote health is not created, even if they are effective.

Advocating for a health promotion program based on health theory that champions health equity and uses evidence-based interventions requires calling on someone with power to take action. That power can derive from different sources—from an elected or legal mandate or from popular support and the power of numbers. In a particular setting (such as a school, workplace, health care organization, or community) power is held, for example, by owners, stockholders, chief executive officers, boards of directors, superintendents, program directors, foundation staff members, government workers, and politicians such as local, state, and federal legislators.

Advocacy is about affecting the larger environment of public policy, and raising awareness of a single program is insufficient to create lasting social change. Public policy must be shaped in a way that will sustain change across institutions. For example, advocates might aim for passage of a public policy that creates safe housing through testing and removal of lead-based paint, but advocates might also make the point that community members need to get informed about safe housing issues and lead paint poisoning prevention, communicate with elected officials, and vote.

Advocacy during program implementation has roots in a number of the health theories. Community mobilization theory supports advocacy through its focus on individuals' taking action organized around specific health issues at a site. Social network and social support theory, with its emphasis on relationship building based on mutual support and shared interest, reinforces for advocates the importance of building social support and networks when advocating. The more people involved with advocacy, the better. Furthermore, communication theory, the diffusion of innovations model, and social marketing all help to shape how and with whom program staff, stakeholders, and participants talk in order to champion a program.

Green and Kreuter (2010) have discussed the necessity of creating healthy environments in which behavior change can occur. In his "Health Impact Pyramid," Frieden (2010) discusses how broad, societal change can have the most influence on the public's health. While it is important to improve individual health behavior, it is more likely that change will occur when conditions are favorable for such improvement (e.g., you'll ride your bicycle to work if there are safe bike paths). Advocacy efforts also include calls for environmental change. Thus, your organization may advocate for individual smoking cessation, but your efforts also include advocacy for tobacco taxes and smoke-free environments.

As part of implementing a health promotion program, the program staff may develop an advocacy agenda and strategy. The agenda is part of the program's action plan, just as an evidence-based health intervention is. One of the most important parts of effective advocacy is having a clear vision of the big issue the program addresses, what has to change, and a plausible plan of action for making the changes. Five key questions can help show the way:

1. **What action—one that is feasible—will actually solve the health problem?** What action needs to happen? Is it a new *law*, regulation, funding, service, or research initiative? The action needs to be compelling in order to get people interested in working for it. It also needs to be small enough that the program can achieve at least part of the action within a year or two, to keep people interested. Whatever the action, state it clearly and succinctly. Often such a statement is thought of as a program action (or behavioral) objective (discussed in Chapter 5) that directs and shapes a program's advocacy. It would be titled the *advocacy action objective*.

2. **Who needs to take action?** Who actually has the authority to make the change? For example, can a mayor, city council, or state or federal agency or legislature effect the desired change? Who needs to be wooed because they can influence those with authority? For example, can members of the media or specific citizen groups help advance the cause?

3. **What does your audience need to hear?** What advocacy message will move all those people to make the change? An effective advocacy message has two parts: an appeal on the merits ("This bill is important because . . .") and an appeal to self-interest ("Hundreds of voters want to know how you'll vote on . . .").

4. **Who is best to share the message with your audience?** What messengers can be recruited, and who will be most persuasive? An advocacy campaign needs a mix of messengers—people who can speak from personal experience, people with recognized authority, and others who might have some special pull with the people you are trying to reach.

5. **What actions will you use to make your point?** What will people be asked to do to deliver the message? The options are many: people are asked to lobby officials politely or protest in front of their offices, get an article in the newspaper, or attend a town meeting. Generally, the best actions to advocate are those that require the least effort and confrontation but still get the job done.

✳ Advocacy as a Professional Responsibility ✳

Advocacy for funding, legislation, regulations, governmental infrastructure, services, or research ensures successful health promotion programs. Researchers assert the importance of combining programs and advocacy in order to best serve the needs of the public (Christoffel, 2000; Roe, Minkler, & Saunders, 1995). Clearly, the importance of advocacy to health promotion programs is profound. Health advocacy is defined as "the processes by which the actions of individuals or groups attempt to bring about social and/or organizational change on behalf of a particular health goal, program, interest, or population" (Joint Committee on Health Education and Promotion Terminology, 2002). In short, health advocacy creates environments in which health promotion programs are successful.

Engagement in advocacy has long been suggested as a professional responsibility of health professionals (Freudenberg, 1982; Ogden, 1986; Steckler & Dawson, 1982). The Institute of Medicine report *Who Will Keep the Public Healthy?* contains a call to action for advocacy around health policy issues (Institute of Medicine, 2003). *Healthy People 2020* stresses the importance of developing policies that aid in achieving the goals and objectives of the *Healthy People 2020* initiative (U.S. Department of Health and Human Services, n.d.). The Galway Consensus Conference Statement lists advocacy as one of the areas of core competency necessary for engaging in successful health promotion practice (Allegrante et al., 2009). Health promotion practitioners clearly need to be effective advocates for a piece of the resource pie for their profession and for the people they work to help (Radius, Galer-Unti, & Tappe, 2009).

For many people working in health promotion programs, the acquisition of advocacy skills seems difficult and just one more thing among many that they need to know. Health promotion specialists are busy with the daily reality of implementing interventions, mobilizing and organizing stakeholders, and writing and revising policies. They often feel that the extra time and energy to advocate for their program just is not there. However, this view is shortsighted. Health promotion programs require supportive and receptive environments in order to achieve long-term sustainability. Focusing only on health promotion interventions and policies leaves out part of the work involved in the planning, implementation, and evaluation of successful health promotion programs; advocacy is part of the work.

Examples of Successful Health Policy Advocacy ✳

Public health measures such as improvements in clean air and water, proper sanitation, and adequate and nutritious food have significantly increased longevity and lessened human suffering. In 1999, the Centers for Disease Control and Prevention listed the top 10 advances in public health in the 20th century (Centers for Disease Control and Prevention, 1999). It is safe to say that many of these advances, including vaccinations, improvements in motor vehicle safety, safer workplaces, better food safety, and recognition of tobacco as a health hazard are attributable not only to scientific discoveries but to advocacy for education and policy change. In the following examples, note how advocacy was used to contribute to these advances.

Mothers Against Drunk Driving (MADD) was founded by Candy Lightner after her daughter was killed by a drunk driver. The driver of the automobile was a repeat offender, and MADD used a media advocacy campaign to educate the public about the dangers of drunk driving. This advocacy raised public consciousness about the threat of drunk driving and spurred lawmakers to initiate more legislation to curb this danger. MADD's media advocacy has been recognized as the impetus that inspired action that decreased fatalities resulting from drunk driving (DeJong, 1996).

The March of Dimes (originally known as the National Foundation for Infantile Paralysis) is an example of a voluntary health organization that achieved its goal. Founded in 1938 by President Franklin D. Roosevelt, it began as a campaign to collect money toward research to find a cure for polio and toward care for those suffering from the disease. All individuals residing in the United States were asked to voluntarily give one dime toward the effort. In 1958, 3 years after the Salk vaccine was introduced to the general public, the March of Dimes changed its focus, becoming an organization dedicated to preventing birth defects, premature birth, and infant mortality (March of Dimes, n.d.); the March of Dimes had achieved its goal of finding a vaccine for polio. As times have changed, many organizations such as the March of Dimes have applied their efforts not just toward soliciting donations for research but also toward advocacy for more funding for research in their chosen areas. Today's March of Dimes works in the areas of research, education, community services, and advocacy (March of Dimes, n.d.).

The strides made in legislation to control tobacco use are credited largely to the advocacy of researchers, activists, health practitioners, and nonprofit organizations. Long-term efforts to educate and heighten awareness about the harmful effects of tobacco have resulted in increased legislative activity in the area of tobacco control. It is interesting to note that these efforts have been accentuated by researchers' and advocates' efforts to heighten awareness about not only the health impact but also the economic costs of tobacco use (Givel & Glantz, 2004). As a result, significant legislation has been passed that limits tobacco manufacturers' contact with children, confines the use of tobacco products in public settings, and protects the worker from the health consequences of secondhand smoke. Advocacy techniques coupled with researchers' conclusions and recommendations have been used to decrease smoking in the United States (Chaney, Jones, & Galer-Unti, 2003).

Not all advocacy efforts are as well documented or as noticeable as the ones we have just described. Nutrition advocates have been responsible for a fair amount of legislation designed to protect and strengthen the healthful food supply in the United States. These advocacy efforts led to sweeping reforms in federal policy such as Public Law (P.L.) 101-535, commonly known as the Nutrition Labeling and Education Act of 1990, which mandates nutrition labels on packaged foods. This law represented a major victory for dietitians and consumers who had heavily advocated for the addition of this educational tool.

Some policy advocacy results in changes at state and local levels. Tip O'Neill, former speaker of the U.S. House of Representatives, has been credited with stating, "All politics is local." That is also true for many types of health policy, as one can see in the wide variance, for example, in *ordinances* that restrict the purchase of guns in municipalities, designate speed limits in states, direct alcohol sales, and ensure swimming pool safety.

At times, ordinances formulated for use in one area rise to the state or national level. This frequently occurs when a local news story gets attention in the national media (for example, through an article in a national newspaper or a story in an online source or National Public Radio). Increasingly, a news story will catch the fancy of a legislator, a legislative body, or the constituents of another state. In this age of rapid media transfer and multiple media outlets, news of unusual or important ordinances is quickly disseminated to other municipalities.

Becoming Fluent in the Language of Advocacy

In order to build skills in advocacy, it is necessary to learn the terminology of advocacy. Table 7.1 lists some key advocacy terms. The terms reflect the interactions of organized political and government structures in the making and administering of public decisions for a society. Advocates and lobbyists

Table 7.1   Key Advocacy Terms

Term	Definition
Advocacy	The processes by which individuals or groups attempt to bring about social or organizational change on behalf of a particular health goal, program, interest, or population
Appropriations	Legislation that designates or appropriates funding to a program
Authorizations	Legislation that sets policies or programs
Bill	A proposed law presented for approval to a legislative body
Direct lobbying	Communication with a legislator or a member of a legislator's staff that gives a viewpoint on a specific piece of legislation
Electioneering	Persuasion of voters in a political campaign
Grassroots lobbying	Any attempt to indirectly influence legislators by motivating members of the public to express specific views to legislators and legislative aides
Law	A local, state, or federal bill that has been passed by a legislative process (for example, a federal law passed by the U.S. Senate and the House of Representatives and signed by the president)
Lobbyist	An individual hired to represent the legislative interests of an organization (or related group of organizations) to members of a legislature
Media advocacy	Strategic use of news media and, when appropriate, paid advertising to support community organizing to advance a public policy initiative
Ordinance	A statute or regulation, usually enacted by a city government

have the task of getting the public involved in the decision-making and administration processes and influencing the decisions made within them.

Legislative advocacy is, essentially, advocating for or against bills, ordinances, and laws. A bill is a piece of legislation that has been introduced as a proposed law. At the federal level, when a bill has been approved by the Senate and the House, it is signed into law by the president. Information about the process through which bills are formulated and processed through Congress are found at the House of Representatives website (see Table 7.2). The Library of Congress has created a website (http://thomas.loc.gov) to aid in tracking legislation. States vary widely in their processes of passing a bill to create a law. In order to find information about government procedures, go to the state or municipal websites that are easily found through a search engine. Table 7.2 lists some useful websites that pertain to advocacy for health promotion programs including where to access statistics and examples that will prove useful in the development of advocacy materials.

Municipalities typically pass ordinances, which are enforced within the confines of the city. So an ordinance that applies within the confines of one town may not exist in the next town over. This is often confusing to

Table 7.2   Advocacy Organizations and Websites

Organization	URL	Brief Description
American Public Health Association	http://www.apha.org/policies-and-advocacy/advocacy-for-public-health/advocacy-activities	Provides advocacy tips, examples, and instructions for carrying out advocacy work
Centers for Disease Control and Prevention—The Community Guide	http://www.thecommunity guide.org	Encourages the use of evidence-based research for policy decisions, program planning, and research design
County Health Rankings and Roadmaps	www.countyhealthrankings.org	Provides per county and per state information on a variety of health factors
Library of Congress	http://thomas.loc.gov	Provides access to bill histories, resolutions, House and Senate committee reports, and the Congressional Record
Midwest Academy	http://www.midwestacademy.com	Provides online training and information for activism
Research America	http://www.researchamerica.org	Provides advocacy tips and public opinion polls
Society for Public Health Education	http://www.sophe.org/ChronicDiseasePolicy/Full_Guide.pdf	Manual provides guidelines for working with state and local policymakers
Trust for America's Health	http://healthyamericans.org	State-by-state health data on specific health issues and relevant policy and funding information
University of Kansas—The Community Toolbox	http://ctb.ku.edu/en	Provides information on community building and advocacy; maintained by the Work Group for Community Health and Development at the University of Kansas
Federal Government	http://www.house.gov http://www.senate.gov http://www.whitehouse.gov	Official sites of the U.S. House of Representatives, U.S. Senate, and White House that provide information about elected officials, staff, committees, legislative initiatives, and procedures utilized in formulating and funding public laws

people. One town may allow drivers to use cell phones while an adjacent community requires a hands-free device. Driving across the city limit, then, while talking on a cell phone, might result in a fine.

Two types of legislative processes are of significant interest to us. An authorization is a law that authorizes a program. An example of this, as previously discussed, is P.L. 101-535. The legislative history of the *bill* is available at http://thomas.loc.gov. Knowing the numbering system for public laws is helpful in gaining a clearer understanding of them. Congress meets in two-year terms. The first number in the P.L. number is the number of the Congressional session. Thus, the 101 means that the bill was enacted during the 101st Congress. The second number is the number of the law passed in that two-year session. In our example, 535 is the number of the law.

Appropriations differ from *authorizations* in their emphasis. Whereas authorizations set policy or programs, appropriations designate money for specific purposes. The federal government and state legislatures have clear deadlines for their budget approvals. Unlike bills, which are debated throughout the legislative calendar, appropriations occur at a set point in the legislative calendar. It is a good idea to keep an eye on these funding cycles in order to know when arguments for funding for health promotion programs will be most effective.

Influencing the legislative process occurs in a variety of ways. Different types of lobbying might be used to influence passage of a bill or approval of an appropriation. In the following section, the legal and employment ramifications of participation in lobbying are discussed.

Legalities of Health Advocacy

Advocacy and lobbying involve some legal issues. Health advocacy might take the form of delivery of general information and educating the public about a topic. For instance, an opinion piece about the dangers of hepatitis C and how it is transmitted is an important form of advocacy. Such an opinion piece might be written, for example, if there is a current attempt by a local governing body to enact an ordinance regulating tattoo parlors in the community. The piece is not written either for or against the ordinance; instead, the piece advocates for healthy and safe practices. There are no restrictions on this type of advocacy behavior.

The U.S. tax code exempts certain types of organizations from federal taxation of income. All of these organization types appear in Section *501(c)(3)* of the Internal Revenue Code. Organizations must apply for tax-exempt status; if they receive this status, they are often referred to as 501(c)(3) organizations. Organizations receiving tax-exempt status are primarily schools, colleges, universities, religious organizations, and charitable organizations (for example, community health organizations as discussed in Chapter 1). Many health promotion programs are initiated by 501(c)(3) organizations or government agencies.

The IRS is very clear about banning the involvement of tax-exempt organizations in electioneering. *Electioneering* is defined as any attempt to persuade voters in a political campaign. For instance, making telephone calls that actively try to persuade people to vote a particular way on Election Day is electioneering. Organizations with 501(c)(3) status are barred from electioneering activity by tax law, and they cannot actively work for a candidate or a political party, nor can they support or oppose a candidate for political office (Vernick, 1999) or intervene in partisan elections. This regulation covers all houses of worship in America. Thus the law is clear that tax-exempt institutions cannot engage in electioneering; however, their ability to legally participate in lobbying is a little less clear.

Lobbying occurs when an attempt is made to influence legislation. The tax status of an employer determines whether employees may lobby and to what extent employees may engage in specific activities.

Basically, there are two types of lobbying: *direct lobbying* and *grassroots lobbying*. These distinctions are important; definitions for both are provided in Table 7.1. In direct lobbying, individuals make contact with a legislator, a member of the staff of a legislator, or a government official who is involved in formulating legislation. A request is made, for instance, that a senator vote yes on a bill. This request is direct lobbying because it is an attempt to directly influence legislation (Vernick, 1999). In grassroots lobbying, the public is encouraged to approach legislators about a piece of legislation—for example, when members of an organization contact members of the public through a call to action that urges them to ask a government official to vote in a certain manner (Vernick, 1999). There is a complicated formula for the percentage of time that employees of a tax-exempt organization can spend on lobbying. Organizations need to be certain that they are in compliance with lobbying restrictions. Failure to comply may result in extra taxes or loss of tax-exempt status. Employees of tax-exempt organizations consult their employer about the policies of their organization.

Advocating While Maintaining One's Job

Advocacy activities on the part of employees is encouraged or discouraged, depending on the employer. Government employees must be exceedingly careful about advocacy work because of the need for employees of the government to avoid any appearance of bias. Employees of 501(c)(3) organizations need to be careful to stay in compliance with IRS rules that their organization must follow in order to maintain tax-exempt status. If you are encouraged as an employee and even as a private citizen to engage in advocacy activities, be certain to stay within your employer's guidelines.

Supervisors need to be informed when employees are engaging in advocacy efforts outside of regular work duties. Although the First Amendment to the U.S. Constitution ensures individuals' right to advocate (the right to free speech), there are no protections from firing if these activities put the employing agency at risk or harm the functioning of the agency.

Once the employer has been informed about the employee's intention to engage in advocacy work, care is taken to be certain that work and after-work advocacy activities are kept separate. When speaking in public, making a phone call, or sending a written communication, be certain that everyone is informed that advocacy work is being performed by you as a private citizen. For example, if you are speaking before the city council on restricting the sale of alcohol, you might say, "My name is _____. Some of you may know me as the head of the student health center. Today, however, I am expressing my personal views on the subject of bar hours." Note that, in general, as a person's visibility increases, people will increasingly tend to see that person's private remarks as opinions of the employing agency. There may come a point at which the public is unable to differentiate between an individual's personal remarks and his or her position in the agency. Take this factor into account and be pragmatic when making decisions about engaging in advocacy work.

Additional precautions are taken when engaging in advocacy work outside of an employing agency: do not use work titles, work stationery, work phones or fax machines, work e-mail or Internet systems, your work address, or a work cell phone or business card when you are acting as a private citizen. In the event that someone sends an e-mail to you at work, for instance, asking that recipients of the e-mail contact a legislator to urge passage of a bill, do not respond from the work account. Forward the e-mail to a home account, and use your home account and home computer for private advocacy efforts. If a local reporter calls to ask questions about your involvement in a local campaign, call her back on a private cell phone while on a break from work. Think twice before using your work facilities, workplace communication devices, or your work title.

Forming Alliances and Partnerships for Advocacy

Successful advocacy efforts do not happen in isolation; they are the result of coordinated, collaborative efforts by individuals and organizations working to achieve common goals. Effective partnerships rely on the strengths each individual or organization brings to the group. One partner may have more financial resources; another may have an established network that are easily mobilized. One may have more clout and thus be able to bring attention to the cause.

In addition, each organization's ability to advocate must be considered. As we noted earlier, employees of government agencies are restricted in how much and what types of advocacy and lobbying they are allowed to do. Nonprofit organizations (for example, community health organizations) tend to have fewer restrictions on advocacy and lobbying, and many for-profit organizations have paid lobbyists on staff or under contract.

When recruiting partners to advocate for health, examine what types of resources are needed, identify who or what organizations can bring those resources to the group, and then actively recruit the individuals or organizations. Consider all sectors of the community. Each sector can take an active role in advocating for health. Consider all traditional health allies, but also consider nontraditional partners: businesses, schools, faith-based organizations, youths, health care providers, elected officials, and community leaders. Be sure that partnerships represent the diversity of the community.

Establishing effective partnerships is a lot like establishing an effective relationship with a significant other. Individuals find each other and then spend time learning more about each other, including compatibility issues, commonality of goals, likes and dislikes, what each brings to the relationship (including excess baggage), and the amount of energy each is willing to expend to make the relationship successful and lasting. And like relationships, effective partnerships require care and maintenance.

Many effective public health advocacy campaigns are collaborations between national, state, and local partners. A good example of such a campaign began in 1991 when public health practitioners were encouraged to advocate for policy change as part of the National Cancer Institute's American Stop Smoking Intervention Study for Cancer Prevention (ASSIST) (National Cancer Institute, 2005). ASSIST was a demonstration project designed to bring public and private partners together to advocate for policies to prevent tobacco use and for tobacco control policies. On the national level, ASSIST was a joint effort of the National Cancer Institute (NCI) and the American Cancer Society (ACS). Both organizations had a common goal: to prevent cancer. NCI contracted with 17 state health departments (SHDs) to hire staff and fund interventions, including advocating for policies that had shown promise in reducing and preventing tobacco use. ACS committed resources (time, dollars, and staff) to ASSIST at national, state, and local levels.

As in any relationship, dynamics and challenges had to be recognized and addressed. From the beginning, ASSIST was beset with challenges that may not have been anticipated. The project required two structurally and functionally different types of organizations (SHDs and ACS) to work together. Funding the SHDs and not the ACS units was perceived by some to cause inequity in power. Despite these and other challenges, effective ASSIST partnerships at national, state, and local levels were successful, and today, ASSIST is considered a best practice model for effecting policy change to reduce disease and death.

C. Everett Koop, then U.S. surgeon general, believed ASSIST was successful in advancing his goal for a smoke-free society. In NCI's monograph *ASSIST: Shaping the Future of Tobacco Prevention and Control*, Koop states, "I have seen the important role that ASSIST leaders and coalitions played in advancing smoking cessation efforts and tobacco containment. They were in the vanguard of these efforts and helped to fashion the next phase of comprehensive tobacco control interventions." He further states, "In my estimation, several key points stand out as legacies of ASSIST," including "the strong emphasis on policy and media strategies to shift the focus from the individual to population-based interventions has had a long-lasting impact on behavioral health . . . and the lessons of ASSIST are broadly applicable to many public health disciplines." Koop goes on to say, "The lessons of ASSIST are essential to the tobacco prevention and control movement and, perhaps even more important, to the entire field of public health" (National Cancer Institute, 2005).

Since the end of ASSIST in 1999, the national tobacco control movement has grown to include all 50 states; territories; municipalities; numerous public and private for-profit and nonprofit organizations; and individuals—paid staff and volunteers from all walks of life—and has been successful in advocating for local, state, and national policies to prevent tobacco use, eliminate exposure to environmental tobacco smoke, and help people quit using tobacco.

Advocacy Methods

There are many advocacy methods, and new ways of advocating are being developed as times, technologies, and communication styles change. Only a few years ago, e-mail was not available to the masses, but it is now regularly used in advocacy efforts. Podcasts, blogs, texts, tweets, and the move to more rapid transfer of information offer a host of opportunities for empowerment through advocacy.

Talking Points

One of the first things developed is a list of *talking points*, which can then be used in a variety of advocacy efforts such as a meeting with a legislator, developing a public service announcement, writing a letter to the editor, or making a contribution to a blog.

Talking points are succinct, stay on the topic, and developed with a specific message in mind. Collect and assemble facts on the health problem or issue. Concentrate on short, understandable, manageable facts that will aid a reader or listener in understanding the importance of the problem on a personal or local level. For example, when speaking about lung cancer in Alabama, pull out the figures on cancer in Alabama. Find the percentage of cancer deaths per annum in Alabama, the cost to Alabama for treatment of cancer and loss of revenue due to cancer, the figures that show the impact of cancer on the ability of Alabama facilities to handle all of their patients, and other relevant statistics (see Table 7.2).

Different points might be accentuated for different groups. The development of talking points can actually aid in the development of a strategy for an advocacy campaign. Once the list of talking points is developed, use them in developing the other advocacy methods.

Newspaper Editorial Pages

The print and electronic versions of newspapers' editorial pages include letters to the editor and op-ed articles. Typically, these appear in both print and online versions of most papers, allowing them to be e-mailed to a person, which is a plus. Writing either a letter to the editor or an op-ed requires preparation. Use the talking points in writing your piece. A letter to the editor employs the principles of persuasive letter writing in that it has three basic parts. In the first portion, or introduction, the writer introduces the reader to the problem and provides a *hook* that will encourage the reader to continue reading. The second portion guides the reader through an understanding of the problem or issue. Here, it is wise to use a couple of facts, which are taken from the talking points that have already been developed. The third portion of the letter is a call to action or a suggestion for resolution of the problem. Good guidelines for writing letters to the editor are on the websites of the American Public Health Association (APHA) and the University of Kansas's Community Toolbox (see Table 7.2).

Letters to the editor are regularly read by staffers of legislators. These letters are considered key items in helping federal and state representatives to understand activities in their home district. Be aware that letters to the editor are important forms of advocacy to policymakers. The editorial page (where the letters are found) is also read by the features editors and news editors of the publishing paper and other newspapers. Media coverage is frequently generated as a result of a letter to the editor. Finally, average citizens read letters to the editor.

Another way to reach the audience of the editorial page is an op-ed. An *op-ed* is a short article that expresses the views of the writer on a topic. An op-ed is typically 750 words and may contradict remarks that have been made by the editor. Sometimes opposing views are sought and run on the same editorial page. These persuasive arguments are often written by subject matter experts or well-known writers. Spend a little time perusing the editorial pages of major newspapers to get a sense of the importance of op-eds.

Letters, E-mails, and Phone Calls

A letter to a key policymaker has elements of persuasion similar to those of a letter to the editor or an op-ed piece, but a few additional tips may prove useful. First, be certain to properly address the letter to a congressperson—use *The Honorable* rather than *Mr.* or *Ms.* Second, the letter is short and to the point. Examine your talking points for ideas about how to address concerns and spark the interest of the policymaker or her aide. Third, look at the preceding paragraphs about writing a letter to the editor to aid you in thinking about the construction of a letter to a legislator. The APHA website (see Table 7.2) provides sample letters to congresspersons.

Sometimes it is necessary to send a letter to a policymaker through the U.S. mail. Seek permission to use your organization's letterhead (if appropriate). However, keep in mind that since the anthrax attacks of 2001, U.S. mail is delayed by thorough inspections, so e-mails, faxes, texts, and phone calls are preferred and are more quickly received by staffers. Many websites of individual congress members have messaging capabilities and you can leave your message there. A staff member regularly reads these notes.

Public Service Announcements

Public service announcements (PSAs) are part of the public relations toolbox of health educators. PSAs aid in advertising events but may also advocate a specific perspective or action in regard to a health problem. Some PSAs are used to heighten awareness of a health problem. Radio and television airwaves are owned by the public, and television and radio stations must pay for their use of the airwaves by giving back a certain amount of public service time. So, if there is upcoming legislation that would positively affect HIV funding, for example, it makes sense to write a PSA that will increase visibility about the issue. It is indirect advertising, and the legislation cannot be discussed, but heightened awareness will be helpful in passage of it.

Blogs

Blogs (online diaries or journals), have rapidly evolved to more sophisticated journals. Many blogs provide links to vlogs (video logs), podcasts, and other websites. Blogs tend to provide commentary or news on a particular subject. Many blogs allow the interactive feature of receiving commentary from readers. More and more journalists have blogs, which creates an interesting blurring of the line between objective journalism and subjective chronicling of the issues of the day. Many people read blogs and accept these diary postings as factually correct. Blogs are most effective for communicating with advocates and supporters about current information and resources important to the health-related change and action being sought through the advocacy efforts.

Twitter, Facebook, and Other Social Media

Can you deliver a message and inspire action through a 140-character tweet? Do followers frequent your Facebook page for information about your advocacy efforts? Do you post Instagram photos with advocacy captions? Twitter, Facebook, Snapchat, and Instagram are social media hubs that can assist you in your advocacy efforts. You can get your message out quickly, effectively, and inexpensively.

Think about how you'll use your followers and who you will follow. Optimize your contacts and have them ready to mobilize to action. That means you'll have to keep them "close" by staying in touch and up-to-date about the workings of your organization. Do not bury them in information. Instead, provide them with important news and at the appropriate depth. If you call for action, provide specific and simple directions. For instance, ask specifically for a retweet.

Meetings with Legislators

The classic advocacy method is meeting in person with legislators in their offices. Many believe it is the most effective method. In preparing to meet with a legislator, there are a few things to keep in mind: Consider that dozens of visitors come in to ask for a favor, a vote, or some other action. Everyone has an argument, a cause, and a reason why their request trumps all others. The other visitors may have long-standing connections with the official. (Tips on how to forge such a connection are provided later in the chapter.)

The four P's of marketing (see Chapter 3) provide the basic elements of a marketing campaign. Similarly, we have developed a basic approach to meetings that we call the four P's of advocacy: preparation, prioritization, punctuality, and politeness:

1. **Preparation.** Preparation for meetings with legislators is as thorough as preparation for a job interview. Prepare a set of talking points to inform your conversation. Prioritize the talking points, and leave a list of facts with the government official. Remember to begin the conversation with the most salient point. During the preparation phase, information about the policymaker's viewpoints and personal background may come to

light. If you are advocating for an increase in cancer education funding, it is advantageous to know that the senator's mother has cancer. The best preparation for the meeting, however, occurs far in advance of the actual appointment. Over time, it is wise to aid the policymaker with fact checking and with education and information, by sending him news on triumphs of local and state health programs and apprising him of changes in health activities in the community. The policymaker will view this help as the work of a trusted friend and expert on health.

2. **Prioritization.** Earlier, we mentioned that talking points be prioritized. Change the order of the discussion of the talking points depending on the elected official. The prioritization of talking points in a meeting is informed by viewing the voting record of the elected official. The APHA advocacy website provides the voting records of congressional leaders on health issues (see Table 7.2). Choose the order of talking points to address in your meeting on the basis of research on the official's voting record and personal interests. In persuasive argument, it is wise to consider the audience receiving the message.

3. **Punctuality.** First, be punctual. Arrive early and check in with the assistant. Use this punctuality principle during the meeting. Stay on task; don't overstay your welcome; and be certain to use time to your advantage in advancing your goal. If you are asking for increased funding for school health programs, don't waste time complaining about the potholes in the roads. Talking about the potholes is off point, wastes the elected official's time, and will give the official the option of solving the problem of the potholes rather than increasing funding for school health programs.

4. **Politeness.** An air of politeness is underlying all proceedings of the day. Citizens do pay the salaries of elected officials, but that does not mean that employees should be treated rudely. Don't react in a rude fashion if the official does not respond in the desired way. Make all your points in a dignified, forthright manner, and provide statistics the policymaker can use in his or her decision-making process. It may not appear that the elected official is listening, but that observation could be in error. This meeting may not achieve its desired outcome, but it may aid subsequent successful dealings with this government worker. President Ronald Reagan was known for arguing with Democratic leaders during the day and having friendly dinners with them at night. Holding a grudge rarely helps in any interaction with others, and this is particularly true in politics. When the meeting ends, thank the elected official or aide, send a follow-up thank-you note, and provide promised materials immediately.

Building Relationships with the Media

The best time to begin advocacy efforts is prior to any kind of crisis. It is better to begin building a team of journalists, legislators, and stalwart supporters long before the problem is the issue of the day. Wallack, Dorfman, Jernigan, and Themba (1993), writing about *media advocacy*, inform readers that their advocacy efforts will not be taken seriously unless they take the media seriously. One way to do that is by applying the four P's to interactions with members of the media: be prepared, prioritize all remarks, be punctual, and be polite.

Be certain to contact and compliment a reporter when a good health story appears in the newspaper. When an error is noted, be polite in making the necessary correction, and volunteer to be a fact checker in the future. Make a list of reporters who are friendly to health issues, and work to keep up a relationship with each of those reporters. If contacted by someone in the media, respond immediately. Let reporters know about emerging health issues, and help them to see the local angle. This preparation and politeness will help in future advocacy efforts. Media advocacy will aid in promoting local health programs and in advancing an advocacy agenda (Wallack & Dorfman, 1996).

It is helpful to think like a journalist. Be aware of their need to sell the story to an editor and to the public. Be aware of deadlines, keep the focus of the story on the journalist's priority population, and conform to guidelines. When pitching a story to local media, imagine a 15-second elevator ride in which the health problem or cause must be explained to a stranger. This exercise will help narrow the topic because it will force you to choose your words very carefully. Think about the hook for the story, and succinctly deliver the most important parts of the message. Writing the *elevator speech* will also serve the purpose of framing the issue. Framing the issue, according to Wallack, Woodruff, Dorfman, and Diaz (1999), helps also to identify alternative ways in which to deliver the message succinctly for the greatest impact.

Media is quickly evolving. The media universe has rapidly expanded beyond the traditional outlets. In the past, we might have directed our message to features and news editors. Now, we may find ourselves talking to a top individual blogger or blogging group. How we frame messages and think about capturing interest have not changed much. Instead, there are more places for us to bring our stories and more ways to get the message out. Spend time following a few blog sites to see which ones might have an interest in the story. If you have your own blog (or organizational blog), you have an opportunity to have your site read and work picked up by other media.

Advocacy and Technology

Rapid technology advances and changes in forms of communication have resulted in the use of new techniques that provide opportunities for advocacy and political action that move far beyond the opportunities in print media. The Internet has opened up ways to communicate with diverse audiences. This tremendous ability to communicate with large numbers of people is seen in today's large-scale organizing efforts. Although a great deal of these efforts appear to be top-down organizing (for example, political campaigns), there are signs of grassroots organizing efforts that use the Internet.

Blogs, vlogs, e-mails, Twitter, social networking sites (e.g., Facebook), webinars, and podcasts are ways to reach large numbers of people very quickly. Smartphones and other handheld communication devices are correlated with an uptick in cyber-activism. Advocacy alerts and activities are introduced so quickly after a news event that it is increasingly difficult to discern which came first—the advocacy effort or the issue itself (Galer-Unti, 2010). The next changes in communication technology are for the omniscient to predict. Irrespective of the latest technology, efforts in health advocacy must be led by a skilled, educated, and enthusiastic group of health promotion program staff, stakeholders, and participants.

Summary

Advocacy is a set of actions used by individuals and groups to create support-ive environments for health promotion programs through organizational or legislative change. Advocacy for funding, legislation, regulations, gov-ernmental infrastructure, services, or research aids in ensuring successful health promotion programs. Advocacy is an important part of implementa-tion for a health promotion program and, thus, an important skill in health promotion. When advocacy efforts are successful, awareness of a disease or risk behavior is heightened, funding for health promotion programs is increased, or legislation that creates an environment in which good health can be attained is created.

It is important to engage in advocacy activities that are acceptable to one's employer. Understanding the difference between advocacy and lob-bying and what is acceptable to different employers is critical in protecting employers from difficulties due to tax code violations.

Effective communication and organizing at the program site are fun-damental skills of health advocacy. Communicating with large groups of people is accomplished, for example, through letters to the editor, social media, public service announcements, or blogs. Mobilizing individuals for change is based on communicating with people but also on helping individuals see the relevance of a health topic to their own life. Successful advocacy efforts have education, motivation, and action as critical components of the work.

For Practice and Discussion

1. Go to the website of a community health organization (a 501(c)(3) organization) and locate the mission of the organization. Has the organization defined an advocacy agenda? If the answer is yes, does the advocacy agenda have clear underpinnings in the mission statement of the organization? Have action steps (or activities) been assigned to the advocacy agenda? If the organization does not have an advocacy agenda create one. For both situations (with and without an advocacy agenda) discuss strategies and action steps that will help with the advocacy agenda of the organization.

2. Have you, a family member, or friend ever participated in advocacy work? If so, describe what these advocacy efforts were. Were the efforts successful? How was success evaluated? What observations or tips would you give to others who are interested in performing advocacy work? How might you have improved the outcome?

3. Do you agree that people working in health promotion programs have an ethical responsibility to engage in advocacy work? What is the role of health researchers in advocacy work? Are there ethical considerations for health researchers who want to become involved in advocacy work?

4. Define (using reliable sources) the word *activism*. Can you describe differences between advocacy work and activism? Give examples of different types of advocacy and activism initiatives. Would participation in any of these affect your job security? If so, describe how this work would affect your employment.

5. Consider a health problem in your local community. How would you frame the issue in such a way as to gain maximum media attention? Outline a media advocacy campaign with a timeline. What benchmarks would you use to measure success, and how would successes or failures affect your advocacy strategy? Be sure to use social media in your campaign or fully explain why you have chosen not to use social media.

KEY TERMS

Advocacy	Grassroots lobbying
Advocacy agenda	Hook
Appropriations	Law
Authorizations	Letter to the editor
Bill	Media advocacy
Direct lobbying	Mothers Against Drunk Driving (MADD)
Electioneering	Op-ed
Elevator speech	Ordinance
501(c)(3)	Public service announcements (PSAs)

References

Allegrante, J. P., Barry, M. M., Airhihenbuwa, C. O., Auld, M. E., Collins, J. L., Lamarre, M. . . . Mittelmark, M. B. (2009). Domains of core competency standards and quality assurance for building global capacity in health promotion: The Galway Consensus Conference Statement. *Health Education & Behavior*, 6(3), 476–482.

Centers for Disease Control and Prevention. (1999). Ten great public health achievements—United States, 1900–1999. *Morbidity and Mortality Weekly Reports*, 48(12), 241–243.

Chaney, J. D., Jones, E., & Galer-Unti, R. A. (2003). Using technology in advocacy efforts to aid in tobacco policy and politics. *Health Promotion Practice, 4*, 218–224.

Christoffel, K. K. (2000). Public health advocacy: Process and product. *American Journal of Public Health, 90*, 722–726.

DeJong, W. (1996). MADD Massachusetts versus Senator Burke: A media advocacy case study. *Health Education Quarterly, 23*, 318–329.

Frieden, T. R. (2010). A framework for public health action: The health impact pyramid. *American Journal of Public Health, 100*, 590–595.

Freudenberg, N. (1982). Health education for social change: A strategy for public health in the U.S. *International Journal of Health Education, 24*, 138–145.

Galer-Unti, R. A. (2010). Advocacy 2.0: Advocating in the digital age. *Health Promotion Practice, 11*, 784–787.

Givel, M., & Glantz, S. A. (2004). The "global settlement" with the tobacco industry: 6 years later. *American Journal of Public Health, 94*, 218–224.

Green, L. W., & Kreuter, M. W. (2010). Evidence hierarchies versus synergistic Interventions. *American Journal of Public Health, 100*, 1824–1825.

Institute of Medicine. (2003). *Who will keep the public healthy? Educating public health professionals for the 21st century*. Washington, DC: National Academies Press.

Joint Committee on Health Education and Promotion Terminology. (2002). Report of the 2000 Joint Committee on Health Education and Promotion Terminology. *Journal of School Health, 72*, 3–7.

March of Dimes. (n.d.). *About us*. Retrieved May 25, 2016, from http://www.marchofdimes.org/mission/a-history-of-the-march-of-dimes.aspx

National Cancer Institute. (2005). *ASSIST: Shaping the future of tobacco prevention and control* (Tobacco Control Monograph No. 16; NIH Publication No. 05-5645.). Bethesda, MD: U.S. Department of Health and Human Services, National Institutes of Health, National Cancer Institute.

Ogden, H. G. (1986). The politics of health education: Do we constrain ourselves? *Health Education Quarterly, 13*, 1–7.

Radius, S. M., Galer-Unti, R. A., & Tappe, M. K. (2009). Education for advocacy: Recommendations for professional preparation and development based on a needs and capacity assessment of health education faculty. *Health Promotion Practice, 10*, 83–91.

Roe, K. M., Minkler, M., & Saunders, F. F. (1995). Combining research, advocacy, and education: The methods of the Grandparent Caregiver Study. *Health Education Quarterly, 22*, 458–475.

Steckler, A., & Dawson, L. (1982). The role of health education in public policy development. *Health Education Quarterly, 9*, 275–292.

U.S. Department of Health and Human Services. (n.d.). *Healthy People 2020*. Retrieved May 25, 2015, from www.healthypeople.gov

Vernick, J. S. (1999). Lobbying and advocacy for the public's health: What are the limits for nonprofit organizations? *American Journal of Public Health, 89*, 1425–1429.

Wallack, L., & Dorfman, L. (1996). Media advocacy: A strategy for advancing policy and promoting health. *Health Education Quarterly, 23*, 293–317.

Wallack, L., Dorfman, L., Jernigan, D., & Themba, M. (1993). *Media advocacy and public health: Power for prevention*. Thousand Oaks, CA: Sage.

Wallack, L., Woodruff, K., Dorfman, L., & Diaz, I. (1999). *News for a change: An advocate's guide to working with the media*. Thousand Oaks, CA: Sage.

CHAPTER 8

COMMUNICATING HEALTH INFORMATION EFFECTIVELY

Neyal J. Ammary-Risch, Allison Zambon, and Ellen Langhans

Communication in Health Promotion Programs

Health communication is the study and use of communication strategies to inform and influence individual and community decisions that affect health. It links the fields of communication and health and is increasingly recognized as a necessary element of efforts to improve personal and public health (U.S. Department of Health and Human Services, Health Resources and Services Administration, 2015). It has been described further as "a multifaceted and multidisciplinary approach to reach different audiences and share health-related information with the goal of influencing, engaging and supporting individuals, communities, health professionals, special groups, policy makers and the public to champion, introduce, adopt, or sustain a behavior, practice or policy that will ultimately improve health outcomes" (Schiavo, 2007). Table 8.1 lists the attributes of effective health communication that were identified in *Healthy People 2010*.

Understanding and using principles of health communication, program staff craft and deliver health messages in a way that is meaningful and appropriate for the audience the program is trying to reach. All too often, well-intended and seemingly clear health communications leave unanswered questions that may have unintended negative consequences (Table 8.2). Knowing that people

LEARNING OBJECTIVES

- Discuss the importance of various modes of health communication in the adoption, cessation, and maintenance of individual health behavior.

- Describe health literacy in terms of contributing factors, vulnerable populations, and plain language message construction and format.

- Describe the components of an effective health communication plan from development through implementation.

- Explain why pretesting concepts and materials is important to health information campaign implementation.

Table 8.1   Attributes of Effective Health Communication˙

Accuracy: The content is valid and without errors of fact, interpretation, or judgment.

Availability: The content (whether targeted message or other information) is delivered or placed where the audience can access it. Placement varies according to audience, message complexity, and purpose, ranging from interpersonal and social networks to billboards and mass transit signs to prime-time TV or radio, to public kiosks (print or electronic), to the Internet.

Balance: Where appropriate, the content presents the benefits and risks of potential actions or recognizes different and valid perspectives on the issue.

Consistency: The content remains consistent over time and also is consistent with information from other sources (the latter is a problem when other widely available content is not accurate or reliable).

Cultural competence: The design, implementation, and evaluation process that accounts for special issues for select population groups (for example, ethnic, racial, and linguistic) and also educational levels and disability.

Evidence base: Relevant scientific evidence that has undergone comprehensive review and rigorous analysis to formulate practice guidelines, performance measures, review criteria, and technology assessments for telehealth applications.

Reach: The content gets to or is available to the largest possible number of people in the priority population.

Reliability: The source of the content is credible, and the content itself is kept up to date.

Repetition: The delivery of/access to the content is continued or repeated over time, both to reinforce the impact with a given audience and to reach new generations.

Timeliness: The content is provided or available when the audience is most receptive to, or in need of, the specific information.

Understandability: The reading or language level and format (including multimedia) are appropriate for the specific audience.

Source: U.S. Department of Health and Human Services, 2000.

Table 8.2   Example of the Need for Plain but Comprehensive Health Communication

A 2-year-old is diagnosed with an inner ear infection and prescribed an antibiotic. Her mother understands that her daughter should take the prescribed medication twice a day. After carefully studying the label on the bottle and deciding that it doesn't tell how to take the medicine, she fills a teaspoon and pours the antibiotic into her daughter's painful ear.

Source: Parker, Ratzan, and Lurie, 2003.

are frequently making important and complicated health decisions with only the written or oral instructions of a health professional has added urgency to the creation of effective health communications.

The practice of effective health communication contributes to health promotion and disease prevention. For example, through the training of health promotion staff and program participants in effective communication skills, the interpersonal and group interactions in a program are improved. Collaborative relationships are enhanced when all parties are capable of good communication. Likewise, the dissemination of health messages through health promotion programs and campaigns can create awareness of an issue, change attitudes toward a health behavior, and encourage and motivate individuals to follow recommended health behaviors. While health communication alone cannot change behavior, understanding its role and how its principles are used in a health promotion program will increase the likelihood that a program will succeed.

What Is Health Literacy?

Everyone encounters situations every day where they are responsible for making decisions about their health. They are challenged with seeking and understanding health information, communicating with their providers, managing and monitoring their own diseases, maintaining good health, navigating the health care system, filling out insurance forms, signing informed consent forms, seeking out options of and access to care, acting as caregivers, comprehending medications and correct dosages, or advocating for their health or the health of loved ones. Outside of the health care system, people make many health choices such as what foods to eat, how much to eat, and the amount of time they exercise—the list of health decisions is a long one, and is increasingly complicated with the amount of information available.

With these many challenges, health literacy skills are a major factor in determining a successful outcome. Although experts are still debating the single definition of *health literacy*, the Patient Protection and Affordable Care Act (ACA) and *Healthy People 2010* (U.S. Department of Health and Human Services, 2000) define health literacy as the "degree to which an individual has the capacity to obtain, communicate, process, and understand basic health information and services in order to make appropriate health decisions." Because the word *literacy* is included in the phrase, people often mistakenly think that health literacy is an issue of concern only for those who cannot read or write. However, health literacy expands beyond reading and writing skills to include the ability to comprehend and assess health information in order to make informed decisions about healthy behaviors, self-care, and disease management (U.S. Department of Health and Human Services, Steps to a Healthier US, 2004; Zarcadoolas, Pleasant, & Greer, 2003).

A range of factors contribute to health literacy. They include social and individual factors such as cultural and conceptual knowledge and listening, speaking, arithmetical, writing, and reading skills (Nielsen-Bohlman, Panzer, & Kindig, 2004). Studies have shown that individuals with inadequate health literacy report less knowledge about their medical conditions and treatment, worse health status, less understanding and use of preventive services, and a higher rate of hospitalization than those with marginal or adequate health literacy (Berkman et al., 2004; Nielsen-Bohlman, Panzer, & Kindig, 2004).

Health literacy is often talked about in terms of the individual. However, health care providers, public health professionals, policymakers, and health care and public health systems are also responsible for health literacy. Although individuals' health literacy skills and capacities are linked to their own education level, culture, or language, it is also important to acknowledge the role of the communication and assessment skills of those with whom people interact in regard to their health, as well as the ability of the media, the marketplace, and the government to provide health information in a manner appropriate to the audience (Nielsen-Bohlman, Panzer, & Kindig, 2004). Taking a universal precautions approach—assuming everyone is at risk for not understanding health information—ensures that people of all health literacy levels can benefit from the communication efforts put forth by those who work to improve public health.

Who Is Most Likely to Have Low Health Literacy?

People most likely to experience low health literacy fall into the following groups (Nielsen-Bohlman, Panzer, & Kindig, 2004):

- Older adults
- Racial and ethnic minorities
- People with low education levels
- People with low income levels
- Non-native speakers of English
- People with compromised health status

These populations often have the greatest health care needs and the highest rates of chronic diseases, and low health literacy can limit their ability to comprehend health information, navigate the health care system, or manage their own diseases and conditions.

Low health literacy is particularly common among older adults. The high prevalence of low health literacy in older adults is of particular concern because they are the most likely to have chronic conditions such as diabetes, cardiovascular disease, or cancer. Approximately 51% of older Americans age 65+ have one or two chronic conditions and 41% have three or more (West, Cole, Goodkind, & He, 2014).

Although low health literacy predominantly affects more vulnerable populations, it continues to grow as a problem for all Americans as our health care system becomes increasingly complex and technologically advanced. Even well-educated individuals can have difficulty understanding or acting on health information, for reasons that vary. A person's age, race, ethnicity, language, disability, or even emotional state when hearing or reading health information can affect health literacy.

Literacy and Health Literacy in the United States

The scope of the health literacy problem is far reaching. The National Adult Literacy Survey (NALS) found that approximately 90 million adults, half of the U.S. population, lack the literacy skills necessary to effectively use the U.S. health system (Kirsch, Jungeblut, Jenkins, & Kolstad, 1993). Health literacy issues can affect people of all backgrounds, but it is particularly burdensome for those with low literacy to try to read and understand health-related information. Most health information is written at or above the 10th-grade reading level, yet the average reading level of people in the United States is eighth grade, and 20% of the population reads at or below the fifth-grade level (Kirsch, Jungeblut, Jenkins, & Kolstad, 1993). The NALS also discovered that 50% of African Americans and Hispanics read at or below the fifth-grade level. Given the disproportionate rates of chronic diseases in these populations, the need for clear, easy-to-read health information is evident.

The 2003 *National Assessment of Adult Literacy* (NAAL) included the first-ever—and to date, only—national assessment of health literacy of adults in the United States, based on this definition of health literacy: "the ability to use printed and written information associated with a broad range of goals at home, in the workplace, and in the community (including healthcare settings)" (Kutner, Greenberg, Jin, & Paulsen, 2006). Results were reported in terms of four literacy levels: below basic, basic, intermediate, and proficient. *Below basic* means that the person has, at most, only the most simple and concrete health literacy skills. *Basic* means that the person has the skills necessary to perform simple and everyday health literacy activities. *Intermediate* means that the person has the skills necessary to perform moderately challenging health literacy activities. *Proficient* means that the person has the skills necessary to perform more complex and challenging health literacy activities. Findings indicated that the majority of adults (53%) had intermediate health literacy, meaning that they could do things like determine the healthy weight range for a person of a specific height on a body mass index chart or determine the times when it would be correct for a person to take a prescribed medication after reading the label. About 22% had basic health literacy, meaning that they could do things like read a clearly written brochure and then identify reasons that a person with no symptoms of a specific disease should be tested for it anyway. And 14% had below basic health literacy, meaning that they were able to do things like circle the date on a medical appointment slip or identify how often a person needs to have a specific medical test after reading a clearly written pamphlet (Kutner, Greenberg, Jin, & Paulsen, 2006). This means that the lowest percentage of adults, just 12%, had proficient health literacy skills.

Though the NAAL is, to date, the only national assessment of health literacy specifically, *the 2012 Program for the International Assessment of Adult Competencies* (PIAAC) illustrated that literacy skills of adults did not change much in the previous decade; only 12% of adults had proficient literacy skills, and even fewer (9%) had proficient numeracy skills.

The 2003 NAAL also examined where adults get information about health issues. Kutner, Greenberg, Jin, and Paulsen (2006) found that adults with below basic or basic health literacy were less likely than adults with higher health literacy to get information about health issues from written sources (newspapers, magazines, books, brochures, or the Internet) and more likely than adults with higher health literacy to get a lot of information about health issues from radio and television. These findings are important because they can help to determine the best communication *channels* to use in reaching out to a specific target audience. Written brochures or pamphlets are often not the best way to provide people with health information, particularly those who are more likely to have low health literacy.

Since the NAAL research findings on where adults get information about health issues, there have been many other studies on where adults go to find health information; many studies focus on digital information, given the ubiquity of the Internet and the rise in use of mobile devices like smartphones. Most notable, the Pew Internet Project's research related to health and health care has provided in-depth insight into where and how adults look for health information online. Of the 87% of U.S. adults that use the Internet, 72% have looked online for health information in the past year. These statistics speak to the importance of *eHealth* and creating health literate digital information (Pew Research Center, 2015).

Plain Language and Other Strategies to Improve Health Literacy

Presenting information in plain language (or plain English) is an integral component of improving health literacy. *Plain language* has many definitions, but it is fundamentally defined as communication that the audience can understand the first time they read or hear it. Written material in plain language means that the members of an audience can:

- Find what they need.
- Understand what they find.
- Use what they find to meet their needs.

While definitions vary, the essence of plain language is a focus on the audience, clarity, and comprehension. Using clear and concrete words in a straightforward manner is the best way to organize information, particularly

Table 8.3 Example of Text Before and After Rewriting in Plain Language

Before

The Dietary Guidelines for Americans recommends a half hour or more of moderate physical activity on most days, preferably every day. The activity can include brisk walking, calisthenics, home care, gardening, moderate sports exercise, and dancing.

After

Do at least 30 minutes of exercise, like brisk walking, most days of the week.

health content. Take, for example, the messages in Table 8.3, which shows how information about exercise was rewritten, using clear, concise words.

All people benefit from information in plain language, but it is especially important when communicating with people with low health literacy. *Plain language* refers not only to the specific words that are used but also to *how information is presented*. Figure 8.1 is an example of a health education resource for people with diabetes that uses plain language techniques. Here are a few of the techniques the figure uses to present information that is visually appealing, logically organized, and comprehensible:

- Use ample white space. Break up dense amounts of text. Keep sentences short.

- Use clear headings and bullets. Try using question-and-answer formats with straightforward answers.

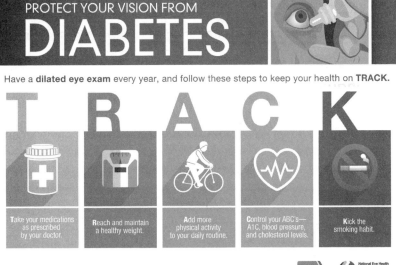

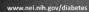

Figure 8.1 Health Education Resource for People with Diabetes That Uses Plain Language Techniques
Source: National Eye Institute, 2015.

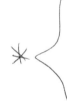

- Use the active voice and strong verbs.

- Avoid medical jargon, and use conversational language.

- Use a design that increases comprehension. Include pictures or graphics that are visually appealing to illustrate examples or important points.

- Supplement written materials with audiovisual materials or conversation.

Since 2010, plain language is the law for federal government communication; all new publications, forms, and publicly distributed documents must be well organized, clear, and concise. Though the law only pertains to government agencies, the guidelines for how to write in plain language are a useful resource and provide examples and tips on using plain language and improving communication. You can find many more examples and tips on using plain language and improving communication by visiting www .plainlanguage.gov.

According to the National Action Plan to Improve Health Literacy (U.S. Department of Health and Human Services, U.S. Department of Health and Human Services, Office of Disease Prevention and Health Promotion, 2010), other strategies to improve health literacy (besides using a universal precautions approach, mentioned earlier) include involving members of the priority audience in the design and testing of communication (called user-centered design), targeting and tailoring communication, and even making organizational changes to address health literacy. Resources such as Health Literacy Online (http://health.gov/healthliteracyonline) and the Clear Communication Index (www.cdc.gov/ccindex) can also help to both create and assess health communication materials.

Many other strategies are effective in communicating with people with low health literacy, particularly people with chronic conditions, whose health relies heavily on their self-care skills and abilities. For example, successful strategies for communicating with people with diabetes have included selecting critical behaviors to focus on; reducing the complexity of information given; using clear, concrete examples; concentrating on single topics at a time; avoiding medical jargon; and using teach-back methods (Rothman et al., 2004). Using teach-back methods in the health care setting are particularly helpful in identifying any misunderstandings a patient may have. In this technique, after patients are given instructions, they are asked to explain back how they'll take a particular medication or follow other instructions. Similar strategies are used in teaching self-care skills for a variety of diseases and conditions in which individuals play a central role. When people are able to fully understand and act on health information, they are better able to manage their conditions and make healthy decisions.

Developing a Communication Plan for a Site

Health communication is an integral part of health promotion programs. It is recommended that each program have a communication plan to guide and develop information exchange between and among the program staff, stakeholders, and participants as the program is implemented. Program staff need to take responsibility for addressing issues of health literacy by communicating with intention and clarity in order to ensure that the program message is received and acted on in a manner that is consistent with the program's goals and objectives. Simply stated, program staff need to make sure that participants are hearing the messages and information that the program wants them to hear and that the information is being understood.

Plans are formal or informal, but the important element is that a health promotion program has a consistent strategy for what information is communicated and how that communication will occur. Here are nine steps to follow in creating effective communication:

Step 1: Understand the Problem

The needs assessment discussed in Chapter 4 is the foundation for the communication plan. It provides a clear picture of the health problem or concern, the program's stakeholders and participants, and the program's priorities (National Cancer Institute, 2001). Likewise, the program's mission, goals, and interventions (see Chapter 5) provide a context and framework for developing materials and deciding what is to be communicated. The final part of this step is a review of existing materials and identification of any gaps in the type of media or communication activities used, *intended audiences* targeted, or messages conveyed. All of these factors are considered and included as part of the communication plan.

Step 2: Define Communication Objectives

Communication objectives define what the staff hope to articulate in a program's health communications. Defining the objectives assists with setting priorities. As Chapter 5 discusses, it is important to set objectives that are measurable and achievable. Table 8.4 provides some examples of well-written communication objectives. In many instances, it is unrealistic to expect a complete change as the result of one program. Objectives are

- Aligned with the program's goals
- Realistic and reasonable

Table 8.4 Sample Communication Objectives

- By the end of the stress management program, 90% of participants at this work site will have received stress reduction brochures and one-page tip sheets.
- After this campaign, 90% of the families with children younger than age 3 in Montgomery County will have received information on childhood immunization.
- By the end of the school year, two public service announcements on physical activity will be developed and viewed in at least three physical education classes at 10 different middle schools in the county.
- After attending a three-session course on self-management of diabetes, 75% of the participants will be able to report their daily blood sugar results via the website or app for the health promotion program.

- Specific to the change desired, the population to be affected, and the time period during which change occurs
- Measurable, in order to track progress
- Prioritized, to aid in allocation of resources (National Cancer Institute, 2001)

Step 3: Learn About the Intended Audiences

The audience may already be defined by the location of the health promotion program, or there are several audiences. The goal in this step is to learn as much as possible about the individuals who make up the target audience in order to tailor the program most effectively. Audience segmentation and formative research can help in this process.

Audience segmentation is the division of priority populations into subgroups that share similar qualities or characteristics (Thackeray & Brown, 2005). Populations are divided into segments according to multiple factors, including geography, demographics, psychographic traits (for example, attitudes, beliefs, self-efficacy), behaviors, and readiness to change (National Cancer Institute, 2001). The goal is to segment the intended population on characteristics that are relevant to the health behavior to be changed and to organize the program's efforts around these groups of similar individuals (National Cancer Institute, 2001; Slater, Kelly, & Thackeray, 2006). For example, the CDC's national tobacco campaign, *Tips From Former Smokers* (www.cdc.gov/tips), segments its audiences. The *Tips* campaign profiles real people who are living with serious long-term health effects from smoking and second-hand smoke exposure. The campaign provides information for general audiences but also provides information on how smoking and second-hand smoke affects specific groups, as well as smoking-related statistics, information, and quitting resources. The messages are tailored for specific audiences, including racial/ethnic minorities, members of the military and veterans, pregnant women, individuals with HIV, and lesbian, gay, bisexual, and transgender individuals.

The goal of *formative research* is to describe the intended audience: who they are, what is important to them, what influences their behavior, and what would enable them to engage in the desired behavior (Thackeray & Brown, 2005). Formative research can also be used to determine how ready the intended audience is to change; what social or cultural factors may affect the program; when and where the audience can best be reached; what communication channels are preferred by the audience; and what learning styles, language, and tone the intended audience prefers (National Cancer Institute, 2001).

Step 4: Select Communication Channels and Activities

To reach your program's intended audience, consider the settings, times, places, and states of mind in which they may be receptive to and able to act on the program's key message (National Cancer Institute, 2001). Then identify the *channels* (routes of message delivery) through which the program's message will be delivered and the activities that are used to deliver it (National Cancer Institute, 2001).

Choosing communication channels to use for your health promotion programs has never been more exciting. New forms of communication technologies are always being developed and health information is increasingly being shared across digital platforms. eHealth, the use of digital information and communication technologies to improve people's health and health care, surrounds people with health information to manage health. It has the potential to improve population health. There are numerous tools and resources that fall under eHealth.

The use of *social media* plays a significant role in health promotion. Tools like Facebook, Twitter, YouTube, and LinkedIn, for example, are used to effectively expand the reach of your health messages, foster engagement with your priority audience, and provide easy access to credible health information. Social media and other emerging communication technologies can connect millions of voices to:

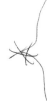

- Increase the timely dissemination and potential impact of health and safety information.
- Leverage audience networks to facilitation information sharing.
- Expand reach to include broader, more diverse audiences.
- Personalize and reinforce health messages to tailor and fit a particular audiences.

- Facilitate interactive communication, connection, and public engagement.
- Empower people to make safer and healthier decisions. (Centers for Disease Control and Prevention, 2011)

As you consider which channels of communication you want to use for your program, keep in mind that you may have to use a combination of channels to create awareness, encourage and motivate individuals, and change attitudes and behavior.

The following channel categories are considered:

Interpersonal channels are more likely to be trusted and put the message into a personal context. These channels include physicians and other health professionals, friends, family, and counselors. Examples of activities or methods for delivering the message within interpersonal channels are one-on-one counseling, telephone hotlines, informal discussions, and personal coaching and instruction. Interpersonal channels are the most effective for teaching and influential, but they are also time consuming and expensive to use and may have a limited reach.

Group channels can reach more of the intended audience while still retaining many of the positive aspects of interpersonal channels. Group channels include neighborhood groups, workplaces, churches, support groups, or clubs. The activities associated with these channels are classroom instructions, large and small group discussions, recreational and sporting events, and public meetings. As with communicating through interpersonal channels, working with groups requires significant levels of effort and may be time consuming and expensive.

Community channels involve working with community groups to conduct activities such as meetings, conferences, and other events to disseminate the program's message. Community channels can reach a large intended audience, may be familiar to the audience, may have influence with the audience, and can offer shared experiences. Community channels can also be time consuming to establish. Another negative aspect is the possibility of losing control of the message if it has to be adapted to fit organizational needs.

Mass media campaigns are a tried-and-true approach that has been used to spotlight many health promotion topics (National Cancer Institute, 2001). Mass media channels include but are not limited to newspapers, magazines, newsletters, radio, and television

(Glanz, Rimer, & Lewis, 2002). These channels offer many opportunities for dissemination of a program's message to individuals and communities.

Education entertainment (a form of health communication in which educational content and information is intentionally incorporated into an entertainment format) is another powerful way to engage an audience, and studies have demonstrated that exposure to health information and behaviors through entertainment media can have strong effects (National Cancer Institute, 2001).

Interactive media, eHealth tools, and social media are communication technologies that are used to reach multiple audiences. These technologies extend both the reach and depth of mass media (Glanz, Rimer, & Lewis, 2002). They include, but are not limited to, webinars, online courses, electronic bulletin boards, newsgroups, chat rooms, blogs, e-mail, text messages, Listservs, podcasts, online videos, and social networking sites (for example, Facebook and Twitter). The types of channels in this category are constantly changing and evolving. The technologies also allow outreach to large numbers of people, are quickly updated with new information, and can provide health information in a graphically appealing and exciting way. Table 8.5 details the Text4baby campaign's use of interactive media and eHealth. Disadvantages of interactive media include expense (for example, the cost of individual electronic devices, user fees such as monthly telephone

Table 8.5   Text4baby: An Example of the Use of Interactive Media/eHealth

Text4baby™ is a free text messaging program for pregnant women and new mothers with an infant up to one year of age, designed to improve maternal and child health (MCH) among underserved populations in the United States. It takes advantage of increasing cell phone ownership in the United States and the increasing popularity of text messaging. It is the first free national health text messaging service, made possible through an arrangement between The Wireless Foundation and most U.S. mobile operators. Text4baby provides evidence-based, critical health and safety information targeted to traditionally underserved pregnant women and new mothers who are in need of services but are often beyond the reach of the health care system.

Since the program's launch in February 2010, more than 830,000 people have ever signed up for Text4baby, however enrollment in the Text4baby program was lower than expected nationally. Regardless, the program had several important findings, including:
- Text4baby subscribers were significantly more likely than women who never heard of Text4baby to report receiving information on high-priority health topics during pregnancy.
- Text4baby subscribers exhibited a significantly higher level of health knowledge than the two other groups of prenatal care users.

Source: U.S. Department of Health and Human Services. Health Resources and Services Administration, 2015.

service charges), unsuitability if the intended audience lacks access to the Internet, and the fact that the intended audience must sign up or search for information on the program in order to receive the message.

Step 5: Develop Partnerships

Employing other organizations as partners is a useful and cost-effective method to broaden the reach of a program. Maibach, Van Duyn, and Bloodgood, (2006) explain that partners can serve as a "powerful and sustainable distribution channel." The foundation of the partnership approach is the value of collaboration between organizations that share common interests and reach diverse audiences in order to achieve outcomes that neither could achieve alone (Hasnain-Wynia, Margolina, & Bazzoli, 2001). Many organizations work with partners or intermediaries in order to reach their intended audience. In addition, partnerships can

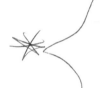

- Provide more credibility for a program's message because the partner organization might be considered a trusted source for the intended audience.

- Increase the number of messages the program can share with the intended audience.

- Provide additional resources.

- Expand support for an organization's high-priority activities. (National Cancer Institute, 2001)

Potential partner organizations are identified and included in the *health communication plan*. Determine the roles that potential partners might play in the program, and include this information as well. Roles might include promoting and disseminating messages and materials, sponsoring publicity and promotion, advertising the program, providing use of communication materials, or evaluating the program.

Step 6: Conduct Market Research to Refine Your Message and Materials

This step includes conducting market research and pretesting in order to determine the activities for each intended audience, messages for each market, and materials to be developed. The next section will go into greater detail on how to develop and test messages and materials.

Step 7: Implement the Communication Plan

In this step, communication activities are integrated into the overall implementation of the health promotion program. At this time, it is important to ensure that all materials and communications that program stakeholders and participants receive are consistent with their level of health literacy. Likewise, it is important that all channels of communication be accessible, supported, and utilized. For example, if cell phone technology such as text messaging is to be used, all program participants need to have a cell phone or access to a cell phone and know how to receive and send text messages.

Step 8: Review Tasks and Timeline

The timeline of the communication plan specifies what needs to be accomplished when. Detailing the tasks enables the work to be assigned and kept on schedule and allows resources to be allocated for each task. The timeline is reviewed and adjusted as the program progresses. The communication plan timeline are incorporated into the Gantt chart for the entire program.

Step 9: Evaluate the Plan

Evaluation of the communication plan is part of the evaluation of a health promotion program (see Chapter 10). Evaluation of a communication plan can focus on a number of issues—for example, utilization and penetration of the program communications (brochures, posters, activity materials, videos, and so on), satisfaction with the communications, or recommendations on how to improve the program materials and information. Table 8.6 provides an overview of communication plans for different sites, including their evaluation.

Developing and Pretesting Concepts, Messages, and Materials

In the preceding section, the steps in developing and implementing a communication plan were explained. The topic of this section is step 6 of the process: conducting market research in order to develop effective messages and materials.

Communicating effectively to an audience (for example, program participants) is a key factor in developing successful health promotion programs. In communicating with the program participants, it is essential

Table 8.6   Examples of the Process of Planning Health Communication in Various Settings

	School	Workplace	Health Care Organization	Community
Partners	Community youth development agencies. After-school programs. PTAs and PTOs. High school and middle school students. Feeder elementary schools.	Managerial staff. Human resources.	All health care providers and staff in clinic. Local grocery store chain. Glucose monitor company's local representative.	Pediatricians. Clinics that serve children. Local McDonald's franchises.
Development and implementation	Create a plan that includes activities across all three grade levels and feeder schools.	Create a staff advisory committee to develop a series of fact sheets and workshops for staff over a 12-month period.	Develop and deliver interactive workshops and webinars. Deliver workshops on a variety of days and times, and offer some in Spanish and Creole. Develop web content and blog posts. Develop eHealth materials including social media messages, e-mails, and text messages.	Work with local pediatrician association, and inform members of places where children can receive free or reduced-cost immunizations.
Evaluation	By the start of the third grading period: Posters developed, tested, and distributed at school and community sites. Two articles in PTA newsletter. Bullying information sheet distributed to 100% of students. Website and eHealth content developed.	By January 15: Stress reduction tip sheets available. Class brochures developed, tested, and distributed. Announcement template for lunch forum developed.	By March 1: Trilingual posters developed, tested, and distributed. Template for personalized invitation developed, tested, and used.	By the first day of school in fall: All materials (articles, ads, fact sheets, and tray covers) developed and tested. By Thanksgiving: All materials distributed in the fall months.

to know how the audience members view their health and what they are being asked to do (or not do). One way to understand different audiences and create programs, materials, and messages that resonate with them is to develop and pretest concepts, messages, and materials to see which ones have the most meaning for them and motivate them to take action.

What Is Pretesting?

Knowing which messages are most salient to the intended audience is one critical component of a successful intervention or program. *Pretesting* is used in developing new materials, revising existing materials, and developing messages and concepts. Pretesting materials and messages can assist in discovering how the audience members will respond to a message, whether they will read the materials and act appropriately, and how the messages will be received.

Why Pretest?

Before describing the steps in detail, it is important to understand why pretesting is important and to consider some challenges or resistant attitudes that might occur when one is advocating for pretesting (National Cancer Institute, 2001). Some may say that pretesting takes too much time and money. But it's just the opposite: if the materials or messages are not pretested, valuable time and financial resources will be wasted on materials or messages that do not resonate with the priority audience. Taking some extra time can actually save time and money in the end. Some say, "I know what a good brochure is and what a bad brochure is, so I do not need to pretest." Because most health promotion implementers are not a part of the priority audience, it is essential to pretest messages and materials to ensure that they will meet communication objectives when they are received by people in the intended audience who may have very different issues and concerns from members of the program staff. Another situation that may arise is that a supervisor might suggest using materials that have been used successfully elsewhere. Again, consider the intended audience. Are there similarities between this audience and the one the materials were created for? More than likely they are different, and because they are different, it is very important to pretest previously developed materials with members of the intended audience.

Pretesting Process

Pretesting is an iterative, data-driven process (Brown, Lindenberger, & Bryant, 2008). The health communication plan is used as a guide through the pretesting process. The purpose of the communication plan is to define the intended audience, the tone of the messages, and the types of materials that will be used. Use the communication plan to help you ensure that pretesting remains on strategy.

The basic iterative steps in pretesting are

1. Review existing materials.
2. Develop and test *message concepts.*
3. Decide what materials to develop.

4. Develop messages and materials.

5. Pretest messages and materials.

6. Revise the materials, then produce and distribute them. (National Cancer Institute, 2001)

Review Existing Materials

Developing materials may be costly and time consuming, so it is best to begin by reviewing all the materials that are currently available. There are many places to look for existing materials, including local and state health departments, professional and voluntary health associations, and federal agencies such as the Centers for Disease Control and Prevention and the National Institutes of Health. Materials produced by federal agencies are in the public domain and are free for anyone to use. To determine the relevance of materials, ask the following questions:

- Are the materials appropriate for the intended audience? Are they culturally appropriate?

- Are the messages consistent with the health communication plan?

- Will the materials meet the communication objectives? (National Cancer Institute, 2001)

When deciding whether to use existing materials, talk with those who developed the materials and determine what permissions would be required for their use or modification, whether they were evaluated for effectiveness, and how effective they were. The answers to these questions will aid in determining whether to use the materials as they are, revise them, or develop new materials.

Develop and Test Message Concepts

Concept development is the process of using the health communication plan (which is often part of the health program's marketing plan) and formative research to generate ideas that are tested and used in developing materials. Message concepts are messages in general form and are intended to present ideas to the audience. Message concepts are not the final messages.

Working with a Creative Team. In developing a concept, the opportunity to work with a creative team may arise. A creative team is a group of graphic artists and multimedia professionals (for example, videographers or filmmakers). The creative team may consist of external consultants, staff members internal to the organization that is creating the program, or both. The key to working with a creative team is making sure to stay on strategy as outlined in the health communication plan. When managing the creative team, it is important to keep in mind the following suggestions:

- Develop a good working relationship with the team, and determine the point person.

- Explain to the team the health communication strategy, including who the intended audience is and what they value.

- Talk about pretesting and how all concepts and materials must be pretested. Explain that you will assist with arranging access to the intended audience for pretesting.

- Ensure that the creative team understands the importance of developing culturally appropriate concepts and materials. (National Cancer Institute, 2001)

Concept Testing. Once several concepts have been developed, test these concepts with the intended audience to ensure that the message appeals to them, that they understand the message, and that they are willing to act on the message. Include the creative team in developing at least two message concepts, but three may be best. It is best to test concepts using a variety of data collection methods, for no one method is optimal (National Cancer Institute, 2001; Salazar, 2004). Focus groups, in-depth interviews, or one-on-one interviews are often used.

Prior to testing the concepts or materials, develop a list of questions for the intended audience. Although every project is different, ask questions that generally help determine the following:

- Comprehension of the behavioral recommendation or call to action

- The ability of the message or materials to attract attention

- The intended audience's ability to recognize the message as relevant

- Cultural appropriateness for the intended audience

- Believability

- Credibility

- Persuasiveness

- Usefulness

- General attractiveness

- Acceptability (Brown, Lindenberger, & Bryant, 2008)

Decide What Materials to Develop

After determining an effective message for the intended audience, begin to consider what format to use to present the message. Some of the decision about format may come from formative research in which audience members reveal which formats they are most likely to look at, read, or listen to. As we discussed earlier, materials are presented in many formats via interpersonal channels, organizational channels, community channels, mass media channels, or interactive channels.

 Develop Messages and Materials

The following guidelines will help ensure that program materials are understood, accepted, and used by the intended audience (National Cancer Institute, 2001).

- **Ensure that the message is accurate.** Make sure that the information provided is factual. It is always good to have the materials reviewed by experts on the topic.

- **Be consistent.** Consistency is critical to a program's success and, ultimately, to its identity. Make sure that the messages in all materials are consistent not only with the communication strategy but also with one another.

- **Be clear.** Keep the message simple and clear. Do not use a lot of technical terms. Make sure that the intended audience's tasks are clear and understandable.

- **Make sure that materials are relevant.** Talk about the program's benefits. The formative or consumer research will provide insight into what the intended audience values.

- **Ensure that materials are credible.** Again, use formative research to guide the decision about whom to use as a spokesperson.

- **Create appealing materials.** Ensure that materials are appealing and eye-catching, so they grab the attention of the intended audience.

 Pretest Messages and Materials

Much like pretesting concepts, it is necessary to pretest draft materials with the intended audience. Some people believe they can skip this step because they have tested the concept and have had professionals review the health content, so to expedite the process, they go from draft material to final production with no review or input from the intended audience. This is a big mistake because one never knows what detail in a finished piece might be problematic to the target audience. In the long run, this round of pretesting will save valuable time and money. Many health education professionals can recall a close call when they were about to skip this step but decided at the last minute to test with the intended audience and found out that they would have had a major flaw in the final material had they not tested the draft first. Testing draft materials is not a step to skip.

Revise and Produce the Materials

After revising the materials and testing them with the audience, send the materials to press and put them to use for the program. Eventually, you will find that developing a set of materials is only the beginning, because as the audience changes, the materials will need to change as well. Thus the process of testing the materials with the audience and making appropriate changes will begin again.

Using Pretesting to Its Fullest

Pretesting is one way to ensure that the intended audience will understand the materials developed and act on their message. It is important to remember that pretesting is not a popularity contest to see which message or type of material the intended audience members like the most or what color they like the best. It is determining what message or what material best fulfills the health marketing and communication plan. Testing at this stage permits you to identify flaws before spending money on final production. To test materials in draft form, use a facsimile version of a poster or pamphlet, a video version of a television PSA, or a prototype of text materials like a booklet. Test these materials with members of the intended audience to accomplish the following:

- **Assess comprehensibility**—Does the intended audience understand the message?

- **Identify strong and weak points**—What parts of the materials are doing their job best—for example, attract attention, inform, or motivate to act? What parts are not doing their job?

- **Determine personal relevance**—Does the intended audience identify with the materials?

- **Gauge confusing, sensitive, or controversial elements**—Does the treatment of particular topics make the intended audience uncomfortable?

Pretesting Example

Guard Your Health is a comprehensive health and wellness program that was established to serve as a central place online for Army National Guard Soldiers and family members to find information and resources on health and medical readiness. The program offers health tips, expert commentary,

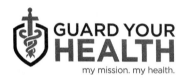
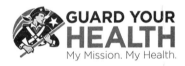
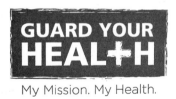
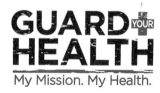

Figure 8.2 Four Test Concepts for a Health and Wellness Program

and community forums on topics such as nutrition, exercise, stress, sleep, dental health, readiness, and family resilience.

During focus groups and intercept interviews, logos for the program were pretested with soldiers, leadership, and administrative staff. They were asked to answer questions about the logos shown in Figure 8.2 and discussed questions such as:

- What colors do you like best?
- Which imagery do you like best?
- Which fonts do you like best?
- Which is your favorite and why?

The soldiers overwhelmingly preferred the "caduceus" and "Minute Man" logos. They felt the "Minute Man" logo was a representation of them and thought "the sword was cool." The bottom left logo was the least well received during testing because soldiers felt it was too feminine and plain. The "distressed" bottom right logo came in second to last. People liked the simplicity of it, but a majority of the younger soldiers did not like the distressed look. Ultimately, the logo with the caduceus was chosen as the symbol for the Guard Your Health program, and soldiers really liked the motto "My Mission. My Health" because it communicated that everyone is responsible for his or her own health, and they understood that maintaining their health is their personal responsibility.

Summary

What and how a health promotion program communicates with its participants and other stakeholders are critical to its success. Plain language is a strategy for developing health promotion resources and materials that are clear, attractive, and easy to understand. Considering the information needs of the program participants and how they prefer to give and receive as well as process health information enhances program effectiveness.

Having a communication plan strengthens a health promotion program. Developing and pretesting concepts, messages, and materials with the intended audience is a critical step in the communication process. Pretesting processes includes developing and testing concepts, deciding what types of materials need to be developed, testing the materials with the priority audience, revising them as necessary, and implementing them. Understanding the role that health communication plays in health promotion will help staff develop effective programs in any setting by understanding the audiences' needs and ensuring that information is provided in a meaningful and appropriate manner. Choosing appropriate communication channels for your audience is also a critical step to help reach people when, where, and how they want to receive health messages.

Health communication alone cannot change systemic problems related to health, such as poverty, environmental degradation, or lack of access to health care, but health communication as part of a health promotion program includes a systematic exploration of all the factors that contribute to health and the strategies that could be used to influence these factors. Well-designed health communications help individuals better understand their own needs so that they can take appropriate actions to maximize their health.

For Practice and Discussion

1. Visit a local market where you shop for food and health supplies (such as prescription drugs, toiletries, vitamins, and over-the-counter medications). Read the labels and instructions on both food and health items. Find an example of an item that uses plain English well to communicate how to prepare and use the item. What makes this a good example? Find an example of an item that communicates poorly about how to prepare and use the item. How can these instructions be improved?

2. You are implementing a new driver safety program to educate drivers about the dangers of texting while driving. You work with the state Bureau of Motor Vehicles and will implement the program in high schools in partnerships with driver education teachers. Describe the approach you will take and how you will develop a health communication plan.

3. Have you ever pretested a message or concept for a health promotion program? If so, describe how you did it. What was the message or concept? Who was the priority audience? How did you go about the pretesting process? What did you learn from the audience? What changes did you make?

4. How would a program's health communication plan differ for, on the one hand, a rural community of 5,000 people (including adults, children, and senior citizens) and, on the other hand, a large urban hospital with 1,500 employees working 7 days a week, 24 hours a day or a school district with 4,000 students in grades from kindergarten to 12th grade? How might the audience segments for each program differ?

5. A manufacturing company is implementing a program to promote physical activity among its 1,000 adult employees at a company site. Prepare a 50-word statement on the importance of physical activity for adults, using plain language.

6. You are working at a student health center at a large university and have been asked to develop and implement a new campaign to promote greater awareness about safer sex habits and STD/HIV prevention, and encourage students to visit the health center to get tested. Describe the communication channels you would choose to reach students and why you chose them.

KEY TERMS

Audience segmentation

Channels

Communication objectives

Concept development

Education entertainment

eHealth

Formative research (or consumer research)

Health communication

Health communication plan

Health literacy

Intended audience

Message concepts

Plain language

Pretesting

Social media

References

Berkman, N. D., DeWalt, D. A., Pignone, M. P., Sheridan, S. L., Lohr, K. N., Lux, L. . . . Bonito, A. J. (2004). *Literacy and health outcomes* (Evidence Report/Technology Assessment No. 87; AHRQ Publication No. 04-E007-2). Rockville, MD: Agency for Healthcare Research and Quality.

Brown, K. M., Lindenberger, J. H., & Bryant, C. A. (2008). Using pretesting to ensure messages and materials are on strategy. *Health Promotion Practice, 9*(2), 116–122.

Centers for Disease Control and Prevention. (2011). *The health communicator's social media toolkit.* Retrieved from http://www.cdc.gov/socialmedia/Tools/guidelines/pdf/SocialMediaToolkit_BM.pdf

Glanz, K., Rimer, B. K., & Lewis, F. M. (Eds.). (2002). *Health behavior and health education: Theory, research, and practice* (3rd ed.). San Francisco, CA: Jossey-Bass.

Hasnain-Wynia, R., Margolina, F. S., & Bazzoli, G. J. (2001). Models for community health partnerships. *Health Forum Journal, 44,* 29–33.

Kirsch, I., Jungeblut, A., Jenkins, L., & Kolstad, A. (1993). *Adult literacy in America: A first look at the National Adult Literacy Survey.* Retrieved from http://nces.ed.gov/pubs93/93275.pdf

Kutner, M., Greenberg, E., Jin, Y., & Paulsen, C. (2006). *The health literacy of America's adults: Results from the 2003 National Assessment of Adult Literacy* (NCES 2006-483). Washington, DC: U.S. Department of Education, National Center for Education Statistics.

Maibach, E. W., Van Duyn, M. A. S., & Bloodgood, B. (2006). A marketing perspective on disseminating evidence-based approaches to disease prevention and health promotion. *Preventing Chronic Disease* [serial online]. Retrieved from http://www.cdc.gov/pcd/issues/2006

National Cancer Institute. (2001). *Making health communications programs work* (NIH Publication No. 02-5145). Retrieved from www.cancer.gov/pinkbook

National Eye Institute. (2015). *Protect your vision from diabetes infographic.* Retrieved from https://nei.nih.gov/nehep/ndm_infocards

Nielsen-Bohlman, L., Panzer, A. M., & Kindig, D. A. (Eds.). (2004). *Health literacy: A prescription to end confusion.* Washington, DC: National Academies Press.

Parker, R. M., Ratzan, S. C., & Lurie, N. (2003). Health literacy: A policy challenge for advancing high-quality health care. *Health Affairs, 22*(4), 147–153.

Pew Research Center. (2015). *Health fact sheet.* Retrieved from http://www.pewinternet.org/fact-sheets/health-fact-sheet/

Rothman, R. L., DeWalt, D. A., Malone, R., Bryant, B., Shintani, A., Crigler, B. . . . Pignone, M. (2004). Influence of patient literacy on the effectiveness of a primary care-based diabetes disease management program. *Journal of the American Medical Association, 292*(14), 1711–1716.

Salazar, B. P. (2004). Practical applications of pretesting health education concepts and materials. *Health Education Monograph Series, 21*(1), 6–12.

Schiavo, R. (2007). *Health communication: From theory to practice.* San Francisco, CA: Jossey-Bass.

Slater, M. D., Kelly, K. J., & Thackeray, R. (2006). Segmentation on a shoestring: Health audience segmentation in limited-budget and local social marketing interventions. *Health Promotion Practice, 7,* 170–173.

Thackeray, R., & Brown, K. M. (2005). Social marketing's unique contributions to health promotion practice. *Health Promotion Practice, 6*(4), 365–368.

U.S. Department of Health and Human Services. (2000). *Healthy People 2010: Understanding and improving health.* Washington, DC: U.S. Government Printing Office.

U.S. Department of Health and Human Services, Health Resources and Services Administration. (2015). *Promoting maternal and child health through health text messaging: An evaluation of the Text4baby program—Final report.* Rockville, MD: Author.

U.S. Department of Health and Human Services, Office of Disease Prevention and Health Promotion. (2015). *Consumer and patient eHealth.* Retrieved from http://www.health.gov/communication/ehealth/

U.S. Department of Health and Human Services, Steps to a Healthier US. (2004). *Prevention: A blueprint for action.* Retrieved from http://aspe.hhs.gov/health/blueprint/blueprint.pdf

West, L., Cole, S., Goodkind, D. & He, W. (2014). *65+ in the United States: 2010 (U.S. Census Bureau, Current Population Reports).* Washington, DC: U.S. Government Printing Office. Retrieved from https://www.census.gov/content/dam/Census/library/publications/2014/demo/p23-212.pdf

Zarcadoolas, C., Pleasant, A., & Greer, D. S. (2003). Elaborating a definition of health literacy: A commentary. *Journal of Health Communication, 8,* 119–120.

CHAPTER 9

WHERE MONEY MEETS MISSION: DEVELOPING AND INCREASING PROGRAM FUNDING

Carl I. Fertman, Karen A. Spiller, and Angela D. Mickalide

Knowing Program Funding

Even if program staff have no interest in or expectation of being involved with the financial aspects of health promotion programs, it is still critical for staff to understand how their decisions affect and are affected by a program's fiscal condition. Therefore, it is extremely important for any individual aspiring to work or working in a health promotion program and organization to know where and how programs get money to operate. Money is also a thread that runs through all of the phases of planning, implementing, and evaluating a health promotion program.

The goal for health promotion professionals is to be able to financially protect, develop, and increase their programs' funding from economic ups and downs and strategically grow and innovate when they're ready. They need to be able to customize their strategies to meet a variety of financial needs, from providing short crash courses in finance essentials to working with organizations very deeply, over many years. Financial awareness is a major portion of running any health promotion program.

Americans spend about $1.65 trillion a year on health care (including health promotion programs). That amount represents 15% of the gross domestic product, the total output of goods and services in the United States. Health care expenses consume one-fourth of the federal budget—more than defense. Americans spend large amounts of money on their health. On the one hand, there is a lot of money involved in and available to health

LEARNING OBJECTIVES

- Compare and contrast funding sources in terms of scope, population, and setting.

- Compare the perspectives of funder staff and program staff on what matters in a program proposal.

- Discuss the factors that motivate funders and how knowing these factors can foster relationships.

- Describe opportunities for health promotion specialists to engage in professional fundraising.

- Identify the challenges and benefits of working with agency volunteers on fiscal management and development activities.

promotion programs as part of the health care industry. On the other hand, there is tremendous competition for the money that is available. Although the general financial condition of health promotion programs is good and improving, serious challenges face individuals who are responsible for the money aspects of programs. And even if staff members are not now responsible for finding the money, they may be someday. It appears that the financial challenges facing health promotion program directors and staffs are universal, cutting across all settings and program types. No matter the setting, the staff (and their programs) most likely to succeed will have some knowledge and expertise in financial management. This observation holds regardless of the size of the programs; it is true for the largest national (and international) programs as well as for programs operating on a shoestring with a few dedicated individuals who donate their time at no cost.

Sources of Program Funding

A program's setting determines what its funding options are. Listed here are 10 sources of money for health promotion programs. Another term for funding money is *revenue*. Typically, a health promotion program receives money and support from a number of the sources in the following list. Likewise, over the phases of planning, implementing, and evaluating a program, funding from different sources will be sought and used. Therefore it is important to explore all available funding options when planning and implementing a health promotion program. Likewise it is important to not only explore but actively pursue a variety of funding sources since economic and political changes occur all of the time. To keep pace with the changes and continue to find funding requires agility and ongoing efforts (relationships) with funding sources.

1. **Public funds** are tax dollars collected and spent by the government to provide the infrastructure for the systems and organizations that operate state and local health and human services. At the federal level, the main organization that coordinates health services is the U.S. Department of Health and Human Services, which includes the National Institutes of Health and the Centers for Disease Control and Prevention. At state and local levels, services and programs use public funds to provide needed services and address health concerns of the local citizenry (National Institutes of Health, 2015). Schools and many hospitals receive public funds to finance their day-to-day operating costs. For example, many schools get money from property taxes as well as tax dollars from their state. A school health promotion program might have its staff (for example, school nurse and health

education teacher) paid for from the public funds while materials and supplies might be from a different source.

2. **Grants** are sums of money awarded to finance a particular activity or program. Generally, these grant awards do not need to be paid back. Federal agencies and other organizations sponsor grant programs for various reasons. Before developing a grant proposal, it is vitally important to understand the goals of the particular federal agency or private organization as well as the goals of the grant program itself (Texas Education Agency, 1999). An understanding of the goals of a grant program are gained through discussions with the person listed as an information contact in each grant description. Through these discussions, a potential applicant may find that in order for a particular project to meet the criteria of the grant program and be eligible for funding, the original project concept would need to be modified. In allocating funds, grantmakers base their decisions on the applying organizations' ability to fit their proposed activities within the grantmakers' interest areas.

3. **Foundations** are entities that are established as nonprofit corporations or charitable trusts with a principal purpose of making grants to unrelated organizations or institutions or to individuals for scientific, educational, cultural, religious, or other charitable purposes. This broad definition encompasses two foundation types: private foundations and public foundations. The most common distinguishing characteristic of a private foundation is that most of its funds come from one source, whether an individual, a family, or a corporation. A public foundation, in contrast, normally receives its assets from multiple sources, which may include private foundations, individuals, government agencies, and fees for service. Moreover, a public foundation must continue to seek money from diverse sources in order to retain its public status.

4. **Client fees** (also known as *fees for services*) are the prices that individuals pay to receive or participate in a service. Often, services are offered at no cost to the recipient because the organization collects revenue from other sources to cover the costs of offering the service or program. Increasingly, however, individuals are being asked to pay some fee for their participation. Public and nonprofit organizations with client fees usually have policies that regulate the fee amounts as well as safeguards to ensure that fees are not a barrier to receiving services.

5. **Matching funds, cost sharing, and in-kind contributions** all refer to monies and resources that are provided by another organization.

Matching funds are monies paid concurrently during the expenditure of an organization's funds for the operation of a program. In cost sharing, monies from another organization have to be spent by the time the program concludes. In-kind contributions are noncash contributions (for example, materials, equipment, vehicles, or food) that are used to operate programs or services.

6. **Collaboration and cooperative agreement** may not directly involve money but rather access and use of resources that are critical to a health promotion program's service delivery and that ultimately save the program's money through not having to duplicate the services of another organization. Collaborations and cooperative agreements are formalized with a document (letter of agreement) detailing the resources, staff, and materials each organization will use in program implementation. Typically, this letter will be signed by each organization's director and will have a stated time frame (for example, 6 months or 1 year). Each organization keeps a copy. Often copies of letters of agreement are provided to funders as part of applications for grants and support. In developing agreements, organizations use their complementary strengths and resources to address a health need that otherwise might go unmet.

7. **Infrastructure (operating, core, or hard) funding** are monies that an organization obtains in order to operate its infrastructure before offering any program, activities, or services. Such monies might pay for the director's salary, staff salaries, rent, janitorial services, clerical staff, or bookkeeping and payroll operations. Some schools and colleges have endowments (funding with specific instructions and criteria for how the money is spent) that are used for the infrastructure costs of health promotion programs that target particular groups of students.

8. **Fundraising** is the process of soliciting and gathering money or in-kind gifts by requesting donations from individuals, businesses, charitable foundations, or government agencies. In the United States in 2014 total giving through fundraising was $358.38 billion (Lilly Family School of Philanthropy, 2015). Some organizations have dedicated fundraising staff. Many organizations rely on their local United Way to raise funds for them. The United Way, a national network of more than 1,300 locally governed organizations, is the nation's largest community-based fundraiser. Local United Way organizations engage their community in order to identify the underlying causes of the most significant local issues, develop strategies and pull together financial and human resources to address them, and measure the results.

In 2013—2014, the United Way system raised $4.1 billion, continuing its status as the nation's largest private charity. U.S. tax laws encourage private citizens to make tax-deductible contributions and donations to tax-exempt organizations (for example, human service, health care, faith-based, and arts organizations) (Forbes, 2015).

9. **Volunteers** are individuals who serve an organization or cause. By definition, a volunteer does not get paid or receive compensation for services rendered. In health promotion programs, volunteers perform many tasks from direct service delivery to service on boards of directors or as program advocates. Popular in many schools are service-learning programs, in which students volunteer in community health organizations as part of their course work. Volunteers provide countless hours of services in health promotion programs through community health organizations.

10. **Health insurance** is a growing source of money for health promotion programs. The majority of Americans have *health insurance* through their employer or the employer of a family member. Government-subsidized or government-provided health care insurance includes Medicare for the elderly or disabled, Medicaid for the disadvantaged, CHAMPUS for military dependents, and medically indigent adult (MIA) programs for the indigent poor at the county level. In addition, in many communities, there are private free clinics that are unaffiliated with any insurance company, plan, or government entity. Key to health insurance being a source of money is that the Affordable Care Act (ACA) established as part of health insurance products the Essential Health Benefit (EHB) package. The ACA directs that the EHB cover at least the following 10 general categories: ambulatory patient services; emergency services; hospitalization; maternity and newborn care; mental health and substance use disorder services, including behavioral health treatment; prescription drugs; rehabilitative and habilitative services and devices; laboratory services; preventive and health promotion services and chronic disease management; and pediatric services, including oral and vision care. Money for health promotion programs from health insurance companies is allotted as part of the revenues generated through the health insurance premiums paid by individuals (and employers). A second source of money from health insurance companies for programs is through reimbursements for professionals who provide health promotion programs, for example, health education specialist, diabetes educators, psychologists, nutritionists, and social workers (Chambliss, Lineberry, Evans, & Bibeau, 2014; Goodman, et al., 2013).

Funding Varies by Program Participants and Setting

At any specific site or in a particular setting, how the money needed to operate a health promotion program gets to the program varies. Table 9.1 shows funding sources for programs that address specific populations in particular settings. The funding for programs at each site shown in Table 9.1 is discussed in this section.

Health promotion programs for adults at workplaces, including small and large businesses, health care organizations, and schools, are increasingly provided as part of their health insurance employee benefits packages. These are negotiated between the insurance company and the organization (for example, a business, school, or hospital). Many people don't realize that health insurance is issued differently for different types of employers and that because insurance is regulated at the state level of government, the laws in regard to health insurance offered by the different types of employers can vary significantly from state to state. Millions of Americans work for small employers, which, for health insurance purposes, are generally those with 50 employees or fewer. Millions of other Americans get their health insurance coverage through large employers. Generally, those are businesses with more than 50 employees. Increasingly, as part of a health insurance benefit, employees at workplaces are offered the opportunity to participate in health promotion programs. The range of health interventions

Table 9.1 Primary Funding Sources for Health Promotion Programs, by Program Participants and Setting

	Program Participants and Setting		
Funding Sources	**Adults at Workplaces (for example, small and large businesses, health care organizations, schools)**	**Children, Teenagers, and Young Adults Attending School and College (K–16)**	**Adults, Children, and Teenagers in Community Settings (for example, preschools, senior centers, recreation centers)**
Public funds		XX	XX
Grants		XX	XX
Foundations		XX	XX
Client fees (fees for services)	XX		XX
Matching funds, cost sharing, and in-kind contributions	XX	XX	XX
Collaboration and cooperative agreement	XX	XX	XX
Infrastructure (operating, core, or hard) funding	XX	XX	XX
Fundraising		XX	XX
Volunteers		XX	XX
Health insurance	XX		

varies according to costs and employee needs. Frequently employers provide in-kind support such as access to classrooms, computers, and organizational e-mail lists in order to circulate program announcements. At some sites, employees pay a small fee for individual program sessions or classes (for example, $5 per session for a 12-session nutrition class held during lunch hour).

Funding for health promotion programs at schools for children, teenagers, and young adults (K–16) have a number of sources (Table 9.1). Schools summarize the different funding sources (or streams) in a single public document called the *school budget*. School districts are required by law to adopt a balanced budget each year. Each state has a legally man-dated school budget cycle (timeline) with legal deadlines, education code requirements, and a budgeting process that districts follow. A district's budget is a record of past decisions and a spending plan for its future. It shows a district's priorities, whether they have been clearly articulated or simply occurred by default. And a district budget is a document that can communicate a lot about the district's priorities and goals to its constituents.

A school district's budget is difficult to understand and even more challenging to describe. Districts have volumes of mandatory reporting forms, accounting procedures, and jargon. School district officials must use responsible fiscal management, make inevitable adjustments to their budget, and comply with the oversight procedures that the states put into place to ensure that districts remain solvent and maintain their financial health. A health promotion program's funding in a school district is found in the district budget. School principals, program directors, and district budget directors are some of the people who are involved in preparing and administering the school budget.

A health promotion program that works in the community and focuses on the community members involves a number of funding sources. Local health departments, which run some community programs, are funded by public dollars. However, many local health departments will use a mix of funding sources to operate a particular program of local interest and need (for example, programs on pregnancy prevention or smoking cessation). Sometimes state or local governments will receive public funds to operate programs mandated by law that have to operate in every community (for example, child protection or breakfast and lunchtime food programs). Many community health promotion programs are operated by community health organizations. Typically, the organization's president, executive director, or program director is responsible for finding the money to operate a program. Community organizations rely on grants, fundraising, service contracts, and health insurance. In both small and large organizations, members of the organization's board of directors (a group of individuals who oversee an organization's operation and mission) might also be involved. Finally, at large organizations there probably are dedicated staff people whose full-time job is to raise money. They have jobs with titles such as director of development, grant writer, special activities and events director, and fundraiser.

Writing a Grant Proposal

An important part of getting funding for a health promotion program is sending a grant proposal to a funder. Typically, this occurs in one of two ways: (1) an organization has a great idea for a new program and sends a proposal to a funder in order to pay for it, or (2) a request for a proposal or grant notice has been made available and an organization tries to adapt an existing idea to fit the funder's program. Another reason that organizations write grant proposals is simply to fund the operation of an organization. Whether one is trying to fund programs or operations, the ability to win grants through proposal writing is critical.

Grant funding is highly competitive. Typically, the proposals are reviewed by the staff of the organization requesting the proposals, experts in the particular program area, and representatives of individuals who might be served by the grant being offered. Proposals are rated and scored according to predetermined criteria.

Even though there are many types of grants available across many different fields, grant seekers all follow a basic process and standards that remain constant across every professional area. Further, many organizations require applications to be submitted online and thus require a certain level of technological skill. To help grant seekers, many organizations, especially national foundations, offer online tutorials for writing a proposal that will fit with their specific goals and objectives in awarding grants. Regardless of the funder, grant seekers must understand how to find funding sources and opportunities, write the grant proposal, deal with the technological aspects of submitting a proposal, and attend to the funder's needs. It is best to embrace the idea that applying for grants involves following a prescribed formula.

Finding Funding Sources and Opportunities

Finding funding sources and opportunities requires these steps:

1. Clarify the purpose of the health promotion program and write a concise statement (that is, a mission statement). Define the scope of work in order to focus the funding search. Identify exactly what items you are seeking funds for.

2. Identify the right funding sources. Do not limit your search to one resource. Foundation centers, computerized databases, publications, and public libraries are some of the resources available for you to use in a funding search (Foundation Center, 2016). Look at the federal government's website on grants (http://www.grants.gov) as well as the *Federal Register* (http://www.gpoaccess.gov/fr). The *Federal Register* is the official daily publication where the rules, proposed rules, and notices of federal agencies and organizations appear. The *Federal Register* also includes the announcements of new federal grants, many of which are health focused. The goal is to find groups that are interested in the health problem addressed by your health promotion program.

3. Contact the funders. Think of the funder as a resource and a friend who wants to help, if there is mutual interest. Some funders offer technical assistance; others do not. Ask for technical assistance, including a review of proposal drafts. Try to talk with a staff member about what is currently being funded by the group. Ask for an annual report. Ask for names of organizations that have previously been funded. Talk with people from those organizations.

4. Acquire proposal guidelines. Read the guidelines carefully, and then read them again. Ask the funder to clarify any questions that you have about the guidelines. Pay attention to the technical details (for example, page length, font size, number of copies, instructions for electronic and hard-copy submissions).

5. Know the submission deadline. Plan to submit the proposal on or preferably before the deadline. Be realistic about whether you have the time to prepare a competitive proposal that meets the deadline.

6. Determine personnel needs. Identify required personnel both by function and, if possible, by name. Contact project consultants, trainers, and other personnel to inquire about their availability; acquire permission to include them in the project; and negotiate compensation. Will staff actually be available to implement the program if it is funded?

7. Assess the feasibility of writing and submitting the proposal, of winning funding, and of fully implementing the program if it is funded. Writing proposals is hard work and takes time. There are a lot of unknowns, but going through these steps will help program staff to make an informed decision about which funding opportunities to pursue.

Writing Process

The time frame for writing a grant proposal varies. For federal grants, it can take 3 to 6 months to write a grant proposal, and another year or so from the time it is sent until it might get funded. Local community foundations and United Way might announce funding opportunities and proposal guidelines at the beginning of a month with a due date for a finished proposal 1 month later and may expect that funded programs will be implemented 1 or 2 months after that.

Before writing the grant proposal, form an internal working committee. Key stakeholders and individuals (often members of the advisory board discussed in Chapter 1) who will be involved with the funded project are included on the working committee. Next, consider asking objective and experienced individuals who have worked in the particular health area or with the funding organization to share their experiences and recommendations about what would be of interest to the funder. After consulting with these individuals and creating an outline of the agreed-on project details, the committee can draft a short description of the specific aims of the program. Using this strategy will make composition of the proposal easier. And although one or two people may be responsible for writing the proposal, the committee can provide feedback throughout the writing process.

As in any writing assignment, it is important to consider the audience that one is writing for. In grant applications, it is often best to use a balance of technical and nontechnical writing because the reviewers at the grant-making organization may not be familiar with the terminology used in your field. Further, most reviewers will just scan your application, and they may not be familiar with theories and methods used in your field. For these reasons, consider separating technical and nontechnical information in the parts of the application that reviewers will most likely read—the abstract, significance, and specific aims. More detailed information can be included when you are explaining program interventions. Some grant-writing specialists suggest that proposal writers begin each paragraph simply and then progress to more complex information or that writers alternate paragraphs that have less and more technical information (National Institutes of Health, National Institute of Diabetes and Digestive and Kidney Diseases, n.d.). Ultimately, as the grant writer, it is your decision as to how to include both broader, less technical descriptions and more technical information in a proposal. Keeping your audience in mind will help you decide which writing strategies to use.

If the staff of the health promotion program do not have the writing skills to create a structured, concise, and persuasive application with attention to specifications and a reasonable budget, consider asking for help from experienced grant writers. Some schools, hospitals, and community health organizations hire outside contractors as writers or editors. Whoever writes

Table 9.2   Overview of a Grant Proposal

Component	Description	Number of Pages
Executive summary	Umbrella statement of your case and summary of the entire proposal	1 page
Statement of need	Why the project is necessary	2 pages
Project description	Nuts and bolts of how the project will be implemented and evaluated	3 pages
Budget	Financial description of the project plus explanatory notes	1 page
Information on organization	Organization history and governing structure; its primary activities, audiences, and services	1 page
Conclusion	Summary of the proposal's main points	2 paragraphs

the application must first read the guidelines to learn the specifications, what information is required, and how it needs to be arranged. Standard proposal components are the narrative, budget, appendix of support material, and authorized signature. Sometimes proposal applications require abstracts or summaries, an explanation of budget items, and certifications. Table 9.2 shows a grant proposal's potential components with suggested pages for each component. However the number of pages vary by funder.

First, the executive summary is a brief description of the proposed project. The executive summary is a clear, concise statement of what problem is being addressed, why it needs to be addressed, how it will be addressed, and what will be changed as a result of the program.

Second, the statement of need focuses on the project's purpose, goals, and measurable objectives, and it provides a compelling, logical reason why the proposal is supported). The needs statement gives the project's background, providing a perspective on the conception of the project.

The project description needs to be concise and informative, and it needs to provide a hook for the reviewers in order to stir their interest and draw their attention to what makes your application unique. Make sure that the proposed program is aligned with the purpose and goals of the funding source. Describe your proposed interventions (methods and processes for accomplishing goals and objectives) and activities, the intended scope of work and expected outcomes, and required personnel functions, including the names of key staff members and consultants. Because the reviewers will probably read many similar proposals, a tailored and attention-getting description of the program will interest the funder. In addition, including a method of evaluation with intended outcomes and expectations will appeal to a funder's need for accountability. Prepare a logic model and a Gantt chart to illustrate the project flow, including start and end dates, a schedule of activities, and projected outcomes.

→ The budget portion of the application is a cost projection of how the project will be implemented and managed. Well-planned budgets reflect carefully thought-out projects. Be sure to include only the things the funder is willing to support. Many funders provide mandatory budget forms that must be submitted with the proposal. Don't forget to list in-kind and matching revenue, where appropriate. Overall, it is important to be flexible about a budget in case the funder chooses to negotiate costs.

→ The conclusion is a succinct, crisp restatement of the program purpose, objective, interventions, and evaluation. Conclusions are read by grant reviewers and is always written with these reviewers in mind. The program timeline and requested funding are not typically be included in the conclusion. The conclusion emphasizes the program's impact on the life quality of the priority population. It is one final opportunity to clearly articulate your program and make a pitch for its funding.

In general, follow all instructions in order to minimize the risk of having a proposal returned because it exceeded the page limits or used too small a font. Look for the page and word limits in the grant proposal guide. Make it easy for the reviewers to find material by using strong headings, graphics, and tables. Graphical representations of timetables for experiments can effectively illustrate their flow and time frame. These basic techniques will help keep writing streamlined and well organized so that reviewers can readily glean the information that interests them. In addition, be sure to cite the appropriate references throughout the proposal.

Technological Process

Submitting a grant proposal involves a potentially large number of technical requirements. At one time, the technical aspects of submitting a grant proposal involved the number of pages and number of copies to submit to the funder. However, with increased use of technology (particularly computers and the Internet), submitting grant proposals has become more challenging. It is now common to submit proposals online through sites that require organizational or individual registration and passwords. The sites may require populating (completing) an online form and uploading files and materials in certain formats and with size restrictions. Although graphics, charts, and other visual elements break the monotony of text and can help reviewers grasp a lot of information quickly, they may be difficult to format with word processing software and they may not remain stable across different hardware and software platforms.

Help for technological problems encountered during the submission process may be limited. Typically, funders do not see technical problems as a reason for accepting proposals after the due date for grant submission.

Clearly, technology can make the grant-writing and submission process easier. However, technology can also add barriers to the already time-consuming endeavor of writing a grant, requiring a concentrated effort, commitment, and persistence on the part of grant seekers and grant writers. Thus the commitment of time and resources for writing a grant proposal might need to include some provision for technical training or outside support in order to compose and submit the application.

Meeting the Funder's Needs

Once the first draft of a grant proposal is complete, sharpen the focus of the proposal. Reviewers will quickly pick up on how well the proposal matches the grant requirements. Remember that a proposal has two audiences: some reviewers who are not familiar with health promotion programs and interventions and some who have field experience of health promotion programs and thus have that sort of program knowledge.

Remember the following points:

- All reviewers are important because each reviewer typically gets one vote.

- Typically, there is a primary reviewer (or perhaps more than one) who is knowledgeable about health promotion programs; write to win over that reviewer.

- Write and organize your proposal so that the primary reviewer can readily grasp and explain what is being proposed.

Ultimately, a grant-making organization has the breadth and depth of knowledge, experience, and wisdom to understand and judge a large range of grant applications. Even if a funding organization is not familiar with all the techniques proposed in a grant, its reviewers can and will judge how well a proposal clearly communicates the desire for funding and the need for it. Finally, the following is a list of common reasons cited by reviewers of grant proposals for not approving them:

- Problem not important enough

- Program not likely to produce useful information or address health problem

- Program not based on health theory or evidence, and alternative not considered

- Health promotion interventions unsuited to the objective

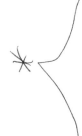

- Proposal addresses a health problem other than the one asked for in the funding announcement

- Technical problems (for example, exceeds page limitations, uses incorrect budget, lacks required information on organization, or lacks endorsement letters from partners)

- Problem more complex than program staff appear to realize

- Lack of focus in program's mission statement, intervention, and evaluation

- Lack of original or new ideas

- Proposed program not appropriate to address the proposed questions

Maintaining Relationships with Funders

All the elements of a personal relationship are present in the relationship between an organization that operates a health promotion program and an organization that funds the program. Expected as part of the relationship are trust, honesty, timeliness, and accountability, as well as transparency in the program's operation and delivery and provision of high-quality services and materials that achieve the program's goals and objectives.

Specific strategies for maintaining a good relationship with a funder include the following:

- Schedule an initial meeting in order to gather information from the potential funder as well as to share information about your organization. Meeting preparation is critical. Prepare a concise, clear document that outlines your program's scope, responsibilities, timeline, and budget. In the meeting, work to establish mutually agreed-on measures of program success right from the beginning. Find out about current programs that are being funded and how program achievements are evaluated. Find out about the stakeholders of the funding organization, including its board members.

- Engage in a frank discussion about funder attributions and recognitions for the health promotion program, and document decisions in writing. For example, would the funder like to have its logo on every brochure, poster, checklist, and webpage related to the program? How will the funder's support be acknowledged in media interviews (for example, "Through our partnership with the Green Foundation, the health department has provided free bike helmets to children in our community."). Are reciprocal links established between the websites of the funder and the health promotion program? Some funders seek constant and highly visible recognition, while others prefer to remain anonymous. To avoid missteps, it is important for health program staff to elicit these funder preferences prior to printing brochures, speaking with the media, or posting content and logos on the program's website.

- If the funder agrees, seek opportunities to leverage its contribution to attract additional funding and funders. Using this strategy can help you expand your health promotion program in several ways—by creating new materials, making additional presentations, achieving greater audience diversity, and penetrating different channels of communication. Some funders may wish to be listed as the founding funder, particularly if their initial contribution launched an organization or major program initiative. The founding funder may permit others to join the donor list, particularly if their brands do not compete. (For example, Nike and Adidas are competing brands, and so are Target and Walmart.) Others may want an exclusive partnership, which the longevity of the partnership and dollar amount contributed may warrant. Remember that loyalty is a two-way street, so it's important to discuss emerging funding opportunities with current funders to ensure that there are no actual or perceived conflicts of interest.

- Keep excellent financial records so that your organization can track income and expenses easily, quickly, and accurately. These records are both computerized and on hard copy in case of technological glitches or natural disasters. Retain this documentation for at least 3 years in order to respond to auditors' requests. Work closely with the finance and administration staff responsible for monitoring the health promotion program's budget to ensure that all reporting requirements are being met. If there are anticipated cost overruns or unexpended funds, communicate these details immediately to the funder and the organization's finance and administration staff so that any necessary adjustments are made prior to the end of the grant cycle.

- Find a champion within the foundation, corporation, or other funding source. Ideally, this individual's role is to institutionalize your health promotion program within the funding organization in order to guarantee its continued support. Examples of helpful actions of a champion include ensuring that senior management is apprised of the health promotion program's achievements, influencing the public relations department to highlight the partnership in media interviews and its annual report, and establishing a cause-related marketing effort with the advertising department, if relevant. Health promotion program staff strive to regularly equip this champion with the necessary tools (for example, the latest educational materials or evaluation reports) to help him or her manage internal relations pertaining to the partnership. In this way, if the champion leaves the funding organization, there will be others there who can adopt a leadership and advocacy role on the grantee's behalf.

 Be willing to admit to the funder when a mistake is made or plans go awry, whether it be an unrealistic timeline, a budgetary miscalculation, a difficulty with program implementation, or neutral or negative results from a program evaluation. The funder might suggest solutions that the program staff have not considered and is willing to invest more resources to rectify the shortcomings. After all, the funder has already made an investment in the health promotion program and is reluctant to see it fail. While no funder wants to throw good money after bad, few funders are willing to lose their entire investment. Honest and frequent communication is the key to winning partnerships.

Fundraising

For health promotion programs operated by a small or large nonprofit organization, another resource that may be available to help with program funding is development staff (sometimes called *development officers*). These individuals have job titles such as fundraising coordinator, development director, or resource developer, and their job is to seek out and manage fundraising efforts for the organization. Development staff responsibilities can include but are not limited to writing grant proposals, researching foundation and corporation requests for proposals, and overseeing or implementing other fundraising strategies. They may work mostly behind the scenes, establishing a structure for effective fundraising.

Development staff are a benefit for health promotion programs. They can provide access to support and resources that might not otherwise be available to programs, due to programs' primary need to focus on implementation. Likewise, health promotion programs are often sought out by development staff, since the programs' focus on improving individuals' quality of life is attractive to funders. Furthermore, development officers like to showcase the impact of an organization's programs on the individuals and groups it serves. Health promotion programs are typically open to visitors, and their work is easily understood by individuals who may not have technical health background or exposure to health programs. Organizations use a variety of fundraising strategies:

Annual giving. An annual giving program is any organization's yearly drive to raise financial support for its ongoing operating needs. Annual giving is about donor acquisition, repeating the gift, and upgrading the gift. Annual giving creates the habit of giving on a regular yearly basis.

Campaigns. Fundraising campaigns have a specific set of defining points that include a specific goal, support of a particular project, and set starting and ending dates. The best way to run any campaign is to begin by defining its mission. After this definition, name the amount needed to achieve the mission, set a deadline, and then determine how donors will be recognized (for example with small gifts or listing in the annual report) (Pelletier, 2007).

Alumni and donor relations. There are a number of key elements in cultivating a long-term and mutually rewarding relationship with a donor. Stewardship relates to resource management, and in the context of a donor's gift, that involves compliance with the donor's wishes with respect to application of the gift, effective management of the resources represented by the gift, and accountability. All donations are acknowledged with a personalized letter of thanks with a charitable donation receipt attached.

Major gifts. Many major gifts are given for a specific purpose, distinguishing them from an annual gift, which is usually unrestricted and available to fund current operations. Major gifts are likely to be given in a restricted manner in order to accomplish a specific purpose that is valued by the donor. Gifts can be solicited for specific purposes, to suit both the organization's needs and the donor's stated preferences.

Planned gifts. When donors plan to give, they can donate a greater, more significant amount than they may have originally thought possible, and for some donors, planning ahead of time is the only way to make a substantial gift. Development officers who deal with planned gifts specialize in handling gifts with tax and estate implications for donors. These include gifts of outright cash and securities; gifts that provide a lifetime income to donors, such as pooled income fund gifts, charitable gift annuities, and charitable remainder trusts; and bequests, gifts of real estate, and gifts of tangible personal property, such as art, jewelry, antiques, and collectibles.

Special event fundraisers. Often called *fundraising benefits*, special event fundraisers are social gatherings that generate publicity for an organization; raise money; charge a fee for attendance but offer some form of entertainment in exchange; and include extravaganzas (gala dinner-dances, concerts, cruises, or major sporting events), events for bargain hunters or gamblers (bingos, raffles, casino nights, garage sales, rummage sales, auctions, flea markets, or bake sales), or educational events (ranging from major speakers who fill large auditoriums to slide shows shown in community centers).

Mass fundraising. Mass fundraising is generated from huge mailings that generate tens of thousands of donors and produce funds with the fewest strings attached. But mass fundraising via mailing and phoning, the pre-Internet techniques, has always suffered from the high cost of raising the money (Thompson, n.d). Recently the Internet has presented a major opportunity and strategy for mass fundraising, with many organizations using a mix of Internet strategies including social networking sites, e-mails, and donations via organizational home pages.

Online crowdsourcing. Over the past five years, mission-driven organizations have set up websites to raise money through social media campaigns (e.g., Indiegogo, Kickstarter, Rocket Hub). This is an exciting trend for small nonprofits with little startup capital, but frightening because there is no promise that money is spent as the donor intended. The benefits are that this strategy is inexpensive, provides an equal opportunity whether the organization is large or small, and has the potential to reach millions simultaneously. The downsides are that no one monitors carefully where the money goes and the contributions tend to be non-tax-deductible. Likewise organizations continue to seek innovative funding strategy using social media (e.g., Twitter, Facebook).

Mobile giving and bidding. Mobile bidding (e.g., auctions) helps protect donors' privacy as it sidesteps the Internet entirely. Donors use their own cell phones, and their credit cards are never out of their hands. After the Haiti earthquake, an individual could simply text $10 to the Red Cross, and many small donors now support the Wounded Warriors Project. This strategy encourages many people to give small amounts of money, but it is harder to retain those donors year after year. As millennials get older, there will be more and more online giving, but it tends not to build loyalty because there is no human interaction. Nothing beats face-to-face communication that helps to maintain the donor relationship. Let's take the example of the ALS Bucket Challenge, which was wildly successful in 2015. Will ALS continue to receive the same amount of support the next year? New tools do not allow us to build a relationship unless we are clever with managing these tools.

Corporate philanthropy. Corporation giving in 2015 was trending upward since the 2009 economic downturn (The Conference Board, 2015). Corporations have always given because they wanted to be good community partners, but now they are becoming more savvy in their philanthropic decision making. The trend is for their staff to show support by volunteering for the organization (e.g., Boys and Girls Clubs) or explicitly recommending that the corporation donate to the cause. Companies are also looking for better mission connections; for example, a pharmaceutical company may not give to the Girl Scouts of America, but may give to the National Safety Council to support a poisoning prevention campaign. Companies now set aside money for small grants programs for general purposes, but larger donations are awarded based on geography or mission. In addition, donations are now more connected to tracking sales.

Working with Board Members

For health promotion programs operated by a small or large community health organization, another resource that is available to help with the funding programs is the organization's board of directors. By law, all nonprofit organizations (such as community health organizations) are required to have a board of directors to oversee the organization's mission, operation, and fiscal management. Most professional fundraisers will say that before boards get involved in fundraising, they must first be involved in the mission and governance of the organization. This involvement with the larger scope of the organization often leads to a more focused commitment to the fundraising program.

Most people do not gravitate to fundraising naturally or easily. It is helpful to involve board members in a process to explore their personal feelings about giving and asking. Most health promotion programs use a variety of methods to ask for money, such as direct mail appeals, special events, pledge programs, or products for sale. Perhaps the hardest way for an organization to raise money is for board, staff, and volunteers to ask people directly for donations (Stoesz, 2015). Experience has shown, however, that it is almost impossible to have a major gifts program without face-to-face solicitation of prospective donors.

The actual fundraising task is immeasurably strengthened when a true partnership between board and staff is in place. Staff members manage the fundraising program, while board members get involved in the elements that suit their interests, skills, and capabilities. A good fundraising plan is

Table 9.3   Board and Staff Members' Fundraising Responsibilities

Board Members

Provide input on the fundraising plan

Organize and participate on fundraising committee

Identify and cultivate new prospects and donors

Ask peers for donations

Always be an advocate for the agency

Make introductions for staff to follow up

Accompany staff on key visits to funders

Help with expressions of thanks when appropriate

Staff Members

Accompany board members on key visits to funders

Help with expressions of thanks when appropriate

Research new and existing donors

Write stories about the impact of a program on program participants

Write grant proposals

Accompany board members on solicitation visits

Take care of all logistics related to fundraising activities

Develop a funding strategy incorporating all funding types and sources, keeping board members apprised of the status of all funded programs and grants

explicit about both board and staff responsibilities. Table 9.3 lists *board and staff members' fundraising responsibilities.*

Asking a person for money face to face is an acquired skill. Few people love to do it initially. And being hesitant about asking for money is common. People hesitate to ask for money for a wide variety of reasons. For example, one can look at the role that money plays in American society to understand one source of the anxiety. Most people are taught that four topics are taboo in polite conversation: politics, money, religion, and sex. Many people were also raised to believe that asking people what their salary is or how much they paid for their house or their car is rude. In some families, one person takes care of all financial decisions. It is not unusual, even today, for an individual not to know how much their spouse or partner earns, for children not to know how much their parents earn, or for close friends not to know one another's income.

In working with board members and volunteers to ask directly (in person) for donations, frame the idea of asking in the context of support and urgency in addressing a health problem. Focus the process on how the organization is working to solve the health problem. Money is only one part of the process (but an important one). Be clear that the money is not being sought for personal gain or use but rather to address a human need larger than any one individual.

Summary

Health promotion programs need money in order to operate. Effective programs have staff members who understand the role of money in programs, the sources and types of funding, and the work involved in acquiring, managing, and reporting on program resources. Although talking about money may seem to be at odds with the goals of a health promotion program, in reality, it is a natural part of figuring out the value of health to a business, school, health care organization, or community. Furthermore, the clearer that program staff are about a program's goals and objectives and the effectiveness of the program in meeting those goals and objectives, the better positioned the staff will be to build funders' confidence that a program is effective and worth funding.

For Practice and Discussion

1. Locate a few health promotion programs that receive funding from at least three of the 10 different funding sources listed in this chapter. Compare and contrast the programs. Discuss differences and similarities among the programs.

2. You are working with a community college to develop and implement a student health promotion program. As part of a planned meeting with a school staff member, you will be asked to discuss options that the college might consider in order to fund the health promotion program. Prepare a brief list of available options and examples of funding sources to pursue.

3. Contact the United Way in your area or region. How does this organization raise money, and whom does it fund? What organizations and programs get the most funding? What criteria must a program meet in order to receive funding? Who gets the least funding? Why are there differences in the funding amounts?

4. Staff members who participate in a lunchtime physical activity program sponsored by their employer, a small business, are asked to pay $2 a session. What are the pros and cons of charging fees for participation in a health promotion program? How can the fees be incentives and disincentives?

5. Think of a health project that would benefit your campus or community. Using a proposed budget of $5,000 follow the guidelines on the website https://www.indiegogo.com/ to design a funding campaign to secure the initial funding.

KEY TERMS

Board members' fundraising responsibilities

Client fees

Collaborations and cooperative agreements

Foundations

Fundraising

Fundraising field

Professional Fundraisers

Grants

Health insurance

Infrastructure (operating, core, or hard) funding

Matching funds, cost sharing, and in-kind contributions

Public funds

Staff members' fundraising responsibilities

Volunteers

References

Chambliss, M. L., Lineberry, S., Evans, W. M., & Bibeau, D. L. (2014). Adding health education specialists to your practice. *Family Practice Management*, *21*(2), 10–15. http://www.ncbi.nlm.nih.gov/pubmed/24693839

The Conference Board—CECP. (2015). Giving in numbers 2015 edition. Retrieved from http://cecp.co/pdfs/giving_in_numbers/GIN2015_FINAL_web.pdf

Forbes. (2015). *The 50 Largest U.S. Charities*. Retrieved April from http://www.forbes.com/companies/united-way/

Foundation Center. (2016). *Proposal writing short course*. Retrieved from http://foundationcenter.org/getstarted/tutorials/shortcourse/

Lilly Family School of Philanthropy. (2015). *Giving USA 2015*. Retrieved from http://www.givinginstitute.org/?page=GUSAAnnualReport

National Institutes of Health. (2015, August). *Before you start writing*. Retrieved from http://www.nih.gov/institutes-nih/nih-office-director/office-communications-public-liaison/clear-communication/plain-language/before-you-start-writing

National Institutes of Health, National Institute of Diabetes and Digestive and Kidney Diseases. (n.d.). *Writing a grant*. Retrieved January 30, 2016, from http://www.niddk.nih.gov/fund/grants_process/grantwriting.htm

Pelletier, M. (2007). *The basics of managing a fundraising campaign*. Retrieved from http://www.helium.com/tm/309652/fundraising-campaigns-specific-defining

Stoesz, E. (2015). *Doing good better: How to be an effective board member of a nonprofit*. Pennsylvania: Good Books.

Texas Education Agency. (1999, June). *A grantseeker's resource guide to obtaining federal, corporate and foundation grants*. Retrieved from http://www.birdvilleschools.net/cms/lib2/TX01000797/Centricity/Domain/4393/Components/grant%20primer.pdf

Thompson, M. (n.d.). *Morris continued*. Retrieved December 13, 2007, from http://cagle.msnbc.com/news/DeanMorris/1.asp

PART FOUR

EVALUATING AND SUSTAINING HEALTH PROMOTION PROGRAMS

CHAPTER 10

EVALUATING HEALTH PROMOTION PROGRAMS

Joseph A. Dake and Timothy R. Jordan

Why Evaluate a Health Promotion Program?

Significant amounts of time, money, and human resources are typically invested in developing, implementing, and managing health promotion programs. Everyone involved in the program wants it to be effective in meeting its *goals* and objectives. However, how do funders, program staff members, and other *stakeholders* know whether the program is operating as it was designed? How do they know if the program was effective and actually helped the *priority population*? How do they know if their investments yielded the desired results? The answer to those questions is program evaluation.

At one time, program evaluation was viewed as something that was done to a program. After the program was designed and implemented, a program evaluator would be contacted to assess a program and its participants for the purpose of issuing a pass-or-fail report card to a funder or policymaker, presumably to contribute to a decision about whether to continue funding the program. Evaluation was often viewed by program staff as expensive and intrusive without adding much value to the program.

As a result of this erroneous view, program staff members would sometimes view the program evaluator(s) as intimidating or threatening. Often a "we-versus-they" relationship developed between program staff and the evaluator(s). This type of relationship often excluded other stakeholders and did little to help the program improve in the future.

LEARNING OBJECTIVES

- Compare and contrast the types and purposes of formative and summative evaluation.

- Describe the role of evaluation in shaping program design and implementation.

- Describe shared components of commonly used evaluation frameworks.

- Compare and contrast evaluation designs.

- Describe factors that influence evaluation costs.

- Explain the purpose and structure of evaluation reports.

- Describe ethical considerations in program evaluation.

To some, these old images of evaluation still linger. Today, however, most health promotion experts realize that program evaluation is not threatening and actually adds great value and benefits to programs. Quality evaluation helps to improve programs and increase the odds that the program will help the priority population. It is a continual, collaborative process that starts with program design and includes stakeholders and members of the priority population. Quality program evaluation helps to strengthen program design and implementation while providing constructive recommendations to enhance program effectiveness. Ultimately, quality evaluation allows program staff to demonstrate program outcomes to funders and stakeholders and increases the odds of additional funding and program sustainability.

How Do I Get Started?

Ideally, program evaluation begins prior to program design with the building of a planning team or steering committee. Collectively, the team directs the design of the program and the evaluation. At a minimum the team includes: (1) the program director/administrator, (2) the program evaluator(s) (3) key program staff members (those who will actually be delivering the program) and, (4) several members of the priority population. It may also be wise to include key stakeholders and representatives from collaborating agencies or organizations.

Prior to designing the program and the evaluation, this team works together to answer a series of important planning questions. Answering these questions is likely to require several meetings over a period of weeks. Some questions that would serve as a good starting point include:

- Who (specifically) is the priority population that the program is designed to help?
- Is the priority population represented on this team?
- How will we gain access to them and gain their approval and acceptance for this program and the evaluation?
- Are there other stakeholders or partners who need to be included in the program planning, implementation, and evaluation processes?
- What do the funders, stakeholders, and program planners want to know about this program?
- What is the overall *mission* for this program? Why will this program exist? How will it help the priority population?
- What are the goals or overall desired outcomes for this program? Improved health? Changes in health behaviors?

- If this program is effective, what specific measurable changes in the priority population will we see?

- How can these desired measurable changes be written as *SMART objectives* to align with our program goals?

- What kinds of *activities* would help us meet our SMART objectives?

- What kinds of data are needed to determine whether the SMART objectives were met? How and where can this information be obtained?

- What resources are available for collecting this data, analyzing it, and reporting it?

- When and how often will data be collected to make periodic corrections and revisions?

- What decisions will be made based on the evaluation findings?

- What type of report would be most useful for program planners, funders, key stakeholders, and the priority population?

As you can surmise from the list of questions above, it is critical for both program planners and program evaluators to know the "who," "what," "when," "where," and "how much" before evaluation planning begins.

One of the most critical planning steps is to ensure that the program's mission, goals, objectives, activities, *measures*, data collection, and data analysis methods are tightly aligned and congruent with one another. Figure 10.1 shows a properly aligned program evaluation serves to inform potential modifications to program activities, program objectives, and possibly even program goals. Without proper *alignment* of program and evaluation components, even a high-quality *evaluation design* will not be able to detect and demonstrate the true effectiveness or impact of a program. Including a skilled program evaluator during the development of the program can help to ensure proper alignment.

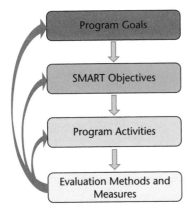

Figure 10.1 Program Evaluation Alignment

Types of Evaluations

The type of information desired determines the type of evaluation that is used. A good understanding of each type is important to properly conduct an evaluation that can answer stakeholders' questions and help make program decisions. The most common types of *program evaluation* are listed below along with some associated planning questions.

Formative evaluations are conducted during program development and implementation. These are useful to help provide the best starting point for the program, to help avoid pitfalls with implementation, and to best guide program improvements during implementation. Formative evaluation involves gathering information and materials during program planning and development to ensure that a program and its corresponding activities are appropriate and acceptable to the priority population. Two subcategories are included as part of formative evaluation: needs assessment and process evaluation.

Needs assessments are a formalized approach to collecting and analyzing data for the purpose of identifying the needs and priorities of a group. After the needs assessment, programs are typically designed to address the gap between "what is" and "what should be" for a given priority population. Measuring the existing gap and determining the intrapersonal, interpersonal, institutional, community, and environmental factors that may help or hinder programmatic efforts will help to maximize the likelihood of programmatic success. This could involve assessment of existing programs and policies, existing relevant (secondary) data, and new (primary) data from the priority population and key stakeholders. The results from this step of an evaluation are used to make any necessary changes to the program or to the implementation plan to help ensure the greatest likelihood for a strong start to the program. A strong program implementation helps to ensure that the evaluation results represent the actual impact of the programming.

Common questions to guide the needs assessment phase of evaluation (before the program is implemented):

- What do potential participants desire in the health promotion program?
- What are the known health needs of the priority population?
- What factors impact these health needs?
- What gaps exist in programming or services to address these needs?
- What other programs have been implemented in the past with this population?

- Were these past programs successful? If yes, why? If no, why not?
- How will program participants be recruited?
- What barriers exist that would prevent a potential participant from enrolling/ participating? (e.g., perceived need, timing of program, transportation, child care challenges, bad experience with similar programs, language issues, trust concerns, perceived susceptibility to or severity of the health issue, etc.)
- What resources exist in the community that would support enrollment in the program?
- What incentives would increase program participation?

Process evaluation is about systematically gathering information *during* program implementation. A strong evaluation assesses a program from start to finish, including how the program was implemented. Process evaluation is used to describe and evaluate the reach of the program, recruitment and retention methods, perceptions of program quality, program acceptability, barriers to program engagement, fidelity of implementation (i.e., to what degree did program implementation adhere to the written design), and any other question that pertains to how the program is being implemented. When problems result during implementation, it can impact the effectiveness of the programming. Thus, identifying and correcting these issues as early as possible can help to ensure that time and resources are not being wasted.

Common questions to guide process evaluation:
- Did the program meet its recruitment and enrollment goals? If not, why not?
- Was there significant drop out of participants? If so, why?
- Who participated in the programming? Was this the desired population to be reached?
- How engaged were the program participants?
- Did the participants understand all of the programming? Were there parts that were confusing?
- Did the participants find the programming useful? What did they find beneficial/ problematic?
- What would the participants change to make the program better or more useful?

- Was the program implemented and conducted as designed (with fidelity)?

- Was the program conducted the same across each site and by each person? What differences existed?

- Were there problems or concerns among those implementing the program (space issues, environmental concerns, size of groups, program materials, etc.)?

- How would staff members change the program to make it better?

Overall, a well-designed and well-monitored process evaluation can help a program director understand the elements that contributed to a health promotion program's success. A good process evaluation can also identify how to improve a program to better achieve intended results. A high quality process evaluation helps evaluators identify external factors that limited program effectiveness and impact.

Summative evaluations determine the short- and long-term changes that occurred as a result of the program. Summative evaluation demonstrate the magnitude of the impact of the program, to show accountability for resources invested in the program, and to provide strong data to be used to make important decision (e.g., to expand, replicate, modify, or terminate an existing program). Generally, summative evaluations assesses the degree to which the SMART objectives and program goals were met. Two subcategories are included as part of summative evaluation: impact evaluation and outcome evaluation.

Impact evaluation methods are used to measure the immediate effects of a health promotion program and the extent to which the program's objectives were attained. The primary question in an impact evaluation is, "What was the program's immediate effect on the participants?" Impact evaluation typically occurs soon after a program concludes (from 0 to 6 months) and focuses on changes that are measurable during the program term (e.g., knowledge, attitudes, skills, behaviors).

Impact evaluation is the most common type of summative evaluation because of the common need to have answers soon after the completion of a program. For example, funders often want results quarterly and at the end of each year. If short-term results are needed, health promotion professionals need to consider outcomes that change during a short period of time. For example, it would not be realistic for a worksite smoking cessation program to show a reduction in lung cancer or for a school-based healthy eating campaign to show a reduction in students'

BMI within 6 months. For such programs more realistic short-term results would include self-reported smoking cessation (or biochemical verification) or an increase in self-reported fruit and vegetable consumption. These are the types of results that are more appropriate for shorter term measurement.

With impact evaluation, there is a wide range of potential measures that are used. These measures vary in how strongly they are associated with real, tangible health behavior change or health status improvements. To determine the strength of the linkage between a potential measure and health—let's say knowledge and health behavior change—the program evaluator consults the published research literature. When possible, the program evaluator measures the actual behaviors that have been proven to be strongly and positively associated with the desired change in health behavior or health status. Examples of good measures in the area of heart disease are healthy eating and exercise behavior. In the area of HIV prevention/reduction, a good measure would be regular condom use.

In some cases, measuring actual behaviors are a challenge during the timeframe for program evaluation. In such cases, using health behavior theories and models to help guide the evaluation is useful. Choosing a model or a theory that has been proven to explain and/or predict a given behavior is an effective alternative to actually measuring the behavior of the priority population.

For example, if time and money are in short supply and you are interested in improving the rates of mammography among African American women, you may want to use the Integrated Behavioral Model and measure program participants' attitudes, perceived norms, personal agency beliefs, and behavioral intentions regarding mammography rather than following participants over the next 3–5 years to see if they actually get a mammogram. Although measuring these psychological variables is not as strong as measuring actual behaviors or longer-term health outcomes such as breast cancer mortality, they are usually better measures than developing something new that is not based on existing research.

Common questions to guide impact evaluation:

- What theories or models have been proven to explain or predict the desired behavior or health status improvements in this priority population?
- What changes took place in the knowledge, perceptions, beliefs, or attitudes that have been shown to predict the desired behavior?

- What behavior change took place that leads to the desired heath status outcomes?
- Are there differences in outcomes based on participant characteristics (age, race/ethnicity, sex, geographic location, level of participation, or other potential factors)?
- Are there differences in outcomes based on differences in programming across sites?
- Can the results be attributed to the program alone or are there other factors that may have resulted in change?
- How can we rule out external factors or other plausible explanations for the change that we detected?
- Given the intermediate effects on the priority population, do the results justify the past and future investments of time, money, and staffing?

Outcome evaluation is a natural extension of impact evaluation and focuses on longer-term (greater than 6 months) outcomes that may result from a health promotion intervention. Outcome evaluation may look at the same factors assessed during impact evaluation but follow program participants for a longer time period to determine the sustainability of the behavior change or to determine longer-term health status outcomes. Participants may also be followed for a longer period of time to assess whether the theoretical constructs that you measured predict actual behavior change (i.e., did women's attitudes toward mammography actually predict their mammography behavior).

When time and resources permit, outcome evaluation can measure actual health status and economic outcomes that may result from a given health promotion program. Such longer-term outcomes may include things like a decrease in mortality due to heart disease, decrease in violent crime, weight loss, decreased incidence of HIV, decreased hospital admissions due to opioid overdose, or an increase in mammography screening. In general, changes in vital statistics for a priority population (e.g., morbidity, mortality, incidence, and prevalence) can only be measured via high-quality, long-term outcome evaluations. Such evaluations require significant resources and the ability to wait for a longer period of time (years) before expecting change to be detectable. Furthermore, the longer the duration of the program evaluation, the more likely that intervening variables can confound the results, which then requires stronger research designs (e.g., control groups).

Additional questions to guide outcome evaluation:

- Did the program achieve is stated goals?
- How did the program impact health status outcomes for the priority population?
- How did the program impact incidence, prevalence, morbidity, and mortality within the priority population?
- How many injuries could be prevented, lives saved, or years of life added as a result of the program being more widely implemented?
- What was the return on investment for this program?

Related Strategies

An area related to evaluation that is receiving increased attention in the health care and educational industries is *improvement science*. This is a newly developing discipline with a focus on learning from strong research and evaluation designs which can then be used in a timely manner to make an impact on the population of interest (Marshall, Pronovost, Dixon-Woods, 2013). The researcher/evaluator of the particular program or intervention that used a strong research design (e.g., randomized control trial) can take the findings from the program or intervention to recommend changes in practice which can maximize the positive outcomes for the population of interest. While this is not necessarily different from quality program evaluation, the focus is slightly different. Improvement science focuses on timely feedback and practical application of *quality improvement* findings.

An example of this is the CDCs new 6|18 Initiative: Accelerating Evidence into Action (Hester, et al., 2016). This is a major federal effort to engage key health care, public health, and academic stakeholders to demonstrate the ability to accelerate stakeholder implementation of selected evidence-based interventions focused on six priority issues (www.cdc.gov/sixeighteen):

- Reduce tobacco use
- Control high blood pressure
- Prevent healthcare-associated infections
- Control asthma
- Prevent unintended pregnancy
- Control and prevent diabetes

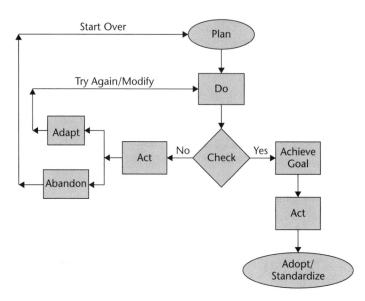

Figure 10.2   Flow Chart of PDCA Cycle
Source: Gorenflo and Moran, 2010.

In the area of public health, improvement science is also being addressed. The Public Health Foundation has quality improvement as one of three focus areas and promote a process of rapid quality improvement (Gorenflo & Moran, 2010). They recommend this be accomplished through a PDCA (or PDSA) (Figure 10.2):

Plan: This first phase is to ① identify and prioritize improvement opportunities, ② to clarify the purpose, identify the priority population, and select measurable objectives, ③ describe the existing processes to better understand where improvements could be made, ④ collect baseline data, ⑤ identify causes of the problem, ⑥ identify possible improvements, ⑦ articulate the effect that is expected as a result of the potential changes, 8) develop an action plan.

Do: This phase is to ① implement the recommended improvement(s), ② collect data, ③ document problems that result from this modified intervention or process.

Check/Study: Analyze the evaluation results against the stated objectives and document lessons learned.

Act: This phase is to rapidly act upon what has been learned. This may include ① adopting the improvements if they met or exceeded the expectations, (2) adapting the intervention based on the information learned from the evaluation and trying again, or (3) abandoning the intervention or particular improvement strategy if the evaluation results suggest that there was nothing gained and adaptations are unlikely to have an impact.

Another variant in evaluation is *developmental evaluation*. This approach focuses innovative programs in their earliest stages of development which may not be well suited for traditional evaluation methods. Developmental evaluation (DE) is well suited for helping to understand complex or changing environments. Similar to improvement science, DE pays particular attention to continuous quality improvement. However, DE typically has strong integration among program staff and program evaluators and is particular well suited for the following five purposes (Fagen et al., 2011):

Ongoing development: Adapting an existing program to changing conditions

Adaptation: Adapting a program based on general principles for a particular context

Rapid response: Adapting a program to respond quickly in a crisis

Preformative development: Readying a potentially promising program for the traditional formative and summative evaluation cycle

Systems change: Providing feedback on broad systems change

Evaluation Terms

A number of terms are used in discussing health promotion program evaluation, regardless of the evaluation type. These terms are important to understand to ensure the greatest odds of a high-quality evaluation.

Quantitative methods involve the gathering and analysis of numerical data. The evaluator determines what quantitative data are needed to assess whether the program's SMART objectives were met. Quantitative methods are commonly used in conducting evaluations of health promotion programs. Examples of quantitative data include the number of participants in a weight management program, responses to Likert scale items in an electronic survey of participants' attitudes toward exercise behaviors, and comparing pretest and posttest scores of adolescents' perceptions toward condom use before and after a pregnancy prevention program. Quantitative methods are very useful because many funders and stakeholders desire data to be described numerically.

It permits an understanding of the degree of change among program participants. Numerical data are required for calculating inferential statistics and reporting whether changes were statistically significantly different. Quantitative data are also used to generalize to a larger population. Because of these benefits, quantitative data are often required for program funding and help with describing impact in an *evaluation report*. The weakness of quantitative data is that it often does not provide insight into "why" a program was (or was not) successful. Such data are typically derived from biometric measurements (e.g., BMI, % of body fat, strength), questions from surveys, or from population-based vital statistics (e.g., prevalence rates).

Qualitative methods involve the gathering of nonnumerical data via such methods as interviews, focus groups, and open-ended survey questions. This type of data often provides a greater understanding of the impact of the program based on insights from key stakeholders (the most important of which are program participants). Qualitative data can help get at the "why" that was missing in quantitative data. While some qualitative data are converted into numerical forms for quantitative analyses, the primary purpose of this method is to gain a depth of understanding that is not possible with most *quantitative methods*. Qualitative data collection techniques allow program participant to share their thoughts, perceptions, challenges, concerns, and so on that would not be possible on a written survey that features closed-ended questions. Obtaining qualitative data from the priority population is especially useful during formative evaluation to help better understand the needs of the priority population.

Mixed methods involve a combination of qualitative and quantitative data collection methods. A mixed method approach is usually the best option for a quality program evaluation because it helps evaluators get closer to the truth. A mixed-methods approach eliminates many of the limitations of doing either quantitative or qualitative alone. This method is best at getting at both the "what" and "why" that is critical in program improvement. Commonly, in mixed methods program evaluation, qualitative methods are the predominant (but not sole) method used during formative evaluation and quantitative methods are the predominant (but not sole) method during summative evaluation. An example of an important function of qualitative evaluation during outcome evaluation would be to understand why the program was impactful to some but not others. Being able to learn during an interview or focus group what led one subset of the priority population to have great results while another subset had poor results would help to provide the necessary feedback for additional program improvements

Reliability refers to the ability of evaluation data collection instruments/tools to provide consistent results each time they are used. Use of reliable instruments is integral to a quality program evaluation. Data collection tools are pilot tested prior to use to establish their reliability.

Validity refers to the ability of evaluation data collection instruments/tools to accurately measure what the evaluator wants to measure. Use of valid instruments is also integral to a quality program evaluation. Data collection tools are pilot tested prior to use to establish their validity.

Cultural relevance means that the evaluation methods and materials, including the measurement tools, have been developed with consideration of the cultural traits of the priority population (e.g., race, ethnicity, religious beliefs, language, socioeconomic status, family style, values). This includes the idea of cultural acceptability in which program participants feel that the methods and materials of the program and its evaluation are appropriate and respectful of the nuances of the priority population. The best way to ensure that the methods and materials of the program and its evaluation are culturally relevant and culturally acceptable is to include members of the priority population on the planning/steering committee. Qualitative methods used during the formative stages can help to ensure a more culturally relevant/acceptable program and a greater likelihood of program impact.

Evaluation Frameworks

Evaluations are guided by a *framework*. Another word for framework is *process*: a consistent approach, structure, and format that helps program participants, staff, and other stakeholders understand the thinking that went into the evaluation, the type of questions asked, how the information was collected, and the type of report that might be expected. There are a number of published frameworks, some of which focus on particular topic areas such obesity prevention (Leeman et al., 2012). This section will discuss two general frameworks.

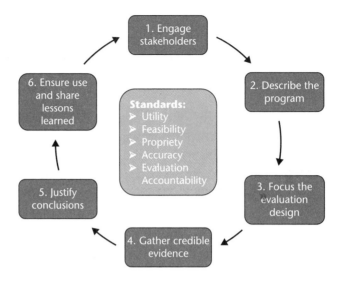

Figure 10.3   Evaluation Framework of the Centers for Disease Control and Prevention with Joint Committee on Standards for Educational Evaluation Standards

CDC Evaluation Framework

The evaluation framework of the Centers for Disease Control and Prevention (2012) is widely used for evaluations of health promotion programs (Figure 10.3). There are six steps which build upon one another, and all of the steps are founded on five standards released by the Joint Committee on Standards for Educational Evaluation (Yarbrough, Shulha, Hopson, & Caruthers, 2011).

Steps:

1. **Engage stakeholders**, especially those involved in program operations (for example, collaborators, funding officials, and staff); those served or affected by the program (for example, clients, neighborhood organizations, academic institutions, elected officials, and opponents); and primary users of the evaluation results. They all have an investment in what will be learned and what will be done with the information.

2. **Describe the health promotion program**, including its mission, goals, SMART objectives, and activities; the need or problem addressed; the expected effects of the program on the need or problem; the intervention strategies and activities; the human, material, and time resources available; the program's stage of development; the program's social, political, and economic context; and a logic model that describes the projected sequence of events for bringing about change.

3. **Focus the evaluation design** in order to assess the issues of greatest concern to stakeholders while using time and resources efficiently,

accurately, and ethically. Specifically, a focused evaluation design takes into consideration the evaluation's purpose, the users who will receive the results, and how the evaluation will be used. Evaluation design also focuses on developing answerable evaluation questions, developing reasonable evaluation methods, and having agreements on the roles and responsibilities of those conducting the evaluation.

4. **Gather credible evidence** that is accurate and will be perceived by stakeholders as believable and relevant for answering questions about the program and its implementation or effects. Stakeholders who were involved in planning the evaluation and gathering data are more likely to accept the evaluation's conclusions and to act on its recommendations.

5. **Justify conclusions**, including recommendations, by ensuring that they are linked to the evidence gathered and to explicit values or standards that were set with the stakeholders. Following this strategy will enable stakeholders to use the evaluation results with confidence.

6. **Ensure use of the results and share lessons learned** by having a strong and participatory evaluation design; preparing stakeholders to use the results by exploring the possible positive and negative implications of the findings; promoting stakeholder feedback by holding periodic discussions during the evaluation process and routinely sharing interim findings, provisional interpretations, and draft reports; following up with the stakeholders by advocating for use of the findings when decisions about the program are being made; and disseminating the findings through full disclosure and impartial reporting in a report that is tailored to the audience and that explains the evaluation's focus, its limitations, and its strengths and weaknesses.

Standards

In addition to its evaluation framework, the CDC also recommends that program evaluations adhere to specific professional standards. The CDC adopted these standards from the Joint Committee on Standards for Educational Evaluation. These standards help program planners and program evaluators to answer an important question: *"Will this program evaluation be effective?"*

The 30 professional standards for program evaluation are categorized into four groups:

1. Utility Standards: Will the program evaluation serve the information needs of the intended users?

2. Feasibility Standards: Will the evaluation be realistic, prudent, diplomatic, and frugal?

3. Propriety Standards: Will the evaluation be conducted legally, ethically, and with due regard for the welfare of those involved in the evaluation, as well as those affected by its results?

4. Accuracy Standards: Will the evaluation reveal and convey technically accurate information about the features that determine worth or merit of the program being evaluated?

To assess the quality of the evaluation design and results, program planners and program evaluators use these standards during the design phase of the evaluation and after the evaluation is completed.

RE-AIM Evaluation Framework

The *RE-AIM evaluation framework* recognizes the importance of both external validity (reach and adoption) and internal validity (effectiveness and implementation) in the evaluation of program interventions (Gaglio & Glasgow, 2012). It is useful in estimating public health impact, comparing different health policies, designing policies for increased likelihood of success, and identifying areas for integration of policies with other health promotion strategies. There are five steps to the model:

1. **Reach:** The portion and representativeness of the program participants relative to the priority population.

2. **Effectiveness:** Focused on the greatest impact on the primary outcomes and the fewest negative side effects.

3. **Adoption:** The portion and representativeness of the health promotion settings and program staff such that the program could be conducted in many other settings.

4. **Implementation:** The ability to consistently and reliably deliver the program in various settings without undue costs.

5. **Maintenance:** The program includes strategies to ensure long-term improvements.

Evaluation Design

Once the evaluator knows the theory or model upon which the program was designed, the type of evaluation, and the evaluation framework that will be used, attention is focused on the evaluation design. The decision on which evaluation design to use will depend on the answers to a number of important questions:

- How much time do you have to conduct the evaluation?

- What resources are available to conduct the evaluation?

- Do you have the ability to randomly select participants and randomly assign them into intervention and control groups?

- If not, do you have access to a group that is very similar to program participants that you could use as a control or comparison group?

- When can you collect the evaluation information? Before the program begins? During implementation? Or after the program ends?

- How many individuals (program participants, stakeholders, staff) will be involved in the evaluation?

- What kinds of data driven by the SMART objectives are needed?

- Is it important to generalize your findings to a larger population or other populations?

The greater the desired level of validity and reliability of the results, the greater the need for a stronger evaluation design. There are numerous research designs that are used in evaluation. The choice of design will largely depend on the availability of various resources. Basically, the differences lie in the type of sampling and group assignment (e.g., random versus convenience), whether (and what type of) a comparison group is available, how many times data will be collected, and when the data will be collected.

The evaluation designs that are the weakest involve a single assessment immediately after the program (posttest) without a comparison group. The strongest design is a randomized control study (participants are randomly selected and randomly assigned into an intervention and control group). The latter is rarely done because of lack of available funding, lack of resources, and due to the fact that health promotion programming is not as well suited for this design as clinical trials.

The following are some examples of research designs used in evaluation grouped in order from weakest to strongest.

1. **Posttest only for the program group:** This is the simplest and weakest of the designs. It assesses program participants only at the end of the program, usually immediately after. The reason this is the weakest design is that there is no opportunity to measure change in participants over time after they enroll in the program. In some cases, retrospective pretesting is done (Nimon, 2014) to help gauge participants perceptions of change.

2. **Pretest and posttest only for the program group:** This builds upon #1 in that there is a baseline measurement prior to participants being exposed to the program. Having a baseline measure (pretest) and a follow-up measure after the program is completed (posttest)

allows evaluators to measure change over time. As with the posttest-only design, it is not possible with this design to attribute any detected changes to the program. Changes may have been caused by other external factors (exposure to other programming in the community/agency/school, policy changes that took place during your program, or news events that triggered change among the participants). Without a control or comparison group, it is simply not possible to rule out other plausible explanations for changes over time that have been detected.

3. **Time series:** This is a continuation of #2 but measures multiple times prior to the program starting and multiple times throughout and after the program. This is a stronger design because it allows an analysis of trend data. This can help to better isolate the time of any changes that are detected and helps to rule out that change was caused by an external event. While this is much stronger than #1 or #2, the lack of a control or comparison group still limits the program evaluator's ability to say with confidence that detected results were due to the program.

4. **Pretest and posttest with a control or comparison group:** Having a control or comparison group significantly adds to the strength of any evaluation design. This is because changes that are seen in the program group but not seen in the control or comparison group provide stronger evidence that the program actually caused those changes. There is however, an important condition. Those in control or comparison groups need to be as similar as possible to the program participants. Best efforts are made to ensure that variables that might influence program results (demographics, geographic location, previous exposure to programs, perceptions/attitudes of the participants, etc.) are similar between the comparison and program group. The strongest method to accomplish this is to use random selection and random assignment into the two groups. If random selection is not possible, then random assignment into the two groups is a good step. While this is the best method to ensure a strong program evaluation, it is not often used in health promotion programming due to an inability to randomly select and assign. Furthermore, using a control or comparison group is often more expensive because of the additional costs associated with identifying, recruiting, and assessing an additional group of people.

5. **Time series with a control or comparison group:** This is the same as #4 but with the added strength of multiple measurements over time.

Data Collection and Analysis

After the decisions about evaluation type, framework, and evaluation design have been made, the evaluator's focus turns to collecting the desired information (data) that is needed to answer the questions developed during the formative and summative evaluation planning, including the criteria for success pertaining to the program's measurable objectives. Much of the data collected during program evaluations is the information needed to determine whether the program met its stated SMART objectives (See Chapter 5).

Data collection involves the process of collecting, managing, organizing, analyzing, synthesizing, and summarizing the data in order to make sense of them and answer the evaluation's overall questions. Quality data are needed to have a quality program evaluation. Quality data comes from proper alignment among program components and program evaluation components. When proper alignment is present, higher quality data are available to the program evaluator.

Quality data does not come about by "throwing together" a quick survey or other data collection tools. Valid, reliable, and high-quality data collection tools take time to develop and pilot test. High-quality data collection tools and methods are essential to obtaining high-quality data. Because there is not always the time needed to develop and pilot test newly designed data collection tools, using valid and reliable tools (e.g., surveys) that have already been created and published can save a lot of time and resources.

There are excellent resources available to health promotion program evaluators that can help provide guidance with program evaluation methods and data collection tools. These same resources are also helpful during program planning and development to determine what has already been shown to be effective. Searching through various registries of best practices and evidence-based programs helps to avoid "re-creating the wheel" and rather start from a foundation of someone else's success. Links to several best practice websites are noted below.

EVIDENCE-BASED PRACTICE WEBSITES

Registries of Programs Effective in Reducing Youth Risk Behaviors

http://www.cdc.gov/healthyyouth/adolescenthealth/registries.htm

HHS Teen Pregnancy Prevention Evidence Review

http://www.hhs.gov/ash/oah/oah-initiatives/teen_pregnancy/db/tpp-searchable.html

National Registry of Evidence-Based Programs and Practices

http://www.nrepp.samhsa.gov/

Healthy People 2020 Evidence-Based Resources

http://www.healthypeople.gov/2020/tools-resources/Evidence-Based-Resources

Research-Tested Intervention Programs

http://rtips.cancer.gov/rtips/index.do

The Guide to Community Preventive Services

http://www.thecommunityguide.org/index.html

Guide to Clinical Preventive Services

http://www.uspreventiveservicestaskforce.org/Home/GetFileByID/989

Promising Practices Network: Programs That Work

http://www.promisingpractices.net/programs.asp

NACCHO Model Practice Search

https://eweb.naccho.org/eweb/DynamicPage.aspx?site=naccho&webcode=mpsearch

Evaluation Reports

An evaluation report is commonly used to report the results of a program evaluation. Evaluation reports are typically provided to funders, program leaders and staff members, and other vested stakeholders. While reports can have different styles, it is important that they provide userfriendly information to the relevant audiences in a timely fashion. The timing of formative or process evaluations is important. Quick feedback during the formative evaluation phase is typically needed to help program staff implement the program or make any needed adjustments to implementation.

In contrast, summative evaluations are typically written and presented at the end of a program year. In some cases, funders will require quarterly or mid-year status reports. In all cases, evaluators and program staff members participating in the evaluation must keep the reporting needs of the stakeholders in mind. The following are basic sections of an evaluation report:

Cover page. At minimum, a cover page will include a *title* for the evaluation, the *date* the report was completed, and the *author* (or authors). Ideally, a reader will know the evaluation's focus and recognize its timeliness after just a quick glance at the cover page. Evaluation photos or organizational logos are often used on the cover page to help convey the evaluation's topic and to spark interest. Contact information or funder information might also be included on the cover.

Table of contents. A single page delineating where each section starts will be useful (especially for longer program evaluation reports).

List of tables or figures. If the report includes tables or figures, it is a nice touch to include the title of each table/figure and the page upon which it will appear in the report. Think of this as the table of contents for tables and figures.

Executive summary. As the name implies, this section summarizes the evaluation report for the "executive," which today really means readers with little time who need to quickly know the main points. Given that this describes the vast majority of people, a well-written executive summary can greatly increase the utility of the report. An executive summary must concisely address the evaluation's purpose, methods, and key findings or recommendations.

Introduction and evaluation questions. This section provides important background information and frames the overall report. The introduction explains why the evaluation was undertaken, by whom, and for whom. In addition, the specific questions the evaluation was designed to address must be clearly stated. The method or approach of an effective evaluation always follows from the question (or questions) that it is trying to answer. Well-defined and compelling questions are essential to a good evaluation report. The introduction also typically provides a description of the program or intervention that is being evaluated.

Methods. The methods section describes how the evaluation was carried out. Typically, the greatest detail pertains to the evaluation design, the sources of information used, and how this information was collected and analyzed. For example, this section will describe how data collection tools such as surveys or in-depth interview guides were constructed and pilot tested, how respondents were selected or sampled, and the analysis techniques that were used.

Results. Evaluation results consist of the presentation of data that were analyzed. It is often helpful to program leaders and stakeholders for the program evaluator to re-state the program's SMART objectives and use the results of data analysis to describe the degree to which the program met its objectives. The use of tables, graphs, and charts in this section is useful to represent the results of data analysis in an easy-to-understand format.

Findings and recommendations. This section describes what was learned through the evaluation. In this section, the answers to the original evaluation questions are given. This section also typically includes acknowledgment of limitations that may have influenced the evaluation's results and findings. Recommendations are the future actions suggested by the findings; this section is tailored to the evaluation's intended principal audience. In the traditional program evaluation paradigm, recommendations were often generated by the external evaluator as his or her "expert" suggestions to the program director and staff members. However, in more participatory evaluation approaches, diverse program stakeholders and direct participants in the program are involved in the development of recommendations based on the findings.

References. Include all references noted throughout evaluation report.

Evaluation reports take different shapes and forms based on the audience for the report and how the report will be used. Aim for a document that is short enough to be read in one sitting at the time it is received or viewed and attractive enough that the reader will want to take time to look through it. If the report is lengthy and visually unappealing, it will likely be thrown on the "to read" pile and may never be read. Often it is helpful to prepare one or two pages of *evaluation highlights* that provide an overview of the evaluation and the significant findings. Always consider how the evaluation findings will be used. Ask what questions the evaluation is answering. Make sure these answers are clearly stated in both the brief evaluation highlights and the full evaluation report. Providing an electronic copy in addition to a hard copy is useful for ease of sharing the results among stakeholders. Furthermore, program evaluators need to be prepared to present the evaluation results to audiences using well designed and attractive visuals (e.g., PowerPoint Presentation).

Implementing an Evaluation

The nuts and bolts of doing an evaluation may include finding and working with an evaluator and dealing with costs, time frame, and participant rights.

Finding and Working with an Evaluator

Most program directors do not have the time, training, personnel resources, or desire to carry out a formal evaluation. Therefore, it is not uncommon for funding agencies (federal, state, and foundations) to require that program directors hire an external, third party, evaluator. An external evaluator may be requested because of potential bias that could be introduced if an agency conducted its own program evaluation. If that were the case, some would likely question the validity of the findings due to potential conflicts of interest. Having program directors or staff members conduct an evaluation of their own programs certainly increases the odds of intentional or unintentional bias being introduced, especially if one's job or funding is riding on the results. Even if a program conducted its own unbiased evaluation, the perception of possible bias would still exist, which would likely jeopardize the effective dissemination of results and limit the organization's ability to seek additional funding based on the findings.

Thus, selecting a program evaluator is an important task for program directors and administrators. A good evaluator provides timely program information to refine and keep a program on track. In addition, a good evaluator accurately documents the program's experiences and effectiveness. This information is useful to a program's stakeholders and for seeking future funding.

The degree to which an evaluator is involved may vary, depending on financial resources, but at a minimum, an evaluator is hired to identify the appropriate evaluation design and methods and how the data is collected and analyzed. Ideally, the program evaluator is brought in prior to the program planning phase so that he/she can assist the program planners with writing high-quality SMART objectives and properly aligning program components with program evaluation components.

Evaluators are found at universities and colleges and through the American Evaluation Association and its network of state and regional affiliates. In addition, some foundations and agencies—such as the W. K. Kellogg Foundation, the Robert Wood Johnson Foundation, and federal and state departments of health and human services—maintain directories of evaluators. Another way to find evaluators is through word of mouth from colleagues who work in similar programs.

Although an evaluator is usually not considered a member of the program staff, he or she is considered an important member of the program team who has various responsibilities. The following list shows a number of the responsibilities of a good evaluator. As part of the budget and contracting process, the amount of time the evaluator will need for each activity would be estimated and planned for in the budget:

- Help program staff and relevant program stakeholders to identify best practices.
- Collect and synthesize past program evaluation results.

- Search for examples of evaluation methods that have been used in similar programs with similar priority populations.

- Collect evaluation tools that have been used in programs identified as best practice.

- Attend program meetings or conference calls.

- Assist program staff and stakeholders with creating strong linkages among and between program mission, goals, SMART objectives, program activities, evaluation measures, and data collection methods.

- Help program staff and relevant program stakeholders design the evaluation.

- Design and pilot test the data collection methods and instruments in collaboration with program staff and key stakeholders.

- Monitor the implementation.

- Oversee the collection of data or collect program data.

- Enter program data into statistical software applications or train program staff to do so.

- Provide oversight of the database, even if program staff may enter the data.

- Analyze the data or subcontract and provide oversight of the analysis.

- Write the evaluation report.

- Present findings to stakeholders.

Evaluation Costs

The cost of a program evaluation is related to a number of factors and typically ranges from 5% to 20% of the program budget (Kellogg Foundation, 1984; Substance Abuse and Mental Health Services Administration, 2015). The lower end of this scale is typically reserved for very large and expensive programs in which the program evaluation is fairly basic. The higher end of the scale is typically reserved for demonstration projects for which program evaluation is one of the primary goals of the funding and is used to determine the effectiveness of the given health promotion program. While a common "rule of thumb" is that 10% of the budget be allocated to program evaluation (Blome, 2009), there is a wide variance based on many factors, including the following:

- The education, experience, and track record of the program evaluator
- The level of technical expertise needed
- The size and complexity of the program being evaluated

- The number of sites in which the program is taking place
- The evaluation design
- The frequency of data collection and analysis
- The program's internal resources and expertise
- Travel needs
- The need to detect small changes in program outcomes

It is important to note that underfunding a program evaluation can lead to a weaker evaluation design or to the hiring of an inexperienced evaluator. Underfunding program evaluation can therefore lead to poor alignment, lack of congruence among program components, and weak outcomes data. This may result in the inability to demonstrate program impact and increased difficulty in obtaining future funding.

Time Frame for Evaluation

If the purpose of evaluation is program improvement, then the evaluation needs to continue as long as the program stakeholders seek to improve the program. *Continuous program improvement* is often the stated purpose of evaluation, and if it is, then evaluation in some form continues as long as the program operates.

However, program evaluations are rarely funded for the life of a program. Sometimes the evaluation is funded for only the first 2 or 3 years of a program, and often this time frame is not long enough for the program to demonstrate some of its longer-term outcomes. Given this reality, programs build evaluation into the program infrastructure in order to ensure a continual flow of information back to the stakeholders.

Ethical Considerations

Health promotion program evaluators engage in their craft considering what is in the best interest of the priority population and the program's key stakeholders. Throughout the evaluation process, the health promotion professional follows the Code of Ethics for the Health Education Profession (Coalition of National Health Education Organizations, 2002). Three articles within the Code of Ethics relate to the development and implementation of a program evaluation:

- Article I: Responsibility to the Public
- Article III: Responsibility to Employers
- Article V: Responsibility in Research and Evaluation. This article describes that health education/promotion professionals conduct

research and evaluation in accordance with federal and state laws and regulations, organizational and institutional policies, and professional standards. It is further broken into seven sections (Coalition of National Health Education Organizations, 2002):

Section 1: Health Educators support principles and practices of research and evaluation that do no harm to individuals, groups, society, or the environment.

Section 2: Health Educators ensure that participation in research is voluntary and is based upon the informed consent of the participants.

Section 3: Health Educators respect the privacy, rights, and dignity of research participants, and honor commitments made to those participants.

Section 4: Health Educators treat all information obtained from participants as confidential unless otherwise required by law.

Section 5: Health Educators take credit, including authorship, only for work they have actually performed and give credit to the contributions of others.

Section 6: Health Educators who serve as research or evaluation consultants discuss their results only with those to whom they are providing service, unless maintaining such confidentiality would jeopardize the health or safety of others.

Section 7: Health Educators report the results of their research and evaluation objectively, accurately, and in a timely fashion.

Additionally, the cultural and social competence of an evaluation is characterized by respect and acceptance of the differences found in diverse communities, whether the differences are related to race, ethnicity, socioeconomic status, sexual orientation, disability, age, gender, or other attributes. Sensitivity to diversity is evidenced by the active involvement of staff that are drawn from the program participants and by continual self-assessment of staff attitudes toward cultural and social differences, in order to eliminate bias.

Summary

Program evaluation is a method of assessing whether a health promotion program is achieving the desired results. Program evaluation involves systematically collecting information in order to answer evaluation questions and make program decisions. Evaluation that is integrated into the overall program design from its inception provides continual information for ongoing program modification and decision making in order to strengthen the program. Finally, as part of implementing a program evaluation, program staff and stakeholders must know how to select an evaluator, determine the evaluation's time frame and costs, and take steps to ensure that participant rights are protected.

For Practice and Discussion

1. Why is it important for program evaluators to be involved with program planners and members of the priority population during the design phase of a health promotion program?

2. Compare and contrast formative and summative evaluation. Provide a scenario as to when you would use each type.

3. Discuss why alignment between program mission, goals, SMART objectives, program activities, evaluation methods, and evaluation instruments is critical to a successful program evaluation. What would be some of the likely consequences if a program's activities were not aligned well with the program's SMART objectives?

4. Compare and contrast quantitative and qualitative methods of program evaluation. Describe a scenario in which each type of method would be useful.

5. Describe how the content of a program's SMART objective drive data collection and data analysis. Provide a specific example.

6. Select two programs from those identified in the "Evidence-Based Practice Websites" list. What are the programs' evaluation designs and methods (for example, instruments, focus groups, or observations)? What evidence of the methods' validity and reliability is stated? How are the evaluation findings reported?

7. You are evaluating a faith-based nutrition and physical activity program that takes place within an African American church congregation. There are 300 participants. As part of the initial program phase, each participant completes a confidential health review that includes a physical examination by a physician, blood cholesterol screening, body mass index measurement, and health risk appraisal. Once participants' names are removed, this information is available to you as the program evaluator.

    - What are the ethical considerations in conducting the evaluation?

    - How will you ensure that the evaluation is culturally competent and culturally acceptable?

    - What types of quantitative and qualitative evaluation measurements will you use and why?

8. You are working with a local hospital to evaluate a program to reduce food insecurity among inner city residents. Describe an evaluation design that you could use if there was a limited budget for evaluation (What kinds of data could be collected? How frequently? How strong of a design would it be?). Describe the differences if the funding permitted a much stronger design.

KEY TERMS

Activities	Mixed methods
Alignment	Needs assessment
CDC evaluation framework	Outcome evaluation
Cultural relevance	PDCA/PDSA cycle
Developmental evaluation	Priority population
Ethics	Process evaluation
Evaluation costs	Program evaluation
Evaluation design	Qualitative methods
Evaluation ethics	Quality Improvement
Evaluation report	Quantitative methods
Formative evaluation	RE-AIM evaluation framework
Goals	Reliability
Impact evaluation	SMART Objectives
Improvement Science	Stakeholder
Measures	Summative evaluation
Mission	Validity

References

Blome, J. M. (2009). *Measuring value: Using program evaluation to understand what's working—Or isn't* [Presentation]. Retrieved from http://publications.nigms.nih.gov/presentations/measuring_value/index.html

Centers for Disease Control and Prevention. (2012). *A framework for program evaluation*. Retrieved from http://www.cdc.gov/eval/framework/index.htm

Coalition of National Health Education Organizations. (2002). Code of ethics for the health education profession. *Health Education & Behavior, 29*(1), 11.

Fagen, M. C., Redman, S. D., Stacks, J., Barrett, V., Thullen, B., Altenor, S., & Neiger, B. L. (2011). Developmental evaluation: Building innovations in complex environments. *Health Promotion Practice, 12*(5): 645–650.

Gaglio, B., & Glasgow, R. E. (2012). Evaluation approaches for dissemination and implementation research. In R. Brownson, G. Colditz, & E. Proctor (Eds.), *Dissemination and implementation research in health* (1st ed., pp. 327–356). New York: Oxford University Press.

Gorenflo, G. & Moran, J. W. (2010). The ABCs of PDCA. Public Health Foundation. Retrieved from: http://www.phf.org/resourcestools/Documents/ABCs_of_PDCA.pdf

Hester, J., Auerbach, J., Seeff, L., Wheaton, J., Brusuelas, K., Singleton, C. (2016). CDC's 6|18 Initiative: Accelerating Evidence into Action. National Academy of Medicine. Retrieved from: http://nam.edu/wp-content/uploads/2016/02/CDCs-618-Initiative-Accelerating-Evidence-into-Action.pdf

Kellogg Foundation. (1984). *W. K. Kellogg Foundation evaluation handbook.* Retrieved from https://www.wkkf.org/resource-directory/resource/2010/w-k-kellogg-foundation-evaluation-handbook

Leeman, J., Sommers, J., Vu, M., Jernigan, J., Payne, G., Thompson. D., . . . Ammerman, A. (2012). An evaluation framework for obesity prevention policy interventions. *Preventing Chronic Disease, 9,* 110322.

Marshall, M., Pronovost, P., Dixon-Woods, M. (2013). Promotion of improvement as a science. *Lancet, 381,* 419–421.

Nimon, K. (2014). Explaining differences between retrospective and traditional pretest self-assessments: Competing theories and empirical evidence. *International Journal of Research & Method in Education, 37*(3), 256–269.

Substance Abuse and Mental Health Services Administration. (2015). *Minimizing evaluation costs.* Retrieved from http://www.samhsa.gov/capt/tools-learning-resources/minimizing-evaluation-costs

Yarbrough, D. B., Shulha, L. M., Hopson, R. K., & Caruthers, F. A. (2011). *The program evaluation standards: A guide for evaluators and evaluation users* (3rd ed.). Thousand Oaks, CA: Sage.

CHAPTER 11

BIG DATA AND HEALTH PROMOTION PROGRAMS

Carl I. Fertman, Joseph A. Dake, and Margaret Wielinski

What Is Big Data?

Big data refers to a set of information and data so large and complex that it becomes difficult to process using conventional database management tools (TechAmerica, 2012). Big data describes large and ever-increasing volumes of data that adhere to the following attributes (Zikopoulos, Eaton, DeRoos, Deutsch, & Lapis, 2012):

Volume—ever-increasing amounts

Velocity—quickly generated

Variety—many different types

Veracity—from trustable sources

In the health and health promotion fields the term *secondary data* has long been used to describe large datasets from which analyses are conducted to explore patterns, trends, and associations. The level of complexity of those datasets can vary. Secondary data already exists because they were collected by someone for another purpose. The data may or may not be directly from the individual or population that is being assessed. The databases typically are composed of data from a large number of individuals, clients, patients, or general population members. The trend to use the term *big data* rather than *secondary data* is due to the creation of related datasets (big data), as compared to separate smaller sets (secondary data) with the same total amount of data, allowing correlations to be found that identify trends in the health of individuals,

LEARNING OBJECTIVES

- Define big data for health promotion programs.

- Describe how big data can enhance the impact and sustainability of health promotion programs.

- Present health promotion program big data challenges.

- Discuss health information management and health informatics professionals.

prevent diseases, organize health promotion activities, and determine and improve program outcomes.

Big data for health promotion programs is the combination of all of the varied datasets that are now available to access. Together they create big data that is analyzed as part of health promotion program planning needs assessment processes as well as program evaluation.

Big data is grouped into two categories. *Structured data* is found in existing databases with defined labels and values. In the field of health promotion, this can include primary and secondary health databases, some fields of the electronic health record, biometric data, and utilization data.

Unstructured data is data that does not reside in this standard column and row style of format. Some examples of unstructured data include text heavy documents such as emails, multimedia files, notes within the electronic health record, medical claims, tweets, webpages, reports, and many more. It is estimated that 80% of all data is unstructured (Holzinger, et al., 2013).

The explosion of social media options has increased the availability of potential datasets that could be analyzed: data from Twitter, Facebook, Pinterest, Tumblr, Instagram; location-based data such as Swarm, Foursquare, Uber; and many more. With nearly two-thirds of Americans owning smartphones in 2015 and that number growing rapidly, social media and smartphone data significantly increase the amount of unstructured data that could potentially be available for analysis (Smith, 2015).

In addition to categorizing data as structured or unstructured, data sources are also categorized as internal and external.

Internal Sources of Secondary Data

Working in a particular setting may have the advantage of allowing the use of internal sources of secondary data. All organizations collect information in the course of their everyday operations. Attendance rates, performance scores (grades, annual tests), number of sick days taken, production statistics, sales figures, and expenses are some of the data that might be available. Health data that are collected as a by-product of health services—for example, clinic records, data from immunization programs, data from water pollution control programs, clinical indicators, or data from health office visits and insurance claims—are possible internal sources of secondary data. Much of this information is of potential use in planning and evaluating a health promotion program. Even being aware of people's work schedules or amounts of vacation and sick days might be important in order to know when people work and when they would be available to participate in a program.

External Sources of Secondary Data

Large numbers of organizations provide health data, including national and local government agencies, trade associations, universities, research institutes, financial institutions, specialist suppliers of secondary marketing data, and professional health policy research centers. The main external sources of secondary information are government (federal, state, and local), voluntary health associations, private foundations, national and international institutions, professional associations, and universities. Table 11.1 shows sources of publicly available secondary data.

A series of changes and trends have created the opportunity to use big data in health promotion programs (Figure 11.1). The *demand for big data* is high. Fiscal concerns, perhaps more than any other factor, are driving the demand for big data applications. Huge cost pressure is fueled by a desire for health care system reform, economic growth, and health service delivery innovation. Analyzing and using the data is seen as a means to maximize public health resources and improve the health outcomes of individuals by designing and evaluating health promotion programs that are well matched to the needs of the individuals served by the programs.

Table 11.1 Publicly Available Health-Related External Sources of Secondary Data

Behavioral Risk Factor Surveillance System	http://www.cdc.gov/brfss/data_documentation/index.htm
Community Commons	(http://www.communitycommons.org/)
General Social Survey	https://gssdataexplorer.norc.org/
Health Care Cost and Utilization Data	http://www.ahrq.gov/research/data/hcup/index.html
Henry A. Murray Research Archive	https://dataverse.harvard.edu/dataverse/mra
Joint Canada/United States Survey of Health	http://www.cdc.gov/nchs/nhis/jcush.htm
Medical Expenditures Panel Survey	http://meps.ahrq.gov/mepsweb/
National Ambulatory Medical Care Survey and the National Hospital Ambulatory Medical Care Survey	http://www.cdc.gov/nchs/ahcd/ahcd_questionnaires.htm
National Health and Nutrition Examination Survey	http://www.cdc.gov/nchs/nhanes/nhanes_questionnaires.htm
National Health Interview Survey	http://www.cdc.gov/nchs/nhis/nhis_questionnaires.htm
National Hospital Discharge Survey	http://www.cdc.gov/nchs/nhds/nhds_questionnaires.htm
National Immunization Survey	http://www.cdc.gov/nchs/nis/datasets.htm
National Survey of Children's Health	http://childhealthdata.org/learn/NSCH
National Survey of Family Growth	http://www.cdc.gov/nchs/nsfg/nsfg_questionnaires.htm
National Survey on Drug Use and Health	http://www.samhsa.gov/data/population-data-nsduh/reports
Pregnancy Risk Assessment Monitoring System	http://www.cdc.gov/prams/researchers.htm
Surveillance Epidemiology and End Results Program	http://seer.cancer.gov/data/
U.S. Census	http://www.census.gov/data.html
Youth Risk Behavior Surveillance System	http://www.cdc.gov/healthyyouth/data/yrbs/data.htm

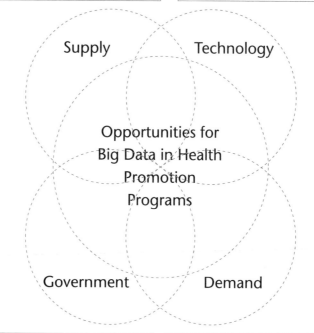

Supply of relevant data at scale, for example:

- Health program and population data accessible with electronic health records and information exchanges
- Community, workplace, and school data are increasingly aggregated and accessible

Technical capability, for example:

- Significant advances in the ability to combine claims and clinical data and protect patient privacy
- Analytical tools now user friendly and widely available

Supply   Technology

Opportunities for Big Data in Health Promotion Programs

Government   Demand

Government market change, for example:

- Continued commitment to making data publicly available
- Government is encouraging private and public sector groups to create and use compatible standards and systems

Demand for better data, for example:

- Huge cost pressure is fueled by health care system reform, economic growth, and health service delivery innovation
- Analyzing and using data to maximize public health resources and improve the health outcomes

Figure 11.1   Recent Changes and Trends Have Created the Opportunity to Use Big Data in Health Promotion Programs

Source: Adapted from Kayyali, Knott, and Van Kuiken, 2013.

Three factors in particular have contributed to the demand for big data in health promotion programs: supply, technology, and government. A dramatic increase in the supply of data is due to incentives for electronic health record (EHR) adoption in the United States funded by the Health Information Technology for Economic and Clinical Health (HITECH) Act that have pushed health care records that are accessible to users. Likewise increasingly aggregated health data and indicators are available for communities, workplaces, and schools.

The recent technical advances have made it easier to collect and analyze information from multiple sources. Health care systems and insurance companies have digitized records, and pharmaceutical companies have been aggregating years of research and development data into databases. Analytical tools are now user friendly and available and allow wider access and use of the health care system data as well as data from school districts, public health agencies, and human services.

Finally, the U.S. federal government and other public health stakeholders have been opening their vast stores of health care knowledge, including data from public health departments, clinical trials, and information on individuals covered under public insurance programs. At the same time the federal government is encouraging private and public sector groups to create and use compatible programming standards and computer operating systems to increase data use.

Data Mining with Health Promotion Big Data

With the wealth of data that is readily available, the challenge has become how to use data for meaningful insights. *Data mining* is the processing and modeling of large amounts of data to discover previously unknown patterns or relationships (Bellazzi & Zupan, 2008). For example epidemiologists are using combinations of large data sources to examine retail sales data of over-the-counter medications, public health department reports, and tweets sent within a geographic region to better detect infectious disease outbreaks. Behavioral scientists now have access to data from wearable technology that measures fitness, sleep, heart rate, and stress. Natural disasters are being better understood with cell phone data and satellite imagery used to track population movement. The possibilities seem nearly endless.

Because of the surge in the use of big data in the health and health promotion fields, the Institute of Medicine and the Department of Health and Human Services hosted a 2010 gathering of leaders from government agencies, academia, health care settings, social service agencies, and businesses called the Community Health Data Forum. The purpose was to discuss methods to harness the power of information to improve health. This initiative has grown into what is now an annual conference called Health Datapalooza. This is to further development of a strong health data ecosystem to promote innovative use of health data to improve health and health care.

The focus on big data was further supported in 2012 with the Obama administration announcing the launch of a "Big Data Research and Development Initiative" with $200 million in funding through six federal agencies.

The National Institute of Health, through their Big Data to Knowledge (BD2K) initiative is projected to spend nearly $656 million through 2020 focused on development of systems and a trained workforce in biomedical, behavioral, and clinical fields to use big data to enhance the public's health (https://datascience.nih.gov/bd2k).

Sophisticated software allows analysts to sort, combine, and contrast key data elements to help decision makers and program managers take effective actions. Tools such as the National Committee for Quality Assurance's (NCQA) *Healthcare Effectiveness Data and Information Set* (HEDIS) are used in the mining process. HEDIS consists of 75 measures across eight domains of care. Using HEDIS it is now possible to mine the various data sets available to health promotion programs to help uncover problems and focus on areas for improvement. Kirby, Kersting, and Flick (2010) identified seven examples of how data mining is used to evaluate health promotion programs in the workplace by focusing on data now available from health insurance providers to employers.

1. **Determine what diseases and conditions are driving trends.** This entails reviewing an organization's medical and prescription drug claims data to verify which health issues are most prevalent among employees and their families. Using this information, the employer can then tailor the health promotion program to help employees adopt healthier behaviors and reduce costs.

2. **Focus interventions to high-risk segments of the workers and those who need the most care.** Reviewing the severity of employees' diseases and conditions will identify those who have complex needs and require significant care management. The interventions' goals include reducing the rate of hospital readmission and directing care to high-quality, low-cost network providers.

3. **Identify gaps in medical treatment and direct employees to the proper care.** Gaps are discovered by comparing employees' data to HEDIS benchmarks. Where possible, employees and their primary-care physicians are encouraged to reduce or eliminate those gaps.

4. **Identify the best, most cost-effective network providers and guide employees to use them.** Data mining can, for example, pinpoint high-performance, high-quality providers and services. It can also identify providers that offer access to appropriate care and interventions that follow evidence-based guidelines. Workplace health promotion programs can then promote the use of these providers and services by employees who need care.

5. **Improve health habits through wellness, health promotion, education, and care-management programs that increase awareness and engage employees in their own care.** Using data mining, a health promotion program plan can determine if its benefit design is effective in promoting wellness and prevention. The result might be the design of a multifaceted, incentive-based plan that includes design, vendor performance, communications, and incentives that help manage costs.

6. **Measure the performance of vendors and administrators and hold them accountable for quality, cost-effective treatment by comparing their results to national benchmarks.** Health promotion programs can implement performance guarantees for the plan's financial, clinical, operational, and utilization components. For example, utilization performance guarantees can help manage emergency room visits for chronic conditions, such as asthma.

7. **Determine what level of cost sharing improves employee health and cuts costs.** One organization that had an upfront deductible and a copayment for office visits decided to try eliminating both. The next year virtually every employee visited his or her primary care physician and specialists, which doubled the plan's physician and specialist visit rates per 1,000 employees. This improved employee health and reduced long-term costs. The key is to be sure that cost sharing encourages appropriate usage. For example, in a recent study of individuals (employees) who self-referred, 61% visited the wrong specialist. If cost sharing is structured to encourage individuals to visit a primary care physician first, they will select appropriate specialists, which will cut costs and improve results.

Overlaying multiple levels of data such as the seven items with data from other institutions and organizations within a geographical area (e.g., hospital or clinic locations, schools, grocery stores, etc.) can provide a picture of the health concerns that can assist to create and sustain a multipronged (socio-ecological) strategy of interventions and public advocacy to address health concerns that span individuals across sites (e.g., schools, workplace, community, family).

As part of data mining, *visual mapping* of health and community data has grown tremendously in popularity as a vehicle to decipher multiple sources of big data into meaningful outcomes to promote health. Data that has a geographic indicator such as address, census tract, or zip code are used to examine patterns to better understand health issues within a community. This could be mapping existing grocery stores in a large city and combining that with food insecurity data from a local health care system to examine readmission rates based on food insecurity and the proximity to a grocery store. Figure 11.2 illustrates the use of mapping to analyze food deserts in Chicago (Gallagher, 2006). This combination of multiple data sources placed into a visual map can help to examine patterns, find spatial relationships, make predictions based on that data, and develop intervention strategies to address the problem. This same data in tabular form or represented individually would not be as functional or impactful. Mapping software provides users the opportunity to develop maps with multiple layers including social determinants of health (demographic characteristics, poverty, health care coverage or access, racial/ethnic distribution, home types); health system utilization; health insurance claims data; school level data (truancy, dropout, test scores); behavioral surveys; employment or job training data; and anything else in which data is collected with some indication of location.

The level of sophistication needed to use mapping software can vary greatly. This software cannot simply import any kind of data and with drop down menus generate visually appealing maps. The data may need to be converted or manipulated in order to make it functional and this process is complicated depending on the data. This can require training that many in the field of health promotion do not get. However, there are online tools that are used with greater ease even though the power of the tool or flexibility of the tool may not be as great.

Health promotion professionals have an ever-increasing number of online tools that have multiple large datasets as their core. The following tools are examples that are used to demonstrate relationships or patterns and to allow merged data comparisons.

County Health Rankings and Roadmaps

The County Health Rankings and Roadmaps (http://www.countyhealth rankings.org/) were developed out of a partnership between the Robert Wood Johnson Foundation and the University of Wisconsin Population Health Institute. The purpose is to combine multiple data sources (National Vital Statistics, Behavioral Risk Factor Surveillance System, health care quality measures) to help compare a given county to others. This ranking system can help local health leaders to prioritize efforts and to add justification for programming or grant writing.

Community Commons

The Community Commons (www.communitycommons.org) is an interactive GIS mapping, networking, and learning utility. It is constantly

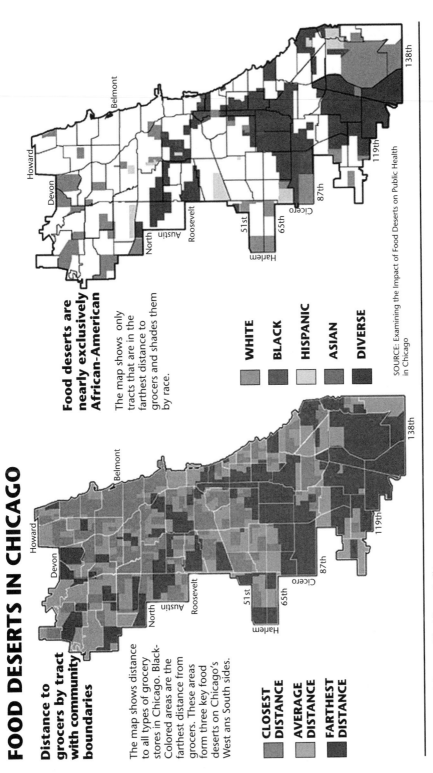

FOOD DESERTS IN CHICAGO

Distance to grocers by tract with community boundaries

The map shows distance to all types of grocery stores in Chicago. Black-Colored areas are the farthest distance from grocers. These areas form three key food deserts on Chicago's West ans South sides.

CLOSEST DISTANCE

AVERAGE DISTANCE

FARTHEST DISTANCE

Food deserts are nearly exclusively African-American

The map shows only tracts that are in the farthest distance to grocers and shades them by race.

WHITE

BLACK

HISPANIC

ASIAN

DIVERSE

SOURCE: Examining the Impact of Food Deserts on Public Health in Chicago

Figure 11.2 Visual Mapping of Food Deserts in Chicago

Source: Gallagher, 2006.

283

expanding with additional data and user-generated tables and maps that are downloaded and changed to reflect a different community of interest. There are numerous databases with information that falls into the following categories: economic, educational, environment, equity, food, and health. These are easily explored using tabular or mapping methods.

Network of Care

Network of Care (http://www.networkofcare.org/splash.aspx) developed out of a partnership between the National Association of County and City Health Officials and NAC to provide local health professionals with tools and data to help promote the health of the community. This includes *Healthy People 2020* indicators, county healthy rankings, death data, population health data, and various health indicators. These data are broken into subgroups and can show the data reported over time. Network of Care also includes CDC effective interventions that are linked to all of the indicators, published articles on the topics, assessments, tests, treatments, medications, action points, support groups, and other resources that would benefit someone in health promotion working in that community. This system is not available in every state, but the number of included states is growing.

Health Landscape

Health Landscape (https://www.healthlandscape.org/) is an online tool to develop maps from publicly available datasets including education, health care, criminal justice, and demographic data. Combining health, socioeconomic, and environmental, and health information allows the user to explore relationships and present combined information in a way that is more meaningful to the reader.

Big Data Enhances the Impact and Sustainability of Health Promotion Programs

Big data enhances the impact and sustainability of health promotion programs by integrating a growing quantity of varied data sources, along with methods to analyze and put it to use, which can lead to improved personal health, health care delivery, and effective health promotion programs. Adams and Klein (2011) suggested three *levels of analytics* to use for health promotion program evaluations, each with increasing functionality and value:

1. **Descriptive**: Standard types of reporting that describe current situations and problems

2. **Predictive**: Simulation and modeling techniques that identify trends and portend outcomes of actions taken

3. **Prescriptive**: Prescribing actions to optimize programmatic, financial, and other outcomes

In particular, health promotion program evaluations use big data predictive and prescriptive analytics as a way to maximize resources and outcomes. To help stakeholders think about the power of big data in the evaluation of health promotion programs, Kayyali et al. (2013) created five evaluation objectives (*pathways*) to guide predictive and prescriptive analyses. Their goal is to produce practical data for stakeholders to use to make decisions about their health promotion program that support individuals' right living, right care, right provider, right value, and right innovation.

1. **Right living.** Individuals must be encouraged to play an active role in their own health by making the right choices about diet, exercise, preventive care, and other lifestyle factors.

2. **Right care.** Individuals must receive the most timely, appropriate health promotion programs and treatment available. In addition to relying heavily on protocols, right care requires a coordinated approach, with all health providers having access to the same information and working toward the same goal to avoid duplication of effort and suboptimal health promotion programs and treatment strategies.

3. **Right provider.** Any health professionals who serve individuals must have strong performance records and be capable of achieving the best outcomes. They need to be selected based on their skill sets and abilities rather than their job titles. For instance, nurses or physicians' assistants may perform many tasks that do not require a doctor.

4. **Right value.** Stakeholders (including program participants, staff and health care professionals and organizations, and community programs) need to continually look for ways to improve value while preserving or improving program quality.

5. **Right innovation.** Stakeholders must focus on identifying new health promotion programs and approaches to program and service delivery. They need to try to improve the innovation engines themselves—for instance, by advancing the offerings of range and types of health promotion programs.

One of the characteristics of big data is that new data is continually becoming available, creating a feedback loop. The concept of right care, for instance, could change if new data suggest that the standard protocol for a particular health promotion intervention does not produce optimal results. And a change in one pathway could spur changes in others, since they are interdependent. An evaluation, for example, could reveal that individuals are most likely to suffer costly complications after back surgery, therefore encouraging more effective and less costly alternative treatments. This finding could influence opinions not only about value but also about the health professionals selected to address musculoskeletal pain and injuries among individuals.

Big Data Challenges

Although the potential value of big data to evaluate health promotion programs is large, *challenges* do exists (Institute for Health Technology Transformation, 2013; Savel & Foldy, 2012). These include integration of disparate sources, consistency/standardization (defined similarly through-out the organization), data fragmentation, trustworthiness (confidence in the data), protection (security of the data), rapid expansion of big data applications, and legal and ethical issues with big data. The challenges highlight a critical need for health promotion program staff and evaluators to understand the data's provenance (i.e., to know the data's origin and purpose) so as to understand its potential contribution and role in any big data processing and analysis.

Integration of Disparate Sources

The sources of big data vary in a number of ways. For example, some data will come from systems that use older technology and software that may or may not be compatible with newer technologies and techniques. In many cases, organizations don't have easy options to upgrade or otherwise adapt their technologies to growing data demands. Organizations are struggling with such questions as how best to determine the value of their data, how to store their data, and how and when to delete and/or archive their data. Related to this is the timeliness or freshness of data at the point of it being used as part of the evaluation. For example, if program participant turnover is high, is it reasonable to make programmatic decisions based on program participants who might not be part of the organization? Finally, understanding how the data is simplified and reduced is important to be able to draw meaningful conclusions and make recommendations.

Consistency/Standardization

Often data is not defined similarly across organizations and even throughout the same organization. For example it might be coded (transformed) for a particular purpose such as for billing. Inaccurate or incomplete data requires having data checked and rechecked before it is used, which is labor and time intensive. Data can exhibit the statistical phenomenon of censoring. For example the first instance of a health concern in a record may not be when it was first manifested (left censoring) or the data source may not cover a sufficiently long time interval (right censoring). Data may also incompletely adhere to well-known standards, which makes combining it from different sources more difficult (Hersh et al., 2013).

Data Fragmentation

The separation, or fragmentation, of data among community organizations, health promotion programs, health systems, public health agencies, and schools, is another significant obstacle to leveraging big data for health promotion. Each entity serves as a single repository, or silo, for information whose purpose is to provide programs, clinical care, scheduling or billing information, or operational information. This continues to be problematic for organizations seeking to get individual systems to communicate with each other easily. It remains especially challenging in smaller organizations with multiple systems and taxonomies that make extracting useful information difficult. The overall result is that organizations end up with little pieces of data from various sources that make it hard to understand how everything fits together.

Trustworthiness

Data trustworthiness or confidence in the data is a major challenge especially with respect to making program and clinical decisions. Most clinical data is stored in "unstructured" form, especially within program notes and EHRs, making it difficult to access for effective analytics. For example, individual providers can read narrative text within a record or report, but most current analytics applications cannot effectively utilize this unstructured data. Most program analytics rely on claims or administrative data. This data consists largely of more structured data but is of limited value in evaluating the efficacy of services and program outcomes (Amarasingham et al., 2010). Emerging big data technology and techniques show promise in helping organizations to process and evaluate data from records, clinic equipment, telehealth devices, and home health monitors.

Protection

Health promotion programs need to diligently focus on protecting and securing four types of data (Ascenzo, 2013; Institute for Health Technology Transformation, 2013).

1. **Personally identifiable information.** The loss of personally identifiable information such as dates of birth, driver's license numbers, and social security numbers is among the greatest of privacy threats. While external threats dominate top-of-mind discussions, information breaches are growing, presenting the potential for significant loss of program participants, incurrence of high compensation claims lawsuits, and permanent damage to reputation.

2. **Clinical data.** Program and electronic health records contain a wide range of individual specific information, including participation, prescription data, service reports, treatment details, and other data. Combined with a policy number, a hacker can use it to receive unauthorized medical care or bill for services never received. The leakage and/or corruption of such information can even result in irrevocable harm to one's personal and professional life.

3. **Financial data.** With banks and individuals getting more proactive about protecting their financial information, the medical industry is becoming an easy target for hackers. The outsourcing of billing activities and increased Internet and mobile involvement in health care create more avenues for potential data theft; the resulting legal consequences and loss of patient trust can taint an organization's brand for life.

4. **Behavioral data.** Behavioral data is the newest and possibly fastest growing in health care, thanks to monitoring devices, GPS tracking, Internet site visits, social media, purchasing habits, exercise activity, and self-reporting. Behavioral data is increasingly becoming the "hot favorite" for cyber thieves as it helps to draw up startlingly accurate representations of human behavior that are of great demand among marketing companies (and also others with illicit intentions). With growing usage of tablets, smartphones, and other mobile devices, this data is becoming more vulnerable to theft.

Rapid Expansion of Big Data Applications

The rapid expansion of big data applications is a challenge for health promotion programs. Accompanying each new big data application development and upgrade are periods of learning about it and determining how to best use it. At the same time pressure exists to use big data to address real health needs and concerns of people. However, the results of this pressure are not always beneficial. For example the Google Flu Project used aggregate Google search queries to estimate influenza trends in multiple countries. The project received early praise because this method was able to more quickly predict flu outbreaks compared to traditional methods. However, subsequent analyses found that there were accuracy problems with the data, and now Google no longer publishes current estimates for flu outbreaks (Walsh, 2014).

Legal and Ethical Issues with Big Data

In the past decade, increased public awareness of professional behavior, coupled with the passage of federal and state legislation controlling the helping professions, has underscored the importance of ethical concerns in health promotion programs. These concerns extend to the use of big data to plan and evaluate health promotion programs. As part of ethical codes for health professionals, increasing attention is now being placed on data use and overuse. For example, using data for other than intended purposes and running analyses for the sake of having data without any clear intent or evaluation questions.

Health Information Management and Health Informatics Professionals: Big Data Professional Fields

In the evaluation of health promotion programs the professionals who work with big data are individuals trained in the fields of health information management and health informatics. Both terms are often used interchangeably even though they are quite different.

Health information management is the accumulation, storage, and accuracy of health data. It is the management of personal health information in hospitals, health care organizations, health insurance providers, and public health programs enabling the delivery of quality services to the public. There is no implication of use of the data beyond viewing individual data records in a digital-based manner. It is simply the access of information. Health information management deals largely with individual-related data. It is responsible for the accumulation, storage and accuracy of individual data (e.g., an individual's program and medical records); it operates the domain of medical records, billing and data regulatory compliance; and it focuses on records management, terminology, coding, transcription, and the business of health care related to medical records management.

Health informatics is a much newer term in the public health and health care industries, and grounded in the history of business intelligence. Health informatics is the utilization of information technologies and information management tactics to enhance process efficiency and reduce costs. Health informatics applies the data gathered and stored through health information management systems and creates knowledge. Health informatics is concerned with the manipulation of organization-wide data to generate reports on outcomes, utilization, and cost to improve program (health promotion) quality and achieve better health care and health outcomes for individuals, families, and communities. It leverages computer systems to help analyze and manage individuals' data. Health informatics professionals have a foundation and background in information infrastructure and architecture, with a focus on database design and programming, information systems design standards and analysis—health systems organization plus the business of health care systems computer information systems.

Increasingly, health information management professionals have been playing a role in health promotion programs and services through their focus on the collection, maintenance, and use of quality data to support the information-intensive and information-reliant health promotion programs and health care systems. They work with clinical, epidemiological, demographic, financial, reference, and coded health care data. Health information administrators plan information systems, develop health policy, and identify current and future information needs. In addition, they apply the science of informatics to the collection, storage, use, and transmission of information. Greater access to data has had a positive impact on health promotion programs. The data helps put preventive plans in place, watch for changes in a certain geographic sites or with demographic groups, as well as report information of interest to the public.

Health information management and health informatics have changed with the increased demand for big data (Figure 11.1), but their main goal is still to analyze, manage, and utilize the information that is essential to individuals' health and ensure that health promotion programs and services can access the information when necessary. Some of the main subdisciplines of health informatics include: biomedical informatics, medical informatics, clinical informatics, nursing informatics, pharmacy informatics, public health informatics, business informatics, and health information management.

Key Health Information Management and Health Informatics Terms

Algorithm. The process for carrying out a complex task, which is broken down into simple decision and action steps. Often assists the *requirements analysis* process carried out before programming.

Clinical data system. Any information system concerned with the capture, processing, or communication of individual (employee) data.

Clinical decision tool. Any mechanical, paper, or electronic aid that collects or processes data from an individual patient to generate output that aids clinical decisions during the doctor-patient encounter. Examples include *decision support systems*, paper or computer *reminders* and *checklists*, which are potentially useful tools in *public health informatics*, as well as other branches of medical informatics.

Consumer health informatics. The use of *medical informatics* methods to facilitate the study and development of paper or electronic systems that support public access to and use of health and lifestyle information.

Decision support system (computer decision aid). A type of *clinical decision tool*: a computer system that uses two or more items of *patient data* to generate case specific or encounter specific advice. An example is a computer risk assessor to estimate cardiovascular disease risk. Evidence-adaptive decision support systems are a type of decision aid with a knowledge base that is constructed from and continually adapts to new research-based and practice-based evidence.

Decision tree. A way to model a complex decision process as a tree with branches representing all possible intermediate states or final outcomes of an event. The probabilities of each intermediate state or final outcome and the perceived utilities of each are combined to attach expected utilities to each outcome.

Individual health record. The primary legal record documenting the health care services provided to a person in any aspect of the health care system. The term includes routine clinical or office records, records of care in any health-related setting, preventive care, lifestyle evaluation, research protocols, and various clinical databases. This repository of information about a single patient is generated by health care professionals as a direct result of interaction with a patient or with individuals who have personal knowledge of the patient.

Primary record. The record that is used by health care professionals while providing care services to review individuals' data or document their own observations, actions, or instructions.

Secondary record. A record that is derived from the primary record and contains selected data elements to aid nonclinical persons in supporting, evaluating, and advancing individual care. Individual care support refers to administration, regulation, and payment functions.

Summary

Big data is used in health promotion programs. Big data refers to a set of information and data so large and complex that it becomes difficult to process using conventional database management tools. Big data is both structured and unstructured and is categorized as internal and external. The demand for big data in health promotion is created by three factors: supply, technology, and government. Data mining is used for processing and modeling of big data to discover previously unknown patterns or relationships. As part of data mining visual mapping of health and community data has increased as a vehicle to decipher multiple sources of big data into meaningful outcomes to promote health. Three levels of analytics are used to enhance the impact and sustainability of health promotion programs each with increasing functionality and value: descriptive, predictive, and prescriptive. And although the potential value of big data for health promotion programs is large, challenges do exist. The professionals who work with big data in health promotion programs are individuals trained in the fields of health information management and health informatics.

For Practice and Discussion

1. What are examples of structured and unstructured big data that is used to plan and evaluate health promotion programs? How does the data differ based on the program site (e.g., workplace, community organization, county public health agency, school, hospital)?

2. Compare and contrast the four visual mapping tools listed in the chapter: County Health Rankings and Roadmaps; Community Commons; Network of Care; and Health Landscape. How would you use them based on a program site (e.g., workplace, community organization, county public health agency, school, hospital)?

3. Propose evaluation questions using the five pathways (right living, right care, right provider, right value, right innovation) suggested by Kayyali and others (2013), which could be used to guide data mining as part of a health promotion program evaluation.

4. Seven challenges exist for using big data in health promotion programs: integration of disparate sources, consistency/standardization (defined similarly throughout organization), data fragmentation, trustworthiness (confidence in the data), protection (security of the data), rapid expansion of big data applications, and legal and ethical issues with big data. The challenges cause program participants to mistrust and resist using the results generated from big data analyses. How do you expect

health information management and health informatics professionals to address the challenges and overcome program participants mistrust and resistance?

5. Algorithms are key in big data for analyzing the health information. In plain language what is an algorithm? What is the relationship between algorithms and data mining?

KEY TERMS

Big data	Levels of analytics
Big data challenges	Pathways of evaluation
Data mining	Secondary data
Demand for big data	Structured data
Health informatics	Unstructured data
Health information management	Visual mapping
Healthcare Effectiveness Data and Information Set (HEDIS)	

References

Adams, J., & Klein, J. (2011). *Business intelligence and analytics in health care—A primer*. Washington, DC: The Advisory Board Company.

Amarasingham, R., Moore, B. J., Tabak, Y. P., Drazner, M. H., Clark, C. A., Zhang, S., . . . Halm, E. A. (2010). An automated model to identify heart failure patients at risk for 30-day readmission or death using electronic medical record data. *Medical Care, 48*(11), 981–988.

Ascenzo, C. (2013). 4 big data threats health org's are socially obligated to safeguard against. Retrieved from http://www.govhealthit.com/blog/4-big-data-threats-health-org%E2%80%99s-are-socially-obligated-safeguard-against

Bellazzi, R., & Zupan, B. (2008). Predictive data mining in clinical medicine: Current issues and guidelines. *International Journal of Medical Informatics, 77*(2), 81–97.

Gallagher, M. (2006). *Examining the impact of food deserts on public health in Chicago*. Retrieved from http://marigallagher.com/projects/4/

Hersh, W. R., Weiner, M. G., Embi, P. J., Logan, J. R., Payne, P. R., Bernstam, E. V., . . . Cimino, J. J. (2013). Caveats for the use of operational electronic health record data in comparative effectiveness research. *Medical Care, 51*, S30–S37.

Holzinger, A., Stocker, C., Ofner, B., Prohaska, G., Brabenetz, A., & Hofmann-Wellenhof, R. (2013). "Combining HCI, natural language processing, and knowledge discovery—Potential of IBM content analytics as an assistive technology in the biomedical field." In A. Holzinger and G. Pasi (Eds.), *Human-computer interaction and knowledge discovery in complex, unstructured, big data. Lecture notes in computer science* (pp. 13–24). doi:10.1007/978-3-642-39146-0

Institute for Health Technology Transformation. (2013). *Transforming health care through big data strategies for leveraging big data in the health care industry.* Retrieved from http://ihealthtran.com/wordpress/2013/03/iht2-releases-big-data-research-report-download-today/

Kayyali, B., Knott, D., & Van Kuiken, S. (2013). *The big-data revolution in US health care: Accelerating value and innovation.* Retrieved from http://www.mckinsey.com/insights/health_systems_and_services/the_big-data_revolution_in_us_health_care

Kirby, M., Kersting, M., & Flick, E. (2010). The benefits of digging deeper: Using data mining to improve employee health and reduce employer costs. *Perspectives, 18*(2). Retrieved from https://chca.memberclicks.net/assets/documents/CCA%20Resources%20-%20The%20Benefits%20of%20Digging%20Deeper.pdf

Savel, T. G., & Foldy, S. (2012). The role of public health informatics in enhancing public health surveillance. *MMWR Surveillance Summary, 61,* 20–24.

Smith, A. (2015). *U.S. smartphone use in 2015.* Retrieved from http://www.pewinternet.org/files/2015/03/PI_Smartphones_0401151.pdf

TechAmerica Foundation. (2012). *Demystifying big data: A practical guide to transforming the business of government.* Retrieved from http://www.techamerica.org/Docs/fileManager.cfm?f=techamerica-bigdatareport-final.pdf

Walsh, B. (2014, March 13). Google's flu project shows the failings of big data. *Time.* Retrieved from http://time.com/23782/google-flu-trends-big-data-problems/

Zikopoulos, P. C., Eaton, C., DeRoos, D., Deutsch, T., & Lapis, G. (2012). *Understanding big data.* New York, NY: McGraw-Hill.

CHAPTER 12

LEADERSHIP FOR CHANGE AND SUSTAINABILITY

Sara L. Cole and David A. Sleet

Catalyzing and Mastering Change

Health promotion programs are designed to promote *change* that improves health. The varied strategies facilitate change, whether it be changes in individual behaviors, policies, or environmental conditions that foster health. People's health is influenced on multiple levels, including the intrapersonal, interpersonal, and population levels, creating the potential for employing many interventions simultaneously (Chapter 1, Table 1.1). The intrapersonal level focuses on individual behaviors, knowledge, attitudes, beliefs, and personality traits. The interpersonal level deals with interactions between and among people—for example, families, friends, and peers. The population level includes institutional factors, social factors, and public policies. Institutional factors are rules, regulations, policies, or informal structures that constrain or promote healthy behaviors. Social factors include social networks and norms among individuals, groups, and organizations. Public policy includes local, state, and federal policies and laws that regulate or support disease prevention practices, including early detection, disease control, and disease management. Focusing on these multiple levels in planning for change is often referred to as taking an ecological approach (Allegrante et al., 2010; Stokols, 1996).

Taking an ecological approach to health promotion presents intervention opportunities that range from promoting changes in individuals' behavior to advocating for changes in social policy and the environment (Liberman & Earp, 2015). At the same time, programs often need to be ready to change directions or strategies quickly to keep up

LEARNING OBJECTIVES

- Explain catalyzing and mastering change to build resources and capacity, including effective leadership.

- Discuss the benefits and process of engaging participants and building support.

- Discuss professional preparation and practice of health education and health promotion professionals through continuing education and credentialing.

- Describe implementation science and its importance to health promotion intervention success.

- Describe how to enhance the impact and sustainability of health promotion programs.

with emerging trends and health and social needs. For health promotion programs, mastering change is a process of supporting and engaging people and resources in the context of an evolving and dynamic environment. This may require enhancing program staff members' skills, finding and developing new networks, and improving the measurement of program outcomes and impacts (Batras, Duff, & Smith, 2014). Increasingly, health promotion programs are also being asked to ensure that the delivery of services are equitable or culturally relevant and that users are "satisfied" with the program.

McKenzie, Neiger, and Thackeray (2009) identified six realities that complicate the ability of health promotion programs to be flexible and agile in their response to change:

1. **Health status can be changed, but it requires hard work and patience**. Health promotion programs contribute to the health of environments, individuals, families, communities, workplaces, and organizations, but it takes time; change is hard work. Addressing health problems is more like a marathon than a short-distance sprint. One example is that it took over 200 years to eradicate smallpox from the earth, and that was after the vaccine had been discovered. While health promotion programs may focus on individual change, important changes in policies, laws, social norms, consumer products, and environments will be necessary to keep everyone safe and healthy.

2. **Building consensus that shapes health promotion programs takes time**. One person does not determine the success of a health promotion program; rather, health promotion programs are the result of input from different groups and individuals—for example, stakeholders, practitioners, and the priority population. The name for this process is *consensus building*: the process of achieving general agreement among program participants and stakeholders about a particular problem, goal, or issue of mutual interest. It is best when it can occur in an environment of frank and honest discussion aimed at hearing and addressing people's concerns. Collaboration with and support of all stakeholders maximizes the process. Engaging stakeholders can facilitate desired environmental changes; however, reaching consensus among these groups often requires compromises—for example, other needs of the target population may need to be met before program goals can be accomplished.

3. **Stakeholder engagement is critical**. Throughout this book the importance of stakeholder engagement has been emphasized. Program participants and staff are key stakeholders, but so are family members

of participants, funders, colleagues, other individuals at a program site, government officials, labor unions, health care groups, or schools, to name a few. Identifying and engaging all the stakeholders can be difficult, but it is critical. It requires dedicated resources—time, money, and people—to find stakeholders and to keep them engaged in the program in a way that supports mutual goals.

4. **The power of various partners to effect change may not be equal, but their contributions are equally important**. For example, a hypertension control program might engage partners from low-income minority communities, community health organizations, faith-based groups, and businesses (for instance, barber shops and beauty shops) as part of a coalition to screen and refer high-risk individuals. While there would be major differences in the size of each group and the resources each could offer, each would contribute in ways that would add value to the program.

5. **Translation of research to practice is necessary, but it is not automatic**. As part of planning, implementing, and evaluating health promotion programs, a cycle of continual feedback between researchers and practitioners is necessary. Just because an intervention has worked in a research study does not mean it will work in a school, workplace, health care organization, or community. Effective health promotion program staff stay current on what research says about effective interventions and, more important, will know or learn how to effectively translate this research into action. This role, which health promotion staff can assume, is sometimes described as being a *knowledge broker* for the setting.

6. **Resistance and reluctance on the part of individuals and organizations is to be expected**. A key focus in health promotion is voluntary action that people take to improve their own health. The needs and past experiences of individuals and organizations will affect their participation in a program. Resistance is expected because change is difficult and maintaining old habits is more comfortable. Likewise, often people know they need to change but they are reluctant due to perceived barriers. Frequently, using the trans-theoretical model stages of change can help program staff to tailor their strategies to overcome resistance and reluctance, thereby improving the health of a priority population.

Peter Senge's book *The Fifth Discipline* codifies many of the experiences of organizations in successfully dealing with change and learning how to change into a set of five practices for building learning capabilities in organizations (Senge, 1990). It is recommended that program staff, stakeholders, and participants be aware of and incorporate the five learning practices (which Senge calls *learning disciplines*) into their daily work.

1. **Personal mastery.** This discipline of aspiration involves formulating a coherent picture of the results that people most desire to gain as individuals (their personal vision) alongside a realistic assessment of the current state of their life today (their current reality). Learning to cultivate the tension between vision and reality can expand people's capacity to make better choices and to achieve more of the results that they have chosen.

2. **Mental models.** This discipline of reflection and inquiry focuses on developing awareness of the attitudes and perceptions that influence thought and interaction. By continually reflecting on, talking about, and reconsidering these internal pictures of the world, people gain more capability in governing their actions and decisions.

3. **Shared vision.** This collective discipline establishes a focus on mutual purpose. People learn to nourish a sense of commitment in a program by developing shared images of the future they seek to create and the principles and guiding practices by which they hope to get there.

4. **Team learning.** This discipline involves group interaction. Attending to group dynamics and processes, staff members can transform their collective thinking, learning to mobilize their energies and actions to achieve common goals and create synergy for creative and thoughtful problem solving.

5. **Systems thinking.** In this discipline, people learn to better understand interdependency and change and thereby learn to deal more effectively with the forces that shape the consequences of their actions. Appreciation of feedback and complexity are important in leading and growing a program.

Engaging Participants and Building Support

Regardless of the program setting (for example, school, workplace, health care organization, or community), effective programs engage people and build support for health promotion. This section discusses six widely used strategies to engage people in health promotion programs: partnerships; coalitions; collective impact; networking, outreach, and referrals; online communities; and community empowerment and organizing. The strategies all have roots in the community mobilization concept of individuals taking action that is organized around specific community issues, particularly health issues (see Chapter 3). The strategies are proactive and focus on building honest, trusting, and respectful relationships in order to maximize individuals' program participation and benefits. The strategies have some commonalities with the advocacy strategies discussed in Chapter 7. Advocacy strategies focus on the broad environment (that is, public policy) but can also be used in local settings to educate organizations. Similarly, the strategies discussed in this chapter, while primarily used to build support within for programs, can also be used to encourage changes in the broader environment. Thus, the five strategies discussed here and the advocacy strategies in Chapter 7 complement one another.

Partnerships

Partnerships improve the health of a community. They encourage people to work together to make a difference. For example, an effort to improve public transportation might involve elected officials, community developers and planners, business people, and those who utilize public transit. Because these partnerships bring people together from different parts of the community, their efforts often have the ability to be successful. Partnerships involve organizations that develop mutually beneficial relationships built on trust and commitment (Table 12.1). Partnerships can extend the reach and effectiveness of a program. In partnerships, the member organizations are generally equal in their relationships and there is mutual agreement on their goals and objectives. When developing partnerships, who needs

Table 12.1   Benefits of Partnerships

Partnerships achieve goals that individual organizations cannot achieve alone by:
- Combining the full force of their members to change local laws, policies, and norms
- Integrating and coordinating prevention services to improve quality and responsiveness
- Minimizing duplication of services
- Fostering diverse ideas and talents
- Mobilizing resources

Partnerships inspire communities to try new approaches by:
- Encouraging the participation of organizations that have never worked together
- Creating unique collaborations among diverse partnership organizations
- Bringing together new talents and approaches to health promotion

Partnerships make it easier for organizations to work together by:
- Helping communities to acknowledge and take responsibility for their health problems
- Motivating organizations outside the health care system to work within it
- Improving communication and trust among groups that might ordinarily compete with each other

Source: Adapted from the Center for Substance Abuse Prevention, n.d.

to be involved? It's important to be as inclusive as possible of all potential partners. This means people and organizations from the various sectors of the community such as schools, business, and government. For example, the Chicago Neighborhood Housing Services has partnerships with banks, other housing organizations, and the city government to develop and support high-quality, safe, and affordable housing for young families and the elderly in Chicago. Sometimes the housing service works alone and sometimes it works with partners. Frequently, Chicago Neighborhood Housing Services and one or more partners will conduct joint projects (that is, partnerships), share resources, and make referrals to each other (Community Tool Box, 2015).

Creating partnerships supports and extends partners' own influence at a site. More work can be accomplished when health promotion programs partner with organizations and agencies to reach a common goal. Forming and maintaining strong partnerships has been shown to increase the efficiency and effectiveness of health promotion programs. For example, partnerships with organizations, agencies, or programs that have a vested interest in the well-being of a community, such as county agencies, senior citizens' centers, unions, chambers of commerce, businesses, Head Start, law enforcement, or schools may help establish or maintain a community-based health promotion program (Community Tool Box, 2015; Harden, 1995).

Partnerships require nurturing, support, and information sharing. Partnering creates an opportunity for program participants and organizations to share their views on health and to learn from one another (Butterfoss, 2007). Above all, partnerships must be mutually beneficial. Developing partnerships with business, industry, public organizations, or nonprofits might provide fertile ground for a program to piggyback a new intervention within an established intervention framework. For example, the Centers for Disease Control and Prevention partnered with Meals on Wheels to provide safety education to homebound older adults when delivering nutritious meals to their homes (Sleet, 2007). Community efforts to prevent youth sports concussions will often times require partnerships between coaches (to remove an athlete from play), athletes (to report a potential concussion), athletic trainers (to recognize symptoms), administrators (to set policies), and parents (to reinforce educational efforts at home) (Centers for Disease Control & Prevention, 2015).

Coalitions

A *coalition* is a formal, long-term alliance among organizations (and individuals too) that are working together toward a common goal (Butterfoss,

2012). Coalition building is important in health promotion. Partnership development and coalition building begin with identifying strengths and challenges, and strategic planning (Butterfoss, 2013).Governance and oversight of the coalition and its work must reflect the collaboration through representatives from many settings, organizations, and individuals (Harden, 1995). In contrast to the partnerships, where partners are generally equal in their relationships and there is mutual agreement on their goals and objectives, a coalition is generally organized by a particular group and that group generally runs the coalition. In addition, coalitions are generally organized for a particular purpose. Coalition members may not necessarily view themselves as active workers toward the goals of the coalition but may want to add their voice and support to a group fighting to address a health issue. Coalition members frequently do not share resources, staff, or materials but may simply write letters, send e-mails, and make telephone calls to key decision makers.

Coalitions can be powerful agents for change. For example, the Steel Valley Coalition Against Drunk Driving was formed to increase the numbers of organizations in support of addressing drunk driving among young people in the small steel towns of southwest Pennsylvania. The Bicycle Coalition of Greater Philadelphia tracks cycling deaths in the Delaware Valley, and each May there is a Ride of Silence to remember the bike riders who were killed in a transit accident in the previous year and to bring attention to the issue (Ford, 2015). At the international level, the United Nations Road Safety Collaboration is an example of a global coalition to reduce the burden of traffic injuries around the world (World Health Organization, 2016).

The development of coalitions is a key ingredient for successful implementation of health promotion programs. The members of a coalition might help decide in which neighborhood to conduct the program, which department at a work site gets to pilot a program, how to address barriers to implementing a program in a particular setting, or what resources the program can gather to improve the chances of success in meeting program goals. Coalitions can not only be an important political force for change but can increase the efficiency of program implementation, improve participant and organization buy-in, and increase capacity. A strong coalition can also increase sustainability by continuing to implement a program long after the original implementers have left.

Benefits of coalitions are numerous, and include strength in numbers, strength in relationships, strength in diversity, and strength in resources. Coalition building and collaboration are not easy. Challenges include the risk of loss of autonomy, competitive edge, and control; conflict over goals and methods; expending scarce resources (time, money, status, data, etc.);

and delay in solving problems (Butterfoss, 2012). There are many opinions about how to successfully employ coalitions to promote health, including a formal community coalition action theory that consists of 14 constructs and 23 testable propositions to increase local support and capacity (Butterfoss, 2007). Ultimately, the program (and its potential health outcomes) must be seen as valuable to each member of the coalition (Harden, 1995). Following are steps to build and sustain an effective coalition from Butterfoss (2007):

1. Clarify/reaffirm vision and mission.

2. Engage community in the coalition.

3. Solidify coalition structure and function.

4. Recruit and retain active, diverse partners.

5. Develop transformational leaders.

6. Market your coalition.

7. Focus on action and advocacy.

8. Evaluate and sustain your coalition.

Collective Impact

Collective impact is a more structured form of *collaboration*. Collective impact is a when a committed group of key leaders and organizations from varying sectors come together for a common agenda for solving a specific social problem. While there are a multitude of examples of partnerships, networks, and other types of combined efforts in public health, collective impact initiatives are distinctly different. Unlike most collaborations, collective impact involves a centralized infrastructure, a dedicated staff, and a structured process that leads to a common agenda, shared measurement, continuous communication, and mutually reinforcing activities among participants (Kania & Kramer, 2011). Informed by lessons shared among practitioners who implement collective impact in the field, the Collective Impact Principles of Practice (Figure 12.1) guides practitioners to successfully put collective impact into action (Collective Impact Forum, 2016).

Since its introduction, collective impact is used as an effective way to improve social and environmental challenges. An example of collective impact is the Elizabeth River Project in southeastern Virginia. For decades, the river was a dumping ground for industrial waste. The project included more than 100 stakeholders, including the city governments of neighboring

Collective Impact Principles of Practice

Design and implement the initiative with a priority placed on **equity**.

Include **community members** in the collaborative.

Recruit and co-create with **cross-sector** partners.

Use data to continuously **learn, adapt, and improve**.

Cultivate leaders with unique **system leadership** skills.

Focus on program and **system strategies**.

Build a culture that fosters **relationships, trust, and respect** across participants.

Customize for **local context**.

Figure 12.1 Collective Impact Principles of Practice
http://collectiveimpactforum.org/resources/collective-impact-principles-practice

communities, the Virginia Department of Environmental Quality, the U.S. Environmental Protection Agency (EPA), and the U.S. Navy, among others. Together, the organizations created an 18-point plan to restore the watershed. Nearly two decades later, more than 1,000 acres of watershed land have been conserved or restored, pollution has been reduced by more than 215 million pounds, concentrations of the most severe carcinogen are significantly reduced, and water quality has greatly improved. The river is not fully restored, but nearly 30 species of fish and oysters thrive in the wetlands, and Bald Eagles nest on the shores (Kania & Kramer, 2011).

"Collective impact takes us from common goals to uncommon results" (Collective Impact Forum, 2014). For organizations who wish to use this approach, The Collective Impact Forum (http://collectiveimpactforum .org) website has a multitude of resources, including articles, stories, an initiative directory, checklists, and more to assist with implementation of this approach.

Networking, Outreach, and Referrals

Networking, outreach, and referrals play an important role in health promotion and social action. Networking allows different groups to work together toward a shared goal by coordinating strategies and pooling resources (Advocates for Youth, 2008). They have their roots in social network and social support theory (discussed in Chapter 3). It is known from research that social networks and social support can influence health (positively and negatively). At least five primary pathways have been identified through which social networks can influence health: (1) provision of social support, (2) social influence, (3) social engagement, (4) person-to-person contact, and (5) access to resources and material goods (Ayres, 2008; Csorba et al., 2007; Twoy, Connolly, & Novak, 2007).

Networking in health promotion is the action of building alliances to address a health problem or concern. It is not about waiting until a problem appears, but rather, deliberate action to know people, resources, and organizations. However, it does not have to be a carefully choreographed process of meeting and greeting people. It is much better done on a more informal basis—but remember that networking is always a two-way street. It must benefit both parties (whether individuals, programs, or organizations) and help them to be most effective, so, as you ask your network for help when you need it, be prepared to return the favor when asked. Networking has the power to bring together stakeholders whose particular focuses have given them different ways of thinking, methods, and strategies for building a smarter and more knowledgeable health care constituency. Responses to the 2014 Ebola outbreak benefitted from the engagement of many sectors at the community level and resulted in more effective disease control (Marais et al., 2015).

Program *outreach* is the intentional sharing of information about a program with specific individuals and groups for the purpose of educating them about the program and for developing support for program participants. Standard materials that might be used for outreach are program brochures, program staff business cards, and flyers. All outreach materials need to contain clear and concise contact information, including names of people to contact, telephone numbers, e-mail addresses, websites, and street addresses (with directions). Typically, these materials will be part of the program communication plan discussed in Chapter 8. Furthermore, these materials are developed following the processes discussed in Chapter 8.

Referral is the process of connecting a person to a program. Program staff identify where potential program participants are and who can direct these individuals to the program. For example, in a school, teachers, nurses, counselors, and parents refer students to health programs. Students might also sign up independently of an adult (a process called *self-referral*). In work settings it is common for a supervisor to refer employees to health programs; in addition, many individuals in work settings self-refer as a result of workplace health screenings. Like networking, referrals are a two-way process. Frequently individuals are attracted to a program but then find that this program does not address their needs. In these situations, program staff can help the individual by making a referral through a network formed by staff of other programs and resources, helping the individual to contact and potentially enroll in a health program designed to address his or her health concern.

Networking, outreach, and referrals are effective means of improving efforts to promote health. Today most people are aware of the impact of technology through sites such as Facebook, Twitter, and LinkedIn, Tumbler, and others which encourage and support social networking. However, going beyond current technology to promote health means that health promotion program stakeholders (including staff and participants) are working across the ecological model of health at all levels to improve their grasp of health problems, pool their knowledge and expertise with others, and jointly develop ways to solve individual health problems across a range of settings (Minkler, et al., 2012). Telephone conversations, meetings, and social gatherings offer opportunities to build a program staff network to bring together organizations, agencies, and people who share interests, can leverage resources, and have staff to create a multidisciplinary team to solve problems.

Online Communities

Using the Internet to form online health promotion communities is another way to create communities. Social networking technologies offer opportunities for information sharing and support. An online community can be a powerful tool for bringing constituents together to share their concern about an issue. The term *online community* represents the concept of convening people in virtual (Internet) space and describes a range of online activities, including electronic collaboration, information sharing, blogs, networking, and web-based discussions, where members can post, comment on discussions, give advice, or collaborate. A number of hosting sites offer, build, and service online communities.

As part of a health promotion program, an online community can be used in a variety of ways in order to:

- Increase the visibility of an issue of concern.
- Mobilize concerned citizens to advocate for a political agenda.

- Facilitate shared learning between constituents, staff, and other like-minded individuals and organizations.

- Support fundraising efforts by connecting with donors or members.

- Announce current events to the public.

- Recruit volunteers for an organization.

- Discuss challenges with colleagues and peers.

Community Empowerment and Organizing

Empowerment is the "social action process for people to gain mastery over their lives and the lives of their communities" (Minkler, Wallerstein, & Wilson, 2008). *Community empowerment* begins with the feeling among individuals at a site that they have the power to make a difference in their situation. Friedman (1992) identified three levels of power that an individual must possess in order to feel empowered: social, political, and psychological. *Social power* is achieved when an individual has access to information, knowledge, and skills. Social power also includes financial resources and participation in social organizations. Once social power is achieved, political power is possible (Friedman, 1992). *Political power* is the power of voice and collective action. This collective voice helps to create change within a community. *Psychological power* is established when an individual feels a sense of personal power or the ability to create change (Friedman, 1992). When all three levels of empowerment are achieved, community mobilization can occur.

Community organizing refers to efforts to involve community members in activities ranging from defining needs for prevention of health problems to obtaining support for prevention programs. All of the strategies discussed in this section (partnerships, coalitions, and so forth) are used to organize people at a site. The process involves working with and through constituents to achieve common goals. Organizing emphasizes changing the social and economic structures that influence health. Organizing can include elements of bottom-up (grassroots or citizen-initiated) strategies and top-down (outside-in or leader-initiated) strategies. In bottom-up strategies, the people at the site define the problems and decide on the solutions, while in top-down strategies, an outside expert (an external or self-appointed leader) facilitates change. Because leaders from the site (for example, school, workplace, health care organization, or community) understand their local culture, politics, and traditions better than outsiders, their participation is essential in tailoring prevention programs to local needs (McKenzie, Pinger, & Kotecki, 2012).

Program staff take a number of steps to empower and organize a group of people in the community. First, the problem or issue is identified, either by people in the community (grassroots) or by a planner or consultant from an agency. Grassroots efforts tend to be more successful, so it is best to let people in the community identify and prioritize their own issues.

If the issue is to be identified by an outsider, he or she must gain entry into the setting, often by approaching a formal or informal leader. The outsider must meet the local leader on his or her own terms (McKenzie, Pinger, & Kotecki, 2012). In one example, health educators at the Central Michigan District Health Department have forged a positive relationship with the Saginaw-Chippewa tribe, allowing the tribal leaders to direct and implement their own programs to improve tribal health. Once access to a population is granted, the people must be organized. Organizing is often initiated by a core group of volunteers who get others involved in the work of the group. Coalitions of groups might be formed to address specific interests. Assets, resources, strengths, and weaknesses are assessed in order to determine the capacity of the organization or community to tackle the problem. Determining priorities and goals helps to move the process along, so that an intervention can be developed and implemented. Partnerships can be formed to work on joint proposals and projects (McKenzie, Pinger, & Kotecki, 2012).

Below is a summary of steps in community organizing: (McKenzie, Neiger, & Thackeray, 2009)

1. Recognize the issue.
2. Gain entry into the community.
3. Organize the people.
4. Assess the community.
5. Determine the priorities and set goals.
6. Arrive at a solution and select intervention strategies.
7. Implement the plan.
8. Evaluate the outcomes of the plan of action.
9. Maintain the outcomes in the community.
10. Loop back.

An example of organizing in a community setting is described by Gielen, Sleet, and Green (2006) in summarizing a successful effort to reduce alcohol-related trauma. A partnership between community organizations and university researchers was formed in order to focus on changes in the social and structural contexts of alcohol use that would facilitate changes in individual behavior. Researchers asked communities to customize and prioritize their initiatives based on local concerns and interests and worked to implement evidence-based prevention policies and activities. Specific components of the mobilization effort were directed toward responsible beverage service and toward preventing drinking and driving, underage drinking, and alcohol access. Coalitions, task forces, and media advocacy were used to raise awareness and support for effective policies among members of the public and decision makers. An evaluation of the impact of the efforts demonstrated significant reductions in alcohol consumed, drinking and driving, nighttime injury crashes, alcohol-related crashes, and alcohol-related assaults (Holder et al., 2000).

Employing empowerment strategies is not without its controversy. Labonte in a classic report from Canada (Labonte, 1993; 1994) argues that empowerment can have the disadvantage of empowering the leaders and not the community. Tengland (2013) compares behavior change approaches to empowerment approaches and finds that behavioral approaches can often lead to "victim blaming" and stigmatization, increasing inequalities in health, whereas empowerment approaches tend to avoid those problems.

Ensuring Competence Through Credentialing

Health educators and community health workers were added to the U.S. Department of Labor in 2012. *Health educators* teach people about behaviors that promote wellness. They develop and implement strategies to improve the health of individuals and communities. *Community health workers* collect data and discuss health concerns with members of specific populations or communities (Bureau of Labor Statistics, 2010).

Community health workers typically have a high school diploma, although some jobs may require a 1-year certificate or a 2-year associate's degree. Community health workers typically have a shared language or life experience and an understanding of the community that they serve. Most states do not require certification of community health workers; however, voluntary certification is available in many states. Requirements vary, but may include completing an approved training program.

Some positions require further education such as a master's or doctoral degree. Graduate programs are commonly focused on community health education, school health education, public health education, or health promotion. Entering a master's degree program requires a bachelor's degree, but a variety of undergraduate majors are acceptable.

Entry-level health educators require a bachelor's degree in health education or health promotion. These programs provide training in theories and methods of health education and help students gain the skills to develop health education materials and programs. Most programs include an internship.

Having program staff with the requisite competencies is an important key to sustaining a high-quality health promotion program. The Institute of Medicine notes, "As weaknesses in the public health infrastructure have become more obvious, the need to certify and credential the public workforce has grown" (Institute of Medicine, 2003, p. 206). Developing and nurturing professionalism in health promotion is a responsibility of program staff, stakeholders, and participants, who need to expect and demand that all staff members hold professional credentials. All health and medical professions have similar credentialing processes. This section details as a model the credentialing process for health educators.

Health education as a profession has moved to credential practitioners in health promotion and health education competencies. *Health education* and *health promotion* (while not synonymous terms) refer to "efforts that enable and support people to exert control over the determinants of health and to create environments that support health" (Allegrante et al., 2009).

The United States has a dual system of quality assurance: individuals can become credentialed as health education specialists, and programs in institutions of higher education are accredited by specific accrediting bodies (Figure 12.2). Health education teachers in public schools are required to have a teaching license from the state in which they are teaching. Health educators working in jobs outside the public school system can obtain a voluntary credential by passing one of two examinations administered by the National Commission for Health Education Credentialing, Inc. (NCHEC). Many health education teachers also obtain this credential.

A *certified health education specialist* (CHES) is a health educator who has successfully completed the entry-level, competency-based exam given by NCHEC. A *master certified health education specialist* (MCHES) is a health educator who possesses both the entry- and advanced-level competencies and sub-competencies of the seven areas of responsibility of a health education specialist. Both CHES and MCHES have met national standards in credentialing and have been accredited by the National Commission of Certified Agencies accreditation since 2008 and 2013, respectively.

The Health Education Specialist Practice Analysis (HESPA) study added the term *health promotion* to the health education model. The reason for the change to "health education/health promotion" was to clarify

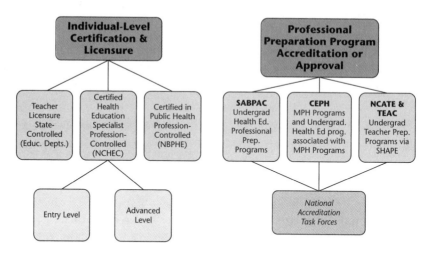

Figure 12.2   Credentialing of Individual Health Educators and Professional Preparation Programs in the United States

Source: Adapted from National Commission for Health Education Credentialing, n.d., and Cottrell et al., 2009.

the role of the health education specialist. NCHEC contributes to health promotion by certifying health education specialists and master certified health education specialists, promoting professional development, and strengthening professional preparation and practice. These objectives are accomplished by creating standards for university programs that train health educators, developing and administering a national exam, and creating continuing education opportunities for health educators (National Commission for Health Education Credentialing, n.d.).

The CHES areas of responsibility on which the competencies and sub-competencies, which vary depending on the level of certification, describe, in general terms, the skill set that is necessary for a certified health educator and useful for just about anyone who is conducting a health promotion program. The CHES areas of responsibility are:

- Assessing needs, resources, and capacity for health education/ promotion
- Planning health education/promotion
- Implementing health education/promotion
- Conducting evaluation and research related to health education/ promotion

- Administering and managing health education/promotion
- Serving as a health education/promotion resource person
- Communicating, promoting, and advocating for health, health education/promotion, and the profession

The basic CHES competencies are to be met by those graduating from baccalaureate and master's degree programs with less than 5years of experience in the field. A written examination is taken, and those passing the examination are known as certified health education specialists. A candidate who wants to take the CHES examination must (1) possess a bachelor's, master's, or doctoral degree from a regionally accredited institution of higher education; (2) have an official transcript demonstrating course titles in health education; and (3) have completed a minimum of 25 semester hours or 37 quarter hours of course work in health education (National Commission for Health Education Credentialing, n.d.).

Individuals having received CHES status must earn 75 hours of continuing education credits every 5 years in order to maintain their certification. Though credentialing is not mandatory for health educators, certification is highly recommended and is often specified as a requirement or a highly desirable qualification on job postings. Credentialing informs potential employers of the skills and competencies they can expect from prospective health education workers.

The NCHEC also implements an advanced level of certification, in response to growing awareness in the field that the entry-level certification was not reflective of the scope of practice of many health educators. The MCHES process was implemented in 2011.

Another credentialing source became available in 2008 to all public health professionals (including health educators) with a master's or doctoral degree from a public health program. This new credential, *certified in public health* (CPH), is accredited by the Council on Education for Public Health (CEPH). The National Board of Public Health Examiners (NBPHE) was created in 2005 to ensure that graduates of CEPH-accredited institutions have the knowledge and skills to be successful in public health. Like NCHEC, NBPHE does this by creating and administering a voluntary exam. To sit for the exam, one must have earned a graduate degree from a CEPH-accredited program or school.

The CPH exam focuses on the five core competencies of public health: biostatistics, environmental health sciences, epidemiology, health policy and management, and social and behavioral sciences (Gebbie et al., 2007). Each of these competencies is important for successful public health (and health promotion) practice, regardless of the individual's specialization or discipline. The CHES and CPH certifications reflect growing expertise and support for high quality health promotion programs and practitioners. They present challenges to practitioners trying to decide the appropriate certification given one's career path and interests (Taub, Allegrante, Barry, & Sakagami, 2009; Dennis, McKenzie, & Chen, 2014).

Implementation Science to Improve Program Effectiveness

Despite the existence of many evidence-based and effective interventions, including those described elsewhere in this book, too often these interventions are not known, not available, not adopted, or not used with fidelity. These are the problems addressed by implementation science. "This situation is equivalent to developing a life-saving medication but not telling physicians or patients that it is available, not packaging the product for public use, not having skilled pharmacists to dispense the medication, and not providing guidance about the management of its effects" (Sogolow, Sleet, & Saul, 2007, p. 493). On the one hand this gap between research and practice is large and continues to be a barrier to program effectiveness. On the other hand new strategies are available that address the challenges of conducting implementation science and creating and sustaining an effective program (Brownson, Colditz, & Proctor, 2012; Jacobs, Jones, Gabella, Spring, & Brownson, 2012.)

A shift has occurred in thinking about intervention research and implementation that recognizes that research doesn't end with the discovery that an intervention works (President's Cancer Panel, 2005). The scientific language and intervention protocols used in the original intervention research must be translated into everyday terms for use by practitioners in the community, and materials must be developed to help guide the end users in adopting and implementing the intervention.

It is recognized that new interventions compete with existing programs for scarce resources. Therefore, in planning the implementation of evidence-based interventions, some attention is paid to the potential barriers in delivering the program. A rationale for changing or starting the program is provided, together with the evidence, materials are prepared to facilitate the delivery, training for those who will implement the intervention is contemplated, and adaptation to cultural differences is considered (without losing fidelity). Administrators and other "gatekeepers" often decide if and how an organization will introduce a new intervention and how they will prepare staff and participants to accept and adopt the new activity or approach. Decisions take place with an eye for costs, staff resources, and acceptability to the priority groups.

There is often an assumption within the public health model that once an effective intervention, say for quitting smoking, has been found, widespread adoption will be automatic. There are many examples of rigorous, expensive, multiyear trials that identified effective interventions that were not feasible to execute in practice. An injury prevention program for schools, for example, may have worked in a controlled research setting in one school, but the 2 hours of classroom instruction required for implementation simply may not be available in other schools. There are several steps that might be carried out to overcome barriers related to implementation success:

• Plan in advance for how the effective intervention might be adapted in other settings.

• Translate the research into practice by attending to the "core elements" that led to success, including key characteristics, resources needed, and staffing.

• Support implementation by appropriate staff selection and training, suitable organizational placement of the intervention, and provisions for technical assistance in implementation.

• Enable widespread use by focusing on leadership, institutional resources, fidelity, strategy development, and infrastructure building.

Enhancing Program Impact and Sustainability

In a time of limited resources, program *sustainability* is important. Sustainability is considered the ability to continue program activities when resources, support, or funding stops. For maximum impact, programs are designed from the start with sustainability in mind. While clearly an ineffective program should not be continued, even effective programs struggle with challenges of sustainability. In a perfect world, a program must be both effective and sustainable to have maximum impact on public health. Both qualities may also be needed to garner continued support and resources. Although there have been examples of programs that were sustained despite evidence that they were not effective, health promotion program leadership requires skill in maintaining and sustaining effective programs (Kahan et al., 2014).

Swerissen and Crisp (2004) suggest that one approach to understanding what it will take to sustain a health promotion program is to consider sustainability in the context of the level of the intervention and the strategies

Table 12.2   Health Promotion Program Interventions and Sustainability Factors

Intervention Level	Intervention Strategies	Program Sustainability
Health promotion interventions for individuals	Focus on information, education, and training in order to promote change in knowledge, attitudes, beliefs, and behavior in regard to health risks such as smoking, eating, physical activity, and injury prevention	Requires a relatively short time frame for initial implementation but ongoing resources if program is to be maintained
Policy and practices of organizations	Focus on organizational change and consultancy in order to change organizational policies (rules, roles, sanctions, and incentives) and practices in order to produce changes in individuals' risky behavior and greater access to social, educational, and health-promoting resources	Requires few ongoing resources once organizational change has been implemented, but a longer-term time frame for establishing the program and a systematic process for withdrawal of resources
Environmental actions and social change at sites	Focus on social action and social planning at existing sites and on creating new sites (for example, organizations, networks, or partnerships) in order to produce change in organizations and redistribute resources that affect health	Often requires significant resources over an extended time frame, but resources may systematically be withdrawn once new sites have been created and resource redistribution occurs
Public advocacy	Focus on social advocacy in order to change legislative, budgetary, and institutional settings that affect community, organizational, and individual levels	Often requires significant resources over an extended time frame, but resources may be withdrawn once institutional change has been achieved

Source: Adapted from Swerissen and Crisp, 2004.

employed. Swerissen and Crisp's levels and corresponding strategies are shown in Table 5.1 in Chapter 5. Table 12.2 adds a new column to Table 5.1 in order to show the four health promotion intervention levels, corresponding strategies, and sustainability factors. For example, programs focused on individual behaviors such as smoking, nutrition, and physical activity have relatively short implementation time frames but require ongoing resources and support. And while health promotion programs dedicated to institutional change through advocacy take a lot of time and resources, once the desired change is in place, it continues to support the desired health behavior after the program has ended. Examples of such programs are those focused on policy, such as legislation that created smoke-free workplaces or policies that enforce lower blood alcohol limits for drivers.

Dutton (2000) has suggested, and we have adapted, some questions that program staff, stakeholders, and participants might ask in order to help sustain an effective program:

> **Do the leaders of the health promotion program have a clear understanding of its impact?** Program staff actively seek information about how well the program is working. Evaluation is ongoing, and

can include process and outcome measures collected at various intervals. Staff seek feedback by talking with participants about their satisfaction with the program, and what could be done to improve their own results. Data from physiologic tests, behavioral risk factors, and attitudes/knowledge can be indicators of program effectiveness.

Do leaders and participants have a shared understanding of the goals and purposes of the program that can be used to monitor, sustain, and improve the program? The program will be most successful when program staff and participants have a similar understanding of what the program is expected to do, and progress toward program goals is measured along the way. If program and participant goals are not being met, changes can be introduced and/or expectations can be modified. Programs improve over time, and feedback can be used to help achieve change.

As new knowledge becomes available, is this knowledge translated into changes that make the program more effective? As new knowledge about what works in health promotion becomes available to staff, stakeholders, and program participants, it needs to be shared widely. It may result in new "best practices" that will require adjustments in the program. Participants will need to know what changes to expect, why change is needed, and any implications that the changes might have on their health improvement and participation. Priorities and implementation strategies may need to be adjusted as a result.

The Center for Civic Partnerships (2015) and Berger and Grossman (2007) describe some tangible strategies for improving sustainability:

- Apply for a grant or contract to broadly disseminate and "scale-up" the intervention.
- Persuade another organization to continue your efforts as part of their program.
- Find a source of public funding, for example through a public health department program.
- Seek in-kind support from community organizations, local organization, and the media.
- Recruit volunteers and student interns.

A program needs a strategy to sustain itself, and while sustainability can never be guaranteed, steps can be taken to make it more likely. In a classic example of failure to plan for implementation and sustainability in a health promotion program, Kok and Green (1990, p. 305) cite findings from a Dutch smoking prevention program for adolescents, "After 4 years of careful and internationally respected research and development, deVries and co-workers presented their program to be implemented nationwide. Now, almost 2 years later, absolutely nothing has happened." Health promotion can learn from this example and invest in specific strategies to improve implementation and sustainability of effective programs.

Summary

Leadership is the responsibility of health promotion program directors, staff, stakeholders, and participants. Leadership in health programs requires an appreciation for the importance of and difficulty in achieving change. Leadership requires skill in developing, maintaining, and sustaining health promotion programs. Some keys to maximizing success are creating a supportive and engaged setting for a program, employing credentialed and qualified staff, and developing a shared understanding of the program's goals, objectives, and strategies.

For Practice and Discussion

1. How has a health promotion program in your community coped with change? What are the effects of the six realities of health promotion programs identified by McKenzie, Neiger, and Thackeray (2009) on a local health promotion program?

2. How might the strategies for engaging participants be applied in different health promotion program settings (e.g., school or a health care organization)? How might a school, work site, health care organization, and community health program differ with regard to empowering them to change?

3. Building culturally competent health promotion programs requires individuals (staff, stakeholders, and participants) to take leadership in sharing their views and thoughts about how well a program is working. How can staff and other stakeholders invite and develop a climate of shared leadership to sustain programs that are culturally competent and that reduce health disparities?

4. Investigate credentialing for other health professions (for example, physicians, nurses, diabetes educators, or physical therapists). What organizations are involved in *individual-level certification and licensure*? What organizations are involved in accreditation of

professional preparation programs? How are these organizations similar to and different from the organizations involved in credentialing and accreditation in health education?

5. What importance does implementation play in a program's success? How can a program intervention succeed in one locale, but fail in another? How can implementation of an effective intervention be improved?

6. How can the staff, stakeholders, and participants of a health promotion program improve the likelihood of sustainability through program outcome and impact assessments? What indicators would characterize success?

KEY TERMS

Certified health education specialist (CHES)	Implementation science
Certified in public health (CPH)	Individual-level certification and licensure
Change	Master certified health education specialist (MCHES)
Coalition	
Collaboration	Mastering change
Collective impact	Networking
Community empowerment	Outreach
Community health worker	Partnerships
Community organizing	Program sustainability
Consensus building	Referral
Empowerment	Sustainability

References

Advocates for Youth. (2008). *Building networks: Collaborating for community education and advocacy*. Retrieved from http://www.advocatesforyouth.org/publications/371-chapter-3-building-networks-collaborating-for-community-education-and-advocacy

Allegrante, J. P., Barry, M. M., Airhihenbuwa, C. O., Auld, M. E., Collins, J. L., Lamarre, M. C. . . . Mittelmark, M. B. (2009). Domains of core competency, standards and quality assurance for building global capacity in health promotion: The Galway Consensus Conference Statement. *Health Education & Behavior, 36*(3), 476–482.

Allegrante, J. P., Hanson, D., Sleet, D. A., & Marks, R. (2010). Ecological approaches to the prevention of unintentional injuries, 76(2), 24–31.

Ayres, C. G. (2008). Mediators of the relationship between social support and positive health practice in middle adolescents. *Journal of Pediatric Health Care*, 22(2), 94–102.

Batras, D., Duff, C., & Smith, B. J. (2014). Organizational change theory: Implications for health promotion practice. *Health Promotion Int.* doi:10.1093/heapro/dau098. First published online: November 14, 2014.

Berger, L. R.,& Grossman, D. C. (2007).Evaluating fidelity and effectiveness of interventions. In L. Doll, S. Bonzo, J. Mercy,& D. Sleet (Eds.), *Handbook of injury and violence prevention*. New York, NY:Springer.

Brownson, R.C., Colditz, G. A., & Proctor, E. K. (2012). *Dissemination and implementation research in health*. New York, NY: Oxford University Press.

Bureau of Labor Statistics. (2010). *21-1094 Community health workers*. Retrieved from http://www.bls.gov/soc/2010/soc211094.htm

Butterfoss, F. D. (2007). *Coalitions and partnerships in community health*. San Francisco, CA: Jossey-Bass.

Butterfoss, F. D. (2012). *Building & sustaining effective coalitions & partnerships* [PowerPoint slides]. Retrieved from http://www.slideshare.net/franbutterfoss/8-steps-for-building-sustaining-coalitions-partnerships-slideshare-pdf-2012-11501130

Butterfoss, F. D. (2013). *Ignite! Getting your community coalition fired up for change*. Bloomington, IN: AuthorHouse.

Center for Substance Abuse Prevention. (n.d.). *What works in prevention* [Pamphlet]. Rockville, MD: U.S. Department of Health and Human Services, Substance Abuse and Mental Health Services Administration.

Center for Civic Partnerships. (2015). *Sustainability toolkit*. Retrieved from http://www.civicpartnerships.org/#!community-building-resources/ci9f

Centers for Disease Control & Prevention. (2015). *HEADS UP to youth sports*. Retrieved from http://www.cdc.gov/headsup/youthsports/index.html

Collective Impact Forum. (2016). *Collective impact principles of practice*. Retrieved from http://collectiveimpactforum.org/resources/collective-impact-principles-practice

Collective Impact Forum. (2014). *What is collective impact?* Retrieved from http://collectiveimpactforum.org/what-collective-impact

Community Tool Box. (2015). *Creating and maintaining partnerships*. Retrieved from http://ctb.ku.edu/en/creating-and-maintaining-partnerships

Cottrell, R. R., Lysoby, L., King, L. R., Airhihenbuwa, C. O., Roe, K. M., & Allegrante, J. P. (2009). Current developments in accreditation and certification for health promotion and health education: A perspective on systems of quality assurance in the United States. *Health Education & Behavior*, 36(3), 451–463.

Csorba, J., Sörfozo, Z., Steiner, P., Ficsor, B., Harkány, E., Babrik, Z., . . . Solymossy, M. (2007). Maladaptive strategies, dysfunctional attitudes and negative life events among adolescents treated for the diagnosis of "suicidal behaviour." *Psychiatria Hungarica, 22*(3), 200–211.

Dennis, D., McKenzie, J., & Chen, W. (2014). *The value of CHES (and now MCHES)?—A commentary.* American Journal of Health Education, 43(3).

Dutton, J. (2000). How do you know your organization is learning? In P. Senge, N. Cambron-McCabe, T. Lucas, B. Smith, J. Dutton, & A. Kleiner (Eds.), *Schools that learn.* New York, NY: Doubleday.

Ford, B. (2015, March 8). An unfinished ride: St. Joseph's Prep grad's death shows safety for cyclists is deficient. Retrieved from http://www.philly.com/philly/sports/An_unfinished_ride.html

Friedman, J. (1992). *Empowerment: The politics of alternative development.* Cambridge, MA: Blackwell.

Gebbie, K., Goldstein, B., Gregorio, D., Tsou, W., Buffler, P., Petersen, D. . . . Silver, G. B. (2007). The National Board of Public Health Examiners: Credentialing public health graduates. *Public Health Reports, 122*(4), 435–440.

Gielen, A. C., Sleet, D. A., & Green, L. W. (2006). Community models and approaches for interventions. In A. C. Gielen, D. A. Sleet, & R. J. DiClemente (Eds.), *Injury and violence prevention: Behavioral science theories, methods, and applications* (pp. 65–82). San Francisco, CA: Jossey-Bass.

Harden, C. M. (1995). Community partnerships: Principles for success. *AHA News, 31*(13), 6.

Holder, H., Gruenewald, P., Ponicki, W., Treno, A., Grube, J., Saltz, R. . . . Roeper, P. (2000). Effects of community-based interventions on high-risk driving and alcohol-related injuries. *Journal of the American Medical Association, 284*(18), 2341–2347.

Institute of Medicine. (2003). *Who will keep the public healthy?* Washington, DC: National Academies Press.

Jacobs, J. A., Jones, E., Gabella, B. A., Spring, B., & Brownson, R. C. (2012). Tools for implementing an evidence-based approach in public health practice. *Prevention of Chronic Disease, 9,* 110324.

Kania, J. & Kramer, M. (2011, winter). Collective impact: Large-scale social change requires broad cross-sector coordination, yet the social sector remains focused on the isolate intervention of individual organizations. *Stanford Social Innovation Review,* 36–41.

Kahan, S., Gielen, A. C., Fagan, P. J., Green, L. W. (Eds.). (2014). *Health behavior change in populations.* Baltimore: Johns Hopkins University Press.

Kok, G., & Green, L. W. (1990). Research to support health promotion in practice: A plea for increased cooperation. *Health Promotion International, 65*(4), 303–308.

Labonte, R. (1993). *Health promotion and empowerment: Practice frameworks. Issues in Health Promotion Series* (HP-10-0102). Centre for Health Promotion (University of Toronto) and ParticipACTION (Toronto, Canada). Retrieved from http://heb.sagepub.com/content/21/2/253.short

Labonte, R. (1994). Health promotion and empowerment: Reflections on professional practice. *Health Education & Behavior, 21*, 253–268.

Liberman, L. D., & Earp, J. L. (Eds.). (2015, April). The evidence for policy and environmental approaches to health promotion. *Health Education & Behavior* (Supplemental Issue), *42*(1).

Marais, F., Minkler, M., Gibson, N., Mwau, B., Mehtar, S., Ogunsola, F., Banya, S. S., & Corburn, J. (2015). A community-engaged infection prevention and control approach to Ebola. *Health promotion international*.

McKenzie, J. F., Neiger, B. L., & Thackeray, R. (2009). *Planning, implementing, and evaluating health promotion programs: A primer* (5th ed.). San Francisco, CA: Pearson Benjamin Cummings.

McKenzie, J. F., Pinger, R. R., & Kotecki, J. E. (2012). *An introduction to community health* (7th ed.). Sudbury, MA: Jones & Bartlett.

Minkler, M. (2012). *Community organizing and community building for health and welfare* (3rd ed.). Piscataway, NJ: Rutgers University Press.

Minkler, M., Wallerstein, N., & Wilson, N. (2008). Improving health through community organizing and community building. In K. Glanz, B. K. Rimer, & K. Viswanath, (Eds.), *Health behavior and health education practice: Theory, research, and practice* (4th ed., pp. 287–312). San Francisco, CA: Jossey-Bass.

National Commission for Health Education Credentialing. (n.d.). *Mission and purpose*. Retrieved January 20, 2016, from http://www.nchec.org/mission-and-purpose

President's Cancer Panel. (2005). *Translating research into cancer care: Delivering on the promise: 2004-2005 annual report*. Bethesda, MD. National Cancer Institute, NIH.

Senge, P. M. (1990). *The fifth discipline: The art and practice of the learning organization*. New York: Random House.

Sleet, D. A. (2007, April). *Unintentional injury prevention: Healthy People 2010 progress review for the Assistant Secretary for Health*. Washington, DC: Centers for Disease Control and Prevention, National Center for Injury Prevention and Control.

Sogolow, E. S., Sleet, D. A., & Saul, J. (2007). Dissemination, implementation and widespread use of injury prevention interventions. In Doll, L., Bonzo, S., Mercy, J., Sleet, &D. (Eds.), *Handbook of injury and violence prevention*, (pp. 493–510). New York, NY: Springer.

Stokols, D. (1996). Translating social ecological theory into guidelines for community health promotion. *American Journal of Health Promotion*, *10*(4), pp. 282–298.

Swerissen, H., & Crisp, B. (2004). The sustainability of health promotion interventions for different levels of social organization. *Health Promotion International*, *19*(1), 123–130.

Taub, A., Allegrante, J. P., Barry, M. M., & Sakagami, K. (2009). Perspectives on terminology and conceptual and professional issues in health education and health promotion credentialing. *Health Education & Behavior*, *36*(3), 439–450.

Tengland, P.A. (2013). Behavior change or empowerment: On the ethics of health promotion goals. *Health Care Analysis*, *24*(1), 24–46.

Twoy, R., Connolly, P. M., & Novak, J. M. (2007). Coping strategies used by parents of children with autism. *Journal of American Academic Nurse Practitioners*, *19*(5), 251–260.

World Health Organization. (2016). *United Nations road safety collaboration.* Retrieved from http://www.who.int/roadsafety/en/

PART FIVE

HEALTH PROMOTION PROGRAMS IN DIVERSE SETTINGS

CHAPTER 13

PROMOTING HEALTH IN SCHOOLS AND UNIVERSITIES

Diane D. Allensworth, Jim Grizzell, Beth Stevenson, and Marlene K. Tappe

Rationale for Promoting Health in Schools and Universities

Preschools, K–12 schools and universities are ideal sites for health promotion because they are efficient places for reaching almost all children, adolescents, and many young adults. There are 75.8 million children and youth enrolled in public and private nursery schools, prekindergarten through secondary schools, colleges, and universities (National Center for Education Statistics, 2013). Students, however, are not the only audience for health promotion activities. Schools also serve as venues for health promotion initiatives for adults—the families of students and particularly the school staff. Schools are a workplace for 9.8 million faculty and staff employed by kindergarten through postsecondary institutions (Snyder and Dillow, 2015). While families of students at all levels are reached through schools, caregivers of preschool children are particularly receptive to learning more about health. Approximately 1 million teachers and caregivers of children aged birth through 5 years are reached through early childhood education programs (NSECE, 2013). Beyond the health benefits that accrue to these adults, these individuals can then serve as healthy role models for children.

Healthier students learn better. Further, students consolidate their health-related behaviors and attitudes as they transition from childhood to adulthood and make lifestyle

LEARNING OBJECTIVES

- Discuss the benefits to faculty, staff, and students of offering health promotion programs in schools and universities.

- Discuss the challenges and opportunities of offering health promotion programs and services in schools and universities.

- Describe current approaches to the design, implementation, and delivery of school and university health promotion programs.

- Describe administrative, clinical, and academic careers in school and university health promotion.

choices that will influence both their current and their future health status. Chronic diseases in adults such as heart disease, cancer, and diabetes are related to behaviors that often are established in youth: tobacco use, physical inactivity, and poor diet. Many youth engage in these three behaviors and three other high-risk behaviors that the Centers for Disease Control and Prevention (CDC) has linked to premature mortality and morbidity in both adolescents and adults: alcohol and other drug use, behaviors leading to intentional and unintentional injury, and sexual behaviors leading to teen pregnancy and sexually transmitted diseases. Although engaging in just one health risk behavior consistently can interrupt a student's progress toward graduating on time (Terzian, Andrews, & Moore, 2011), nearly 53% of adolescents reported engaging in two or more high-risk behaviors, 36% reported engaging in three or more risk behaviors, and 15% reported engaging in five or more risk behaviors (Fox, McManus, & Arnold, 2010). With approximately 40% of premature death and disease occurring because individuals engage in health risk behaviors, it is critical to provide youth with *health education* and other learning opportunities to enable them to develop and apply the health-related knowledge and skills and healthy beliefs, values, and norms they need to practice health-enhancing behaviors.

Health behaviors, health status, and academic achievement are inextricably intertwined. A reduction in health risk behaviors can improve learning and reduce health disparities. The Centers for Disease Control and Prevention (CDC, 2015) notes that one of the major indicators for the overall well-being of youth and a primary predictor and determinant of adult health outcomes is academic success. Conversely, health problems such as chronic illness, physical and emotional abuse, or hunger can lead to chronic absenteeism, inability to pay attention in class, poor test scores, and academic failure (CDC, 2015). Students who receive D's and F's are more likely to engage in high-risk behaviors than students who have mostly A's and B's (see Figure 13.1). Bradley and Greene (2013) found that in 96.6% of the 122 studies they analyzed there was a significant inverse relationship between engaging in health risk behaviors and academic achievement. They concluded that improving health behaviors and increasing academic achievement of students be seen as a composite goal of health and education agencies.

A nationwide survey of K–12 teachers (MetLife, 2012) identified the need for a coordinated approach to promoting students' academic achievement (Table 13.1). Teachers reported that only 56% of students

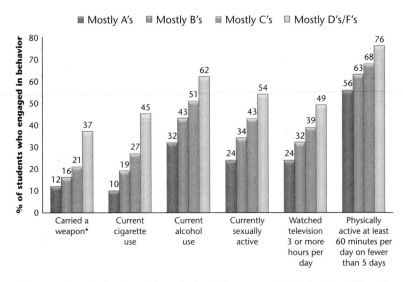

■ Mostly A's   ■ Mostly B's   ■ Mostly C's   □ Mostly D's/F's

*This means that 12% of students with mostly A's carried a weapon and 37% of students with mostly D's or F's carried a weapon. As reported by students.

Figure 13.1 Relationship Between Grades and Risk Behaviors: Percentage of High School Students Who Engaged in Selected Risk Behaviors, by Type of Grades Earned—United States, Youth Risk Behavior Survey, 2009
Source: CDC, 2009.

Table 13.1 Nationwide Survey of K–12 Teachers' Perceptions of Student's Health and Needed Health Services

	Totals (%)	Elementary (%)	Middle (%)	High School (%)
Teachers reporting that mostly/nearly all students . . .				
Arrive at school alert and rested	60	69	62	48
Are healthy and physically fit	56	61	56	51
Teachers strongly agree that school provides support services . . .				
Adequate health services to students	17	19	17	14
Adequate counseling and support for students	22	19	25	23
Healthy food choices for students	11	14	11	8

arrived at school healthy and physically fit. Only 17% of teachers felt that there were adequate *health services* for students and only 22% thought that the counselling and support for students was adequate (MetLife, 2012). When K–12 students receive needed health interventions and services, both academic performance and educational achievement levels improve (Byrk, Sebrig, Allensworth, Luppesca, & Easton, 2010; City Connects, 2012; ICF International, 2010; Moore & Emig, 2014) with the benefits even extending to the next generation (Murray et al., 2006) (see Figure 13.2).

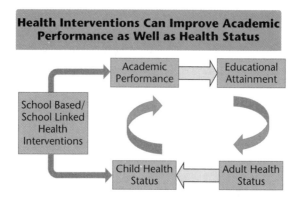

Figure 13.2   Relationship Between Health Status and Academic Performance
Source: Murray et al., 2006.

Evolving Role of Promoting Health in Schools and Universities

The use of schools and universities for health promotion is traced to the colonial period when Benjamin Franklin outlined a plan for education that included recommendations for instruction related to healthy eating, physical activity, and temperance. Further, the landmark public health document known as the Shattuck Report also recommended that children receive health instruction in schools, that sickness among students enrolled in schools and universities be assessed, that proof of vaccination be a requirement for school enrolment, and that sanitary (health) professors in colleges and medical schools be hired.

By the beginning of the 20th century, a variety of other strategies to promote the health of students were found in schools and universities including the use of hygiene textbooks for students as well as health textbooks for future teachers. Additional health promotion strategies in the past century included the appointment of doctors as school sanitarians, development of a system for the medical inspection of schools, screening of students for health problems, use of nurses to supplement the work of doctors in schools, establishment of a school lunch program, and implementation and practice of the professions of school psychology and counselling. Approaches to preschool, including the focus on health, improved greatly with the initiation of Head Start as part of the War on Poverty legislation in 1965. Head Start programs supported comprehensive development of children from birth to age 5 including early learning, health, and family well-being. Over time, many of these initiatives evolved into local, state, and national mandates to promote the health and learning of students in school.

The Coordinated School Health model, which had been promoted since the late 1980s until 2015 by the CDC, advocated the coordination of eight components within the school: health education; *physical education*; *community and family involvement*; health services; *nutrition services*; counselling, psychological, and social services; a *healthy school environment*; and staff health promotion. The Coordinated School Health approach promoted administrative support and commitment, appointment of a school health coordinator, organization of a school health team, utilization of a program planning model, implementation of multiple strategies through multiple components, a focus on students, and professional development for staff. At the district level, the CDC recommended establishing a district/municipality coordinating council consisting of representatives from the district, public health, and health care agencies as well as representatives from other community agencies interested in improving the health and well-being of students. An evaluation of the research on the value of each of the components of coordinated school health by the Society of State Leaders of Health & Physical Education & the Association of State and Territorial Health Officers revealed that each component was associated with improvements in academic achievement and behaviors.

The Whole Child Initiative, which was launched in 2007 by the Association of Supervision and Curriculum Development (ASCD) as a response to the No Child Left Behind legislation of 2001 on only academic achievement, identified a new learning compact that prepared students for college, career, and citizenship. ASCD's goal was to change the conversation from a narrow focus on only academic achievement measured by national test scores to one that promoted the long-term development of students by promoting five tenets. These five tenets hold that each student (1) enters school healthy and learns about and practices a healthy lifestyle; (2) learns in an environment that is physically and emotionally safe for students and adults; (3) is actively engaged in learning and is connected to the school and broader community; (4) has access to personalized learning and is supported by qualified, caring adults; and (5) is challenged academically and prepared for success in college and/or employment and participation in a global environment.

Current Role of Promoting Health: Preschool Through Postsecondary Schooling and Universities

Health Promotion for Early Care and Education

Preschool programs provide *early care and education* for nearly 5 million children ages 3 to 5 and over 2 million children ages birth to age 2

(Mamedova & Redford, 2015). Quality early childhood education addresses developmental and health issues in addition to providing instruction. In 2006 the *National Association for the Education of Young Children* (NAEYC) revised its program standards to help guide development of high-quality programs in preschool and early care settings. The standards: (1) Relationships, (2) Curriculum, (3) Teaching, (4) Assessment of Child Progress, (5) Health, (6) Teachers, (7) Families, (8) Community Relationships, (9) Physical Environment, and (10) Leadership and Management (NAEYC, 2008). Standard 5, Health, requires that "The program promotes the nutrition and health of children and protects children and staff from illness and injury . . . in order for them to "benefit from education and maintain quality of life" (NAEYC, 2008, para. 5). In 2014, the NAEYC revised the criteria related to the assessment of the standards. The three categories of criteria for assessing this standard for program accreditation focus on "Promoting and Protecting Children's Health and Controlling Infectious Disease," "Ensuring Children's Nutritional Well-Being," and "Maintaining a Healthful Environment" (NAEYC, 2015, pp. 42, 53, 57). These categories include criteria ranging from the maintenance of current health records to opportunities for children to engage in large-motor play activities to food safety as well as hand washing practices by both children and staff.

The Community Preventive Services Task Force recommends in the *Promoting Health Equity through Education Programs and Policies* (2015) publicly funded, center-based, quality early childhood education programs. Particularly for low-income children ages 3 to 5 years, based on strong evidence from several research studies that document the effectiveness of programs to promote cognitive development and increase readiness to learn, which is likely to reduce educational achievement gaps, improve the health of low-income student populations, and promote health equity. However, in 2010, less than half of children in families in the lowest income quartile who qualified for these services were enrolled in early childhood education programs because not enough sites are available to meet the demand for these services (Duncan & Magnuson, 2013). The need to focus health promotion in preschools and early childhood populations has increased, in part, from the recommendations found in the Institute of Medicine's report *From Neurons to Neighborhoods*, which substantiated the need for resources and focus on social-emotional and regulatory development of children.

Improving quality in early childhood care and education is an active and growing area. The *Quality Rating and Improvement System* (QRIS) National Learning Network uses a systemic approach to assess, communicate, and improve the level of quality in early childhood and school-age care and education programs. Through QRIS, states define what constitutes a higher quality of care based on designated criteria and use a rating system with a recognizable and understandable symbol to communicate to the public how well participating early care and education programs meet these state criteria. QRIS often link to child care subsidy reimbursement rates, use licensing and administrative regulations as a baseline to define what constitutes improved quality and link to enhanced training, professional development, qualifications, and program accreditation. Health and safety are a part of a state QRIS in 63% of states with QRIS. Since 2010, the number of QRIS operating in states and localities has markedly increased from 25 in 2010 to 38 in 2014 (The Build Initiative & Child Trends, 2014).

The CDC developed a Spectrum of Opportunities for Obesity Prevention in Early Care and Education Settings (see Figure 13.3). Although this figure was developed for obesity prevention, it has relevance for a range of health promotion areas and provides a framework for approaching preschools and early childhood with any health promotion efforts.

Health Promotion for K–12 Students: Whole School, Whole Community, Whole Child Model

The Whole School, Whole Community, Whole Child (WSCC) model is the result of an agreement between ASCD and CDC in 2014 to merge

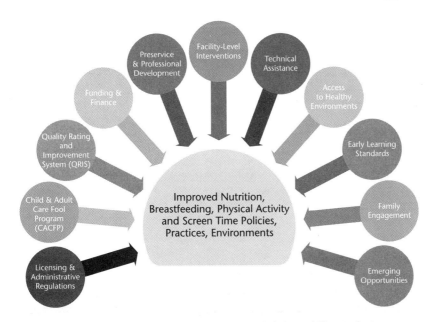

Figure 13.3 Spectrum of Opportunities for Obesity Prevention in Early Care and Education Settings

ASCD's Whole Child Initiative with CDC's Coordinated School Health approach. The WSCC model combines the basic concepts from each original model. The components have been enlarged from eight to 10 by separating two of the original eight CDC components of Coordinated School Health. The component of healthy and safe school environment was separated into social and emotional climate and physical environment, and the component of family and community involvement was separated into family engagement and community involvement. Further, the physical education component was expanded to explicitly include physical activity by being renamed as physical education and physical activity involvement.

The importance of community engagement is evident with community being both a component but also a link and support to every other component (Figure 13.4). The focus of the new model is on the child both as the recipient of services as well as partners in the implementation of the model (Morse & Allensworth, 2015). Research from both the education

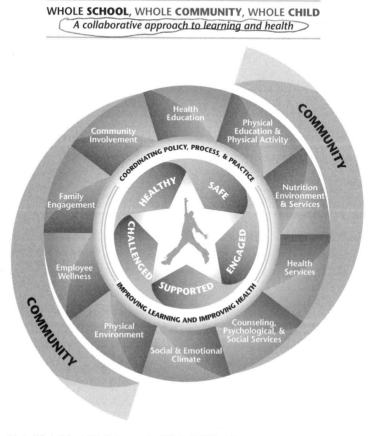

Figure 13.4 Whole School, Whole Community, Whole Child Model

sector (Fletcher, 2005; Toshalis & Nakkula, 2012) and the health sector (Griebler, Rojatz, Simovska, & Forster, 2014; Wallerstein, 2006) support the value of empowering students to become allies, decision makers, and planners in the implementation of those programs addressing their well-being. Various forms of youth engagement such as peer education, peer mentoring, youth action, student voice, community service, service-learning, youth organizing, civic engagement, and youth-adult partnerships have been used effectively to engage students as partners in instructional and health promotion activities. Use of these strategies has improved student self-efficacy, sociopolitical awareness, and civic competence as well as their achievement (McLaughlin, 2000). Guidance on how to implement the WSCC model is available from the CDC website (http://www.cdc.gov/healthyyouth/wscc/index.htm) and the ASCD website (http://www.ascd.org/programs/learning-and-health/wscc-model.aspx).

Although there is enthusiasm about the WSCC model and integrating schools and communities, there also is the recognition that although some communities have outstanding school health initiatives, both the linkages between schools and communities as well as the quality of many of the components within schools are seriously deficient in many schools. All states have some requirements for most components of the WSCC model, the variety of services as well as the quality of services varies considerably as states have responsibility for the education of students within their respective state. For example, 74% of states adopted the National Standards of Health Education yet most schools do not provide health instruction every year to all students as recommended in the standards (Kann et al., 2013). Only 7.5% of K–5 schools nationwide provide the 360 cumulative hours of health education recommended by the National Health Education Standards (Joint Committee on National Health Education Standards, 2007); for grades 6–8 only 10.3% schools nationwide provide the recommended 240 cumulative hours and only 6.5% of high schools provide the recommended 320 cumulative hours of health instruction (U.S. Department of Health and Human Services, 2015). Students need opportunities for health instruction based on the National Health Education Standards. These standards emphasize the CDC's Characteristics of an Effective Health Education Curriculum and delineate the health-related concepts and skills and healthy beliefs, values, and norms students need to engage in healthy behaviors. Additionally, the CDC's *Health Education Curriculum Analysis Tool* (HECAT) published in 2012 is used to support the development, revision, or selection of health education curricula consistent with the National Health Education Standards and CDC's Characteristics of an Effective Health Education Curriculum.

Physical education and physical activity are also a critical component of the WSCC model. Unfortunately, physical education does not fare much better than health education. Nationwide, the percentage of schools in each state that taught a required physical education course in any grade (6–12) ranges from a median high of 94.8% in grade 6 through a median low of 39.5% in grade 12 (Demissie et al., 2013). Even having a course in any one grade does not ensure that the time requirements are fulfilled. For example, only 3.8% of elementary schools, 7.9% of middle schools, and 2.1% of high schools provide the recommended number of minutes of daily physical education (150 minutes per week in elementary schools; 225 minutes per week in secondary schools) for the entire school year for students in all grades (CDC, 2013). Students need opportunities for physical education based on the National Physical Education Standards developed by the Society for Health and Physical Education in 2013. In addition to physical education, students need access to an array of opportunities to engage in physical education and physical activity outside of physical education. Physical education and physical activity initiatives are consistent with the CDC's recommendations for a Comprehensive School Physical Activity Program. An assessment of the local physical education curriculum is guided by the use of the CDC's Physical Education Curriculum Analysis Tool (http://www.cdc.gov/healthyschools/pecat/index.htm).

The most common provider of school health services is the school nurse. Although three fourths of districts had adopted a policy stating that schools will provide for the administration of medications, case management for students with disabilities, CPR, first aid, identification or school-based management of chronic health conditions, and violence prevention; other health services are provided by less than 55% of districts nationwide including instruction on self-management of chronic health conditions such as asthma or diabetes (48.6%); counseling for emotional or behavioral disorders including anxiety, depression, or ADHD (54.3%); and prevention of tobacco use (54.4%) (Brener, Vernon-Smiley, Leonard, & Buckley, 2013). Although most schools nationwide had a part-time nurse to oversee school health services, only 31.5% of these schools had a registered nurse providing health services full time to students. Unfortunately, the recommended ratio of one nurse to 750 students was attained in only 48% of those schools that employ a school nurse (Brener, Wheeler, et al., 2007). Having a full time school nurse providing services to students has been shown to improve attendance of students among poor and minority students (Lwebuga-Mukasa, & Dunn-Georgiou, 2002; Telljohan, Dake, & Price, 2004) and improve case management of chronic diseases (Bonaiuto, 2010).

Both physical health and mental health services expand with the addition of school-based health centers where enrolled students can receive primary care at little or no cost to students at a clinic located within the school. Only 12.5% of districts nationwide have at least one school-based health center that offers both health services and mental health or social services to students (Brener, Vernon-Smiley, Leonard, & Buckley, 2013). School-based health centers are sponsored and managed by community health care centers (33.4%), hospitals (26.4%), local health departments (13.3%), or other community organizations (Lofink et al., 2013). Students using school-based health centers in comparison with nonusers:

- Receive more preventive care visits and screening for high-risk behaviors (American Academy of Pediatrics, Council on School Health, 2012); and

- Have fewer emergency room visits (American Academy of Pediatrics, Council on School Health, 2012).

Systematic Integration of Communities and Their Schools

Emerging research about the value of systematically integrating community health care resources with schools' resources which the new WSCC model promotes is compelling. An analysis of 11 rigorous research studies of schools providing integrated student supports has strengthened the value of community integration of services to student academic achievement. The services that communities have supplied include physical and mental health services, tutoring and mentoring services for students, and connecting the families of students to parent education, family counseling, food banks, and/or employment assistance. While not all communities had supplied every service in the 11 studies, schools providing some combination of services and support found that student grade retention and dropout decreased while attendance, math achievement, reading, and overall GPA improved. Further, this analysis found a return on investment ranging from more than $4 saved for every $1 invested to almost $15 saved for every $1 invested. The researchers noted that integration was key to success—both the integration of supports to meet any one individual students' needs as well as the integration of services into the life of the school (Moore & Emig, 2014).

The Coalition for Community Schools, early in its history, used the term *full service schools*, which signified that these schools linked community agencies to ensure that the physical, social, and emotional needs of students and families were met. Community schools have an integrated focus that promotes early childhood education, a core instruction program that motivates and engages students, family support and engagement, health and social services, and a safe supportive school and community environment. Many school-based health centers are located within community schools.

Another professional organization that promotes similar integrated services is Communities in Schools, which serves elementary through secondary students in 2,400 schools in 25 states. This organization has been recognized by the U.S. Department of Education as the initiative associated with the strongest reduction in dropout rates among all existing fully scaled dropout prevention programs (ICF International, 2010). An evaluation of the Communities in Schools' model confirmed that the more fully and faithfully the model is implemented, the stronger the effects (Communities In Schools, 2011). Communities In Schools programs are based on five basic strategies, which are very similar to those strategies promoted by the Coalition of Community Schools:

1. A one-on-one relationship with a caring adult
2. A safe place to learn and grow
3. A healthy start and a healthy future (Access to health and dental care, food programs, counseling services)
4. A marketable skill to use upon graduation
5. A chance to give back to peers and community

Health-Promoting Universities

Not only has the World Health Organization promoted the concept of *health-promoting schools* but also the concept of *health-promoting universities.* The outcomes or goals of a health-promoting university include improving the health of students, university personnel, and the wider community as well as integrating health into the university's culture, structure, and processes. Originally the key objectives in achieving these goals included the following: promoting healthy and sustainable planning and policy throughout the university; ensuring healthy work environments; providing healthy and supportive social environments for students, staff, and the local community; establishing and enhancing primary health care; facilitating personal and social development among students and staff; ensuring a healthy and sustainable (that is, *green*) physical environment; encouraging wider academic interest in health promotion and research; and creating community partnerships for health (Tsouros, Dowding, & Dooris, 1998). At the 2015 International Conference on Health Promoting Universities a new charter was developed that contained the following two calls to action for health promoting universities (Health Promoting Universities and Colleges, 2015): ① embed health into campus administration, culture, academics, + operations ② lead health promotion action locally + globally

Call to Action 1: Embed Health into Campus Administration, Culture, Academics, and Operations

* *Embed health in all campus policies:* Review, create, and coordinate campus policies and practices with attention to health and well-being so that all planning and decision making takes account of and supports the well-being and flourishing of people, campuses, communities and our planet.

* *Create supportive environments:* Enhance the campus environment as a living laboratory, identifying opportunities that support health well-being, as well as sustainability and resilience in the built, natural, social, economic, cultural, academic, organizational, and learning environments.

* *Generate thriving communities and a culture of well-being:* Be proactive and intentional in creating empowered and connected campus communities that foster an ethic of care and collaboration while incorporating a well-being lens into teaching, learning, research, programs, procedures, services, physical spaces, policies, and decisions.

* *Support personal development:* Develop and create opportunities to build student, staff, and faculty resilience, personal capacity, and life-enhancing skills—and support them to thrive and achieve their full potential.

* *Create or reorient campus services:* Coordinate and design campus services to support and enhance health and well-being, optimize human and ecosystem potential, and promote a supportive institutional culture.

Call to Action 2: Lead Health Promotion Action Locally and Globally

* *Integrate health, well-being, and sustainability in multiple disciplines:* Incorporate and embed an understanding and commitment to health, well-being and sustainability in and across the diverse sectors and disciplines on campus, ensuring that health becomes a foundation for all those involved in teaching, learning, research, and work on campus.

* *Advance teaching, training, and research in health promotion:* Ensure adequate training, learning, teaching, and testing of health promotion;

and develop research partnerships and a research agenda to advance health promotion in higher education and beyond.

- *Lead local and global action for health promotion:* Partner with local and regional communities in order to develop knowledge and action for health promotion, locally, regionally, and globally.

Both the American College Personnel Association (http://www.myacpa .org/commwellness) and the National Association of Student Personnel Administrators (https://www.naspa.org/constituent-groups/kcs/wellness- and-health-promotion) have promoted a variety of wellness activities on campuses for U.S college students.

Resources and Tools

A number of unique resources are available to help in planning, implement- ing, and evaluating health promotion initiatives in school and university settings. Table 13.2 provides illustrious examples of surveys assessing the health status of children and youth, their health risk behaviors, and their ability to access health care, as well as assessing the policies and programs of schools within our country.

Tools

Early Childhood Education

The *Quality Rating Improvement System (QRIS) Compendium* (qriscompendium.org) is a catalog and comparison of quality rating and improvement systems to promote thoughtful design, analysis, and continuous improvement in early care and education systems. The 2014 QRIS Compendium is being used to improve health outcomes in early care and education settings.

Caring for Our Children: National Health and Safety Performance Standards, (http://cfoc.nrckids.org/) developed by the American Academy of Pediatrics (AAP), the American Public Health Association (APHA), and the National Resource Center for Health and Safety in Child Care and Early Education (NRC), provides 686 national standards representing the best evidence, expertise, and experience in the country on quality health and safety practices and policies that are followed in today's early care and education settings.

K–12 Schools

The *Health, Mental Health and Safety Guidelines for Schools* guidelines developed by the American Academy of Pediatrics and their colleagues

Table 13.2   Sources of Data on Health and Health Promotion

Source	What the Source Describes
General	Child data by state, county, city, or congressional district
Kid's Count Data Book	
http://datacenter.kidscount.org/	Information on health status and health care access
National Survey of Children's Health	
http://childhealthdata.org/browse/survey	
Early Childhood Education	State child care center regulations and oversight
We Can Do Better (National Association of Child Care Resource and Referral Agencies, 2011)	
http://www.naccrra.org/sites/default/files/default_site_pages/2013/wcdb_2013_final_april_11_0.pdf	Data on state-funded prekindergarten programs
2014 State Preschool Yearbook	Programs and practices at the state district, school, and classroom level for elementary through secondary schools
http://nieer.org/sites/nieer/files/Yearbook2014_full2_0.pdf	
K–12 Education	Health policies and activities in secondary schools
School Health Policies & Program Survey	
State and district level: http://www.cdc.gov/healthyyouth/shpps/2012/pdf/shpps-results_2012.pdf	
School and classroom level: http://www.cdc.gov/healthyyouth/data/shpps/results.htm	
School Health Profiles Survey	
http://www.cdc.gov/healthyyouth/profiles/index.htm	
Youth Risk Behavior Survey	Health risk behaviors of high school and middle school students
http://www.cdc.gov/yrbs	
College and University	Health status and health behaviors of undergraduate students
ACHA-NCHA Undergraduate Survey	
http://www.acha-ncha.org/reports_ACHA-NCHAII.html	

from numerous other professional health and educational associations recognize that while the primary mission of schools is to educate students, schools also have a responsibility for students' health and safety while they are at school. Guidelines have been developed to address family and community engagement, health and safety education, physical education, health and mental health services, nutrition services, physical environment and transportation, social environment, and staff health and safety (Taras et al., 2004).

The *School Health Index*, developed by the CDC, is a self-assessment and planning tool that schools can use to improve local initiatives related to coordinated school health programs. The School Health Index includes modules linked to each of the components of coordinated school health programs. Each module contains questions to assess school strengths and weaknesses related to the component as well as six specific health topics: safety, physical activity, nutrition, tobacco use, sexual activity, and asthma. Each module also includes a planning activity for school personnel to complete an action plan once they have conducted the self-assessment process.

College and Universities

CAS Professional Standards for Higher Education, 9th edition, developed by the Council for the Advancement of Standards in Higher Education in 2015, identifies 44 sets of professional standards and corresponding self-assessment guides for student affairs, student services, and student development programs in order to foster student learning, development, and achievement.

The Standards of Practice for Health Promotion in Higher Education, 3rd edition (American College Health Association, 2014) provides guidelines for health promotion in the university setting identifying guidelines for assessment and the provision of quality assurance of health promotion in higher education making explicit the scope of practice and essential functions for the field.

Challenges

Although economy of scale is a good reason to implement health promotion programs at early childhood education centers, schools, and universities, such initiatives present challenges—for example, understanding the culture and goals of educational institutions, gaining access to students, and communicating with teachers and faculty in order to gain their support for any health promotion initiative. First and foremost, those from public health or community agencies who wish to provide health promotion programming to students must understand that the chief goal and mission of educational institutions is education and learning—not health. Furthermore, in recent years schools have had added pressure to focus on academics, with the emphasis on accountability for students passing high-stakes state and national tests established by the No Child Left Behind Act; therefore, there is little time left in the curriculum for new health programs, particularly those that might be viewed as not central to the role of schools. So the health promotion program staff who work outside the school or university and want to secure instructional time for health promotion must focus on the educational impact of the intervention and frame the arguments for partnerships in terms of the anticipated educational outcomes (e.g., reduced absenteeism, reduced tardiness, better comport-ment, enhanced time on task, increased achievement, increased graduation rates, etc.) in addition to describing health outcomes and benefits.

Gaining access to students requires respecting the hierarchy in schools. To work with Pre-K students and teachers, one must seek approval of the childhood education center director or for K–12 students, the school principal. To work in more than one school in a district, one must seek the approval of the superintendent. At the district level, also approach the coordinator for health and physical education (and/or the district coordinator for school nursing, and/or the district coordinator for counseling) to secure support for the schools' or the district's participation in a health promotion initiative. Gaining access to students in institutions of higher education often depends on gaining approval at the department level. If access to students in a particular course is required, the department chairperson or individual faculty member is the person to approach for approval. Health promotion program staff who want to work with students directly contact the director of residence halls or the dean of student life for permission.

Communication with education staff needs to be succinct and free of health promotion jargon. Language used by public health officials occasionally differs somewhat from that used by education staff. For example, for health workers, *surveillance* implies assessment of morbidity and mortality, whereas for K–12 educators, it means using a camera to monitor student behavior. Beyond awareness of the occasional definition that differs, health promotion program staff who are approaching education staff from outside need to be prepared to talk about links between the curriculum or lessons they would like to provide and the state/national education standards and performance indicators for the grade level(s) of students who are to be the recipients of the program. Further, the health promotion program staff are able to identify research-based best practices that will be used and the proposed initiative's characteristics that bode well for successful outcomes. See *Speaking Education's Language* (http://c.ymcdn.com/sites/www.chronicdisease.org/resource/resmgr/school_health/nacdd_educationsector_guide_.pdf) for a tutorial that can assist health professionals to work successfully in public K–12 schools.

Career Opportunities

Those individuals interested in working with children and youth could be employed in health departments or other community agencies as well as directly by schools and universities. A wide variety of professional opportunities are available for individuals who are interested in a career in promoting the health and learning of students in school and university settings. Individuals who are interested in teaching students in K–12 settings must pursue degrees that will allow them to meet state standards for teacher certification by completing degrees or programs in early childhood education, elementary education, health education, or physical education. Other school-based or school-linked professionals who directly influence the health and learning of students in Pre-K–12 settings include school principals, superintendents, curriculum directors, school nurses, school physicians, athletic trainers, school food service directors, dieticians, school counsellors, school psychologists, and school social workers. Community health educators who work in health organizations (for example, local affiliates of the American Cancer Society) or agencies (for example, local public health departments) can partner with schools by collaborating individually with school professionals or collectively as members of school health councils or by offering school-based or community-based programs designed to influence the health and learning of youth. In addition, public health educators can work in state agencies and organizations (for example, state or regional affiliates of the American Heart Association) as well as national agencies (for example, the Centers for Disease Control and Prevention) to influence the health and learning of youth. For those interested in employment at the university level, the American College Health Association (2014) has identified competencies as well and the type of positions that are available in *Guidelines for Hiring Health Promotion Professionals in Higher Education* (https://www.acha .org/documents/resources/guidelines/ACHA_Hiring_Health_Promotion_ Professionals_in_Higher_Ed_May2014.pdf).

Summary

Preschools, K–12 schools and universities offer tremendous opportunities for health promotion. The role of schools and universities in promoting and protecting the health of children, adolescents, and young adults has been recognized throughout history. In recent years, however, many initiatives have been put in place to support health promotion activities in school and university settings. Future professionals can take part in a wide variety of partnerships to promote the health of children, adolescents, and young adults. Students who are interested in pursuing careers in health promotion are encouraged to join professional organizations that will support their professional preparation and development as health promotion specialists in school and university settings.

For Practice and Discussion

1. Use the rationale for health promotion in preschool, K–12 schools, and university settings to create a brief (3-minute) presentation to justify the provision of health promotion programs in each of these settings.

2. Think about a specific preschool, elementary school, middle school, high school, or university. Identify and describe the programs, services, and policies that are designed to promote or protect student health in this school or university.

3. Use the Internet to explore three of the organizations that serve professionals who work in early care and education, school or university settings to promote the health of students. For each organization, identify its mission, the professionals that it serves, and its important initiatives.

4. Moore and Emig (2014) identified the major providers of integrated services support. Choose one organization and identify its major services and outcomes. Share within the class.

5. Using the resources and tools described in this chapter, design a 4-hour training session on promoting student health for new community college staff members.

6. Identify and read the national standards of practice for as many components of the WSCC model that are available.

KEY TERMS

Early care and education

Family and community involvement

Health education

Health promoting universities

Health services

Healthy and safe school environment

Mental health services

National Association for the Education of Young Children

Nutrition services

Physical education

Whole School, Whole Community, Whole Child Model (WSCC)

References

American Academy of Pediatrics, Council on School Health. (2012). School-based health centers and pediatric practice. *Pediatrics, 129*, 387–393.

American College Health Association (2014). Guidelines for Hiring Health Promotion Professionals in Higher Education, Second Edition. Retrieved from https://www.acha.org/documents/resources/guidelines/ACHA_Hiring_Health_Promotion_Professionals_in_Higher_Ed_May2014.pdf

American College Health Association (2012). Standards of Practice for Health Promotion in Higher Education, Third Edition, May 2012. Retrieved from https://www.acha.org/documents/resources/guidelines/ACHA_Standards_of_Practice_for_Health_Promotion_in_Higher_Education_May2012.pdf

Bonaiuto, M. M. (2010). Strategies for identifying students in need of school-based asthma services: Challenges and questions that emerged from a rapid evaluation of a school-based asthma program. *Journal of Asthma & Allergy Educators, 1*, 109–116.

Bradley, B. J., & Greene A. C. (2013). Do health and education agencies in the United States share responsibility for academic achievement and health? A review of 25 years of evidence about the relationship of adolescents' academic achievement and health behaviors. *Journal of Adolescent Health, 52*, 523–532.

Brener, N. D., Wheeler, L., Wolfe, L. C., Vernon-Smiley, M., & Caldart-Olson, L. (2007). Health services: Results from the School Health Policies and Programs Study, 2006. *Journal of School Health, 77*(8), 464–485. doi:10.1111/j.1746-1561.2007.00230.x

Brener, N. D., Vernon-Smiley, M., Leonard, S., & Buckley, R. (2013). Health services: Results from the School Health Policies and Practices Study 2012. In Centers for Disease Control and Prevention (Ed.), *Results from the School Health Policies and Practices Study, 2012* (pp. 49–64). Retrieved from http://www.cdc.gov/healthyyouth/shpps/2012/pdf/shpps-results_2012.pdf

The Build Initiative & Child Trends. (2014). *A catalog and comparison of quality rating and improvement systems (QRIS)* [Data System]. Retrieved from http://qriscompendium.org/

Byrk, A., Sebrig, P. B., Allensworth, E. M., Luppesca, S., & Easton, J. Q. (2010). *Organizing schools for improvement. Lessons from Chicago*. Chicago, IL: University of Chicago Press. Retrieved from http://ccsr.uchicago.edu/books/osfi/prologue.pdf

CAS Professional Standards for Higher Education. (2015). CAS professional standards for higher education, 9th edition. Colorado: Council for the Advancement of Standards in Higher Education.

Centers for Disease Control and Prevention. (2009). *Association between health-risk behaviors and academic grades*. Retrieved from http://www.cdc.gov/healthyschools/health_and_academics/data.htm

Centers for Disease Control and Prevention. (2013). Comprehensive School Physical Activity Programs: A Guide for Schools. Atlanta, GA: U.S. Department of Health and Human Services. Retrieved from http://www.cdc.gov/

healthyschools/physicalactivity/pdf/13_242620-A_CSPAP_SchoolPhysActivity
Programs_Final_508_12192013.pdf

Centers for Disease Control and Prevention. (2015). *Health and academics.*
Retrieved from http://www.cdc.gov/healthyyouth/health_and_academics/
index.htm

City Connects. (2012). *The impact of City Connects: Progress report 2012.*
Retrieved from http://www.bc.edu/content/dam/city-connects/Publications/
CityConnects_ProgressReport_2012.pdf

Communities In Schools. (2011). 2009–2010 results from the Communities
In Schools Network. Retrieved from http://www.communitiesinschools.org/
media/uploads/attachments/Network_Results_2009-2010.pdf

Community Preventive Services Task Force. (2015). *Promoting health equity
through education programs and policies: Center-based early childhood education.* Retrieved from www.thecommunityguide.org/healthequity/education/
centerbasedprograms.html

Demissie, Z., Brener, N. D., McManus, T., Shanklin, S. L., Hawkins, J., & Kann, L.
(2013). *School health profiles 2012: Characteristics of health programs among
secondary schools.* Atlanta, GA: Centers for Disease Control and Prevention.

Duncan, G. J., & Magnuson, K. (2013). Investing in preschool programs. *Journal of
Economic Perspectives, 13,* 109–131.

Fletcher, A. (2005). Meaningful student involvement: Guide to students as partners
in school change (2nd ed). Retrieved from http://www.soundout.org/MSIGuide
.pdf

Fox, H. B., McManus, M. A. & Arnold, K. N. (2010). *Significant multiple risk
behaviors among U.S. high school students.* Fact Sheet. National Alliance to
Advance Adolescent Health. March. No. 8. Retrieved from http://osbhcn.org/
files/Risk%20Behaviors%20and%20HS%20Students.pdf

Griebler, U., Rojatz, D., Simovska, V., & Forster, R. (2014). Effects of student participation in school health promotion: A systematic review. *Health Promotion
International.* Retrieved from http://heapro.oxfordjournals.org/content/early/
2014/01/05/heapro.dat090.full.pdf

Health Promoting Universities and Colleges. (2015) *The Okanagan charter
for health promoting universities and colleges.* Retrieved from http://www
.internationalhealthycampuses2015.com/

ICF International. (2010). *Communities in schools national evaluation five year
executive summary.* Retrieved from http://www.communitiesinschools.org/
media/uploads/attachments/Communities_In_Schools_National_Evaluation_
Five_Year_Executive_Summary.pdf

Institute of Medicine (2000). From neurons to neighborhoods: The science of early
childhood development. Washington D.C., National Academy Press.

Joint Committee on National Health Education Standards. (2007). *National health
education standards: Achieving excellence* (2nd ed.). Atlanta, GA: American
Cancer Society.

Kann, L., Telljohann, S., Hunt, H., Hunt, P., & Haller, E. (2013). *Health education. In Results from the school health policies and practices study 2012*. Atlanta, GA: CDC. Retrieved from http://www.cdc.gov/healthyyouth/shpps/2012/pdf/shpps-results_2012.pdf#page=27

Lofink, H., Kuebler, J., Juszczak, L., Schlitt, J., Even, M., Rosenberg, J., & White, I. (2013). *2010–2011 census report of school-based health centers*. Retrieved from http://www.sbh4all.org/school-health-care/national-census-of-school-based-health-centers/

Lwebuga-Mukasa, J., & Dunn-Georgiou, E. (2002). A school-based asthma intervention program in the Buffalo, New York schools. *Journal of School Health, 72*, 27–32.

Mamedova, S., & Redford, J. (2015). *Early childhood program participation, from the National Household Education Surveys Program of 2012*. National Center for Education Statistics. Retrieved from https://nces.ed.gov/pubsearch/pubsinfo.asp?pubid=2013029rev

McLaughlin, M. W. (2000). *Community counts: How youth organizations matter for youth development*. Retrieved from http://www.issuelab.org/resource/community_counts_how_youth_organizations_matter_for_youth_development

MetLife. (2012*). The MetLife survey of American teachers: Teachers, parents and the economy: A survey of teachers, parents and students*. Retrieved from http://www.metlife.com/assets/cao/contributions/foundation/american-teacher/MetLife-Teacher-Survey-2011.pdf

Moore, K. A., & Emig, C (2014). Integrated student supports: A summary of the evidence base for policymakers. *Child Trends*. Retrieved from http://www.childtrends.org/wp-content/uploads/2014/02/2014-05ISSWhitePaper3.pdf

Morse, L. L, & Allensworth, D. D. (2015). Placing students at the center: The whole school, whole community, whole child approach. *Journal of School Health, 85*, 785–794.

Murray, N., Franzini, L., Marko, D., Lupo, P. Jr., Garza, J., & Linder, S. (2006). Education and health: A review and assessment, Appendix E. In Code red: The critical condition of health in Texas. Retrieved from http://www.utsystem.edu/sites/utsfiles/documents/publication/code-red-critical-condition-health-texas/appendix.pdf

National Association for the Education of Young Children. (2008). *Overview of the NAEYC early childhood program standards*. Washington, DC: Author. Retrieved from http://www.naeyc.org/files/academy/file/OverviewStandards.pdf

National Association for the Education of Young Children. (2015). *NAEYC early childhood program standards and accreditation criteria & guidance for assessment*. Washington, DC: Author. Retrieved from http://www.naeyc.org/files/academy/file/AllCriteriaDocument.pdf

National Association of Child Care Resource and Referral Agencies. (2011). *We can do better: NACCRRA's ranking of state child care center standards and oversight*. Retrieved from http://www.naccrra.org/about-child-care/state-child-care-licensing/we-can-do-better-state-child-care-center-licensing

National Center for Education Statistics. (2013). Table 105.30. Enrollment in educational institutions, by level and control of institution: Digest of Education Statistics: 2013. Retrieved May 26 from http://nces.ed.gov/programs/digest/d13/tables/dt13_230.50.asp

National Survey of Early Care and Education Project Team. (2013). *Number and Characteristics of Early Care and Education (ECE) Teachers and Caregivers: Initial Findings from the National Survey of Early Care and Education (NSECE)*. OPRE Report #2013-38, Washington DC: Office of Planning, Research and Evaluation, Administration for Children and Families, U.S. Department of Health and Human Services.

Snyder, T. D., & Dillow, S. A. (2015). Table 105.10. Projected number of participants in educational institutions, by level and control of institution: Fall 2013 *Digest of Education Statistics 2013* (NCES 2015-011). National Center for Education Statistics, Institute of Education Sciences, U.S. Department of Education. Retrieved from http://nces.ed.gov/pubs2015/2015011.pdf or from http://nces.ed.gov/programs/digest

Taras, H., Duncan, P., Luckenbill, D., Robinson, J., Wheeler, L., & Wooley, S. (2004). Health, mental health and safety guidelines for schools. *American Academy of Pediatrics*. Retrieved from http://www.nationalguidelines.org/

Telljohann, S. K., Dake, J. A., & Price, J. H. (2004). Effect of full-time versus part time school nurses on attendance of elementary students with asthma. *Journal of School Nursing, 20*, 331–334.

Terzian, M. A., Andrews, K. M., & Moore, K. A. (2011). Preventing Multiple Risky Behaviors among Adolescents: Seven Strategies. *Child Trends Brief Results to Practice*, September 2011. Publication #2011-24. Retrieved from http://www.childtrends.org/files/Child_Trends-2011_10_01_RB_RiskyBehaviors.pdf

Toshalis E., & Nakkula, M. J. (2012). Motivation, engagement, and student voice. *The Students At The Center Series*. Retrieved from http://www.studentsatthecenter.org/topics/motivation-engagement-and-student-voice

Tsouros, A., Dowding, G., & Dooris, M. (1998). Strategic framework for the Health Promoting Universities project. In A. Tsouros, G. Dowding, J. Thompson, & M. Dooris (Eds.), *Health promoting universities: Concept, experience and framework for action* (pp. 121–137). Copenhagen: World Health Organization.

U.S. Department of Health and Human Services. (2015). Early and middle childhood. *Healthy People 2020*. Retrieved from http://www.healthypeople.gov/2020/topics-objectives/topic/early-and-middle-childhood/objectives

Wallerstein, N. (2006). What is the evidence on effectiveness of empowerment to improve health? Health Evidence Network Report. Retrieved from http://www.euro.who.int/__data/assets/pdf_file/0010/74656/E88086.pdf

CHAPTER 14

PATIENT-CENTERED HEALTH PROMOTION PROGRAMS IN HEALTH CARE ORGANIZATIONS

Louise Villejo, Cezanne Garcia, and Katherine Crosson

Historical Context and Evolution of Engaging Patients and Families in the Design and Delivery of Health Promotion Programs

For centuries, patient instruction and health education have been intrinsic components of the health care process. Even as the institutionalization of U.S. health care in the middle to late 1800s first emerged, the function of educating patients about their illness, family members (caregivers) in the care of the sick, proper sanitation precautions, and disease prevention was as imperative then as now. With the growing prevalence of disability and tuberculosis in the World War II veteran population, patient education as a separate, key component of patient care emerged, with topics expanding from long-standing commitments to educate about disease prevention to include patient understanding of their disease and its treatment. This broadened scope of patient instruction was endorsed in the late 1960s and early 1970s by the American Public Health Association and subsequently mandated by the Department of Health, Education, and Welfare as an essential component of health care in hospitals. Following the American Hospital Association's establishment of the Patient Bill of Rights in 1973, which positioned patient education as an essential part of quality care, other medical, public health, and accreditation associations further

LEARNING OBJECTIVES

- Discuss the historical context and evolution of the design and delivery of patient-centered health promotion programs.

- Identify core components of effective patient-centered health promotion programs.

- Identify and discuss resources and tools for patient-centered health promotion programs.

- Explore the opportunities and challenges of patient-centered health promotion programs.

- Describe health promotion careers in health care organizations.

articulated essential fidelity standards to ensure the provision and quality of patient education.

In the 1980s and 1990s, individuals known as patient advocates began to exert their influence on the health care system. Giving voice to patients, families, and their caregivers, patient advocates worked closely with advocacy groups, relying on their close identification with the patient population to assess informational and educational needs, as well as lobbying on behalf of the patient population for patient-centered services within the health care environment (Davenport-Ennis, Cover, Ades, & Stovall, 2002). The patient rights movement emerged and provided the foundation for social action driving improvements in community health and health policy focused on health system access, cost, and safety. Patient advocates were fervent about the need for change in the health care system and the importance of health care providers listening to patients' concerns, respecting their lifestyles, and partnering with rather than dictating to patients, their families, and their significant others. These clinician-patient communication priorities were coupled with advocacy for delivery system improvements, policy reform, and funding to support patient-centered ways to benefit patients' lives and care. The earliest advocacy groups emerged from advocates keen to improve care and treatment for oncology patients, individuals with HIV/AIDS, and a range of health care issues focused on maternal and child health care. Advocacy group membership broadened over time to include a diverse array of government, private, and public members, together increasing the national awareness of selective health issues, a growth in funding and implementation of research, dissemination of information, and outreach activities. The success of these early groups has resulted in advocacy group expansion to many other health and chronic illness areas (Silberman, Ricketts, & Cohen Ross, 2008).

Current patient engagement practices, based upon a growing evidence base and the advocacy of patient-centered principles and practices, is emboldened by the support of diverse health care agencies and leadership that fuels current and future assurances of a central role for the effective engagement of patients and families. The transformative Institute of Medicine (IOM) report *Crossing the Quality Chasm* (2001), laid the groundwork for absolute qualities necessary for building a high-quality health care delivery system: equitable, timely, effective, efficient, safe, and patient-centered. This report has inspired the tireless work of advocacy, health care, accreditation, certification, and health professional membership associations who have translated these tenets into awareness and skill-building training, research agendas, policy reform, and advocacy efforts to accelerate and advance the practice of patient engagement to achieve these health care goals.

Tools and practices of today's health promotion and wellness programs in health care settings have been strongly influenced by the intersection of advocacy, research, and best practices in patient education, patient engagement, worksite health promotion, and payment reform. All share common confidence that health, health care delivery, research, and system-transforming actions are guided by the principles of "with" patients and not "on" or "for" patients.

Effective Programs in Health Care Organizations

Components of effective institution-wide, patient-centered health promotion programs in health care organizations include

- Involving staff, patients, and families

- Engaging leadership at both the clinical and administrative levels

- Adopting program planning principles

- Designing programs that incorporate evidence-based approaches and best practices

- Using an interdisciplinary, collaborative approach

- Committing to quality performance, improvement, and continual evaluation

There is much health promotion in health care settings shares with both workplace and community-based settings. Unique to health care organizations, however, are health promotion programs that are patient centered and associated with patient education to help individuals and their caregivers understand and participate in decisions about their health, disease, and treatment. These programs support informed decision making and often include skills training needed for individuals' participation in health management, treatment, and recovery. Increased expectations of a partnership role in health care has fueled consumers' demand for personalized health information, tailored health promotion programs, and an increase in self-management strategies.

Patients and their families are increasingly managing their health with the aid of evolving technologies online (Smith, 2011). Despite newly available communication channels, physicians remained the most highly trusted information source to patients, with 62% of adults expressing a lot of trust in their physicians. When asked where they preferred going for specific health information, 50% reported wanting to go to their physicians first. When asked where they actually went, 49% reported going online first, with only 11% going to their physicians first (Hesse et al., 2005).

Patients can access their own health information through *electronic health records* (EHRs) to help support engagement and decision making in their care. The advancement of EHR sharing across different health care settings is slowly emerging, challenged by cost, security, and proprietary concerns. EHRs can include the patients' medical history, medication, allergies, immunization status, laboratory test results, appointments, billing information, and patient education resources. In addition, aggregate EHR data is used by health education specialists to inform and tailor health promotion programming to patient population needs, such as lifestyle counseling support. Adoption, implementation, and demonstrated meaningful use is supported by Medicare and Medicaid Electronic Health Records Incentive Programs (www.cms.gov/Regulations-and-Guidance/Legislation/EHRIncentivePrograms/index.html).

Involving Staff Patients and Families

The first critical component in patient-centered health promotion program in health care is to engage the population you serve. Patient- and family-centered care is "an approach to the planning, delivery and evaluation of health care that is grounded in mutually beneficial partnerships among health care patients, families, and providers." It is built on the four core concepts of dignity and respect, information sharing, participation, and collaboration (Institute for Patient- and Family-Centered Care, 2015). *Patient- and family-centered care* has and will continue to be a transformational force in health care. By creating capacity for patients and families as allies for quality in their health care experience, the driving forces of change can become more patient- and family-centered, applying a more biopsychosocial perspective rather than predominantly system- or clinician-centered (Greene, Tuzzio, & Cherkin, 2012).

This approach strives to maintain a balance between technically competent care and emotionally supportive care. The *patient and family education* programs incorporating a patient- and family-centered approach have demonstrated a greater adherence to treatment protocols, self-care, safe care at home and psychosocial support (Johnson et al., 2008). In addition, there is a need to strengthen the integration of health promotion resources and interventions as integral components of clinical decision making and treatment education for patients and families.

The cost of supporting the integration of the patient-as-advisor into council structures and committees within a health care organization is small considering the benefits. Costs may include training, meeting attendance expenses such as parking and refreshments, and in some organizations, patients/family advisors are hired as staff supporting these efforts. The organization must also have a commitment to educating staff about how to best work with advisors, as well as best practices for patient-centered care. Benefits of patient engagement include knowledge and experiences, reduced health care utilization and costs, and improved health status and behavior (Edgman-Levitan, Brady, & Howitt, 2013). When patients' needs and preferences are at the center of every care decision and action, the patient care experience is greatly enhanced (Stewart et al., 2000).

Engaging Leadership

Another critical component of an effective patient-centered health promotion program in health care settings is the active and involved engagement of both clinical and administrative leadership. It is essential that health promotion and patient education programs be tied to an institution's strategic vision and aligned with improving outcomes. Programs must be presented in such a way that they demonstrate their contribution to improving health outcomes. Specifically, the programs must support patients' understanding of their disease and treatment, adherence to treatment protocols, knowledge building and self-care skills for safe care at home, and asking questions to ensure understanding of the care experience. Clinician and administrator champions committed to the program must be identified and engaged to foster and share stories about programs' successes (American Hospital Association, 2004).

Adopting Program Planning Principles

Health promotion and patient education programs with the greatest promise are comprehensive, use standardized processes, integrate several different modalities to address diverse patient population learning needs, and focus on specific groups—individuals, families, social networks, organizations, and communities. An effective program is well integrated within a clinic-specific or institution-wide strategic plan and tailored to patient care and individual needs. Structured educational interventions and behavioral counseling initiatives in the health care setting have contributed to improved health outcomes and reduced hospital readmissions and overutilization of outpatient services, and resulted in fewer medication errors, increased *patient safety*, lowered health care costs, and supported the adoption of healthier lifestyles and behaviors (Jack et al., 2009). The learning environment is often a teaching room in a clinic, an examining room, or a patient learning center. Hospitals and clinics are recognizing the value of patient and family resource centers in meeting consumer information and support needs. Many health care organizations offer patient family resource centers, online and print educational resources, and televisions and computers for health education programming throughout their facilities. This is in the recognition that a better informed patient leads to improved health outcomes and furthers the incentive for a patient resource center to strengthen a hospital's marketing position (Institute for Patient- and Family-Centered Care, 2015).

Incorporating Evidence into Practice

The ever-evolving research base has strengthened *evidence-based practices* in patient and family health promotion and improved understanding of the links between patient behavior and health outcomes (Table 14.1). Patient-centered health promotion programs in health care organizations are strengthened by accreditation- and certification-driven patient and family education standards. Panels of experts translate research and best practice evidence into practice standards, resulting in high-quality, outcome-oriented patient and family education programs.

The use of decision-aid tools is a highly effective strategy that demonstrates the value of integrating evidence-based practices with patient's personal values (O'Connor et al., 2003). Patient decision aids typically are multimedia tools or booklets designed to communicate the best available

Table 14.1   Standards for High-Quality Outcome-Oriented Patient and Family Education Programs

- Accreditation standards for health care settings developed by the Joint Commission (2015)
- Clinical practice standards promulgated by the U.S. Preventive Services Task Force (2015)
- Patient-centered medical home certification standards (American Academy of Family Practice, 2016; Joint Commission, 2015)
- Institution or system-specific practice guidelines that are defined as part of policy and procedure guidelines within most health care organizations such as the Indian Health Service's Patient Education Protocols and Codes (Indian Health Service, n.d.)
- Tailored disease-specific or practitioner-specific patient- and family-centered care and education guidelines
- American Diabetes Association's National Standards for Diabetes Self-Management Education and Support (Haas et al., 2014)
- Guidelines for Establishing Comprehensive Cancer Patient Education Services (Cancer Patient Education Network, 2013)
- Guide to Patient and Family Engagement in Hospital Quality and Safety (AHRQ, 2013)

evidence on treatment or screening options to patients and their families in ways that encourage them to engage in meaningful dialogue with their health care provider to choose an intervention that is consistent with the evidence and the patient's personal values. These tools support clinician and patient collaboration and are designed to translate the research evidence and help patients apply this information to preference-sensitive health decisions (Elwyn et al., 2006).

Using an Interdisciplinary, Collaborative Approach

An interdisciplinary, collaborative approach is vital to the success of patient-centered health promotion programs. Such programs work in partnership with clinically trained professional teams (e.g., physicians, nurses, social workers, health educators, dietitians, physical therapists, and pharmacists) and patients and their families to guide the development of interventions that will enable patients to manage and live with their disease, adapt new health behaviors, and learn new skills. The American Hospital Association developed a white paper, "Workforce Roles in a Redesigned Primary Care Model," which recommends that all health care professionals are educated within the context of interdisciplinary clinical learning teams, and primary health care is centered around the patient and family in a user-driven design, in all aspects of practice. Health and wellness are intergrated together for patients in a way that provides a sustainable infrastructure of health care for patients and the community (American Hospital Association, 2013).

Interdisciplinary clinical teams help guide health promotion practice at the institutional level by creating, implementing, and supporting institutional priorities for development and management of patient-centered programs. At the program level, clinical managers and staff can provide feedback to the team about the best and most timely way to integrate health promotion interventions with routine patient care. And at the one-to-one teaching level, clinical managers can support training and provide coaching to ensure staff competencies in teaching patients.

The Joint Commission (2015) requires an interdisciplinary approach to patient health promotion and profiles discipline-specific practice standards. Commitment to the use of an interdisciplinary approach helps staff in each discipline to understand the unique role of each team member and address patients' learning needs more effectively through the use of consistent and evidence-based information and practices, creating continuity and quality care experiences for patients and families.

Committing to Quality Performance, Improvement, and Continual Evaluation

The evidence-based principles of education with promising effects on behavior and clinical outcomes include individualization of instruction in order to provide explicit feedback on learning or clinical progress; reinforcement of learning; tailoring of education to the needs, interests, and abilities of the learner; use of multiple communication channels, including information that describes and manages expectations in the care experience; the *teach-back* method and creating capacity for the patient and family engagement to take action or remove barriers to action using tools such as the patient activation measure (Banerjee, MacDougall, & Lakhdar, 2012; Hibbard, Stockard, Mahoney, & Tusler, 2004; Kruis et al., 2013). Professionals involved with patient-centered health promotion programs in medical settings routinely monitor and evaluate behavioral and clinical outcomes.

Improving and sustaining such programs relies increasingly on identifying the key components of an intervention that are effective and being able to demonstrate that effectiveness to leadership. Programs must strive to show their impact on utilization, patient satisfaction, effectiveness, and outcomes. How does the program support institutional initiatives and health care outcomes? Which metrics best demonstrate impact that will generate continued support? How can you track how the program helps the organization meet regulatory requirements? These questions are addressed at the beginning of program planning so they are reflected in program evaluation and used to continually assess and improve the program.

Health Promotion Resources

Over the past 25 years, changes in medical practice and the delivery of health care have dramatically altered how patients and their families receive information, instruction, education, and special support from one another. Additionally, health care team efforts are supported and enhanced by new electronic technologies and strategies that go well beyond the clinician-patient interactions.

Before initiating any planning for health promotion programs in the health care setting, review existing standards, guidelines, and mandates related to health education and health promotion including the following resources:

- *The Joint Commission's R3 Report: Patient-Centered Communication Standards for Hospitals* provides the rationale and references that

The Joint Commission employed in developing the patient-centered communication standards for hospitals. (www.jointcommission.org)

- *The National Culturally and Linguistically Appropriate Services (CLAS) in Health and Health Care* from the Department of Health and Human Services Office of Minority Health. Strategies and plans are included that will guide the implementation of culturally and linguistically appropriate services. (www.minorityhealth.hhs.gov)

- *Institute of Medicine's Roundtable on Health Literacy (2015)* includes 10 attributes that make it easier for those with limited *health literacy* to navigate, understand, and use information and services to take care of their health. (www.iom.edu)

- *Your health care organization's strategic plan and related policies and procedures* addressing health promotion, cultural competency, patient education, and engagement.

- *Plain Language Guidelines* from the National Institutes for Health (NIH). (www.nih.gov/clearcommunication/plainlanguage/index.htm)

- *Readability Tests and Instruments* from the Centers for Disease Control and Prevention (CDC). (www.cdc.gov/healthliteracy/DevelopMaterials/GuidanceStandards.html)

- *The Affordable Care Act* identifies health literacy provisions for research dissemination, shared decision making, medication labeling, and workforce development to improve access to and quality of health care. (http://www.chcs.org/media/Health_Literacy_Implications_of_the_Affordable_Care_Act.pdf)

Another essential step is to review aggregate data that describes patient population demographics, lifestyle behaviors (exercise, smoking, diet, alcohol and drug use), ethnicity, language preferences, health status data, health literacy and *patient activation* and/or self-efficacy information about willingness, and health behavior change attitudes. This data provides a snapshot in time of patients' educational and informational needs, concerns, preferences, readiness to learn, and possible challenges to learning.

For the individual care encounter, there are general and disease- or illness-specific educational needs assessment tools that are very effective in helping patients and their clinical team members focus on what the patient needs to know about their medical condition, health outcomes, and treatment options. One of the most widely used screening tools in the health promotion field is the computer- or paper-based health risk appraisal (HRA). The CDC defines the tool as "a systematic approach to collecting information from individuals that identifies risk factors, provides individualized feedback and links the person with a least one intervention to promote health, sustain function and/or prevent disease" (CDC, 2010).

Equally important in developing programs is to assess health care delivery system properties, such as the availability of health promoting and disease specific education resources in the primary language(s) of the patient populations' served, the availability of interpreter services to assist patients and their families in their care encounter and clinic practices that support patient preferences for a family or trusted friend's presence during the care encounter. It is also critical to foster the strengths and assets of clinician practices that support the patient's communication preferences and learning. For example, how does a health care provider explain complex medical information to individual patients and families with limited English language skills or diminished health literacy? Educators need to pay close attention to special patient subgroups and tailor patient education and health promotion programs to also meet these unique needs, or risk not achieving the desired behavioral outcomes. Also, review best practice and peer-reviewed literature for design, implementation, and evaluation innovations and recommendations.

Focus groups are another way to gather detailed information about individual preferences for learning and cultural beliefs, and identify ways to enhance knowledge and self-management skills for specific medical conditions (Krueger & Casey, 2014). Additionally, engaging the organization's leaders, administrators, members of boards, and Patient and Family Advisory Council members in a program design committee in program development is especially valuable for program design ideas and to garner support for operational resources such as staffing, space, and curriculum materials.

Using needs assessment information gleaned from aggregate health record, HRA data, and focus groups, educators must involve patients, families, clinicians, and administrators in establishing specific objectives for the education program's audience, defining the educational approach, and designing or selecting appropriate teaching tools. Additionally, the information is useful in discerning how to best introduce the health promotion program in the health care setting, train educators to deliver the program, and identify educational approaches that are most effective.

There are many educational approaches employed to assist patients and families learn new behaviors and skills and to eliminate actions that are not health promoting. One-on-one instruction, group classes, peer and provider counseling, and prescribed viewing of videotapes or computer-based education programs followed by question and answer sessions with health care providers is current practice. There is growing evidence that clinician use of *motivational interviewing (MI)* during a care encounter can

Table 14.2   Selecting Appropriate Educational Resources for Patient Audiences

Agency for Healthcare Research and Quality's Patient Education Materials Assessment Tool (PEMAT)
www.ahrq.gov/professionals/prevention-chronic-care/improve/self-mgmt/pemat/index.html
Health Information Technology (IT) Literacy Guide www.healthit.gov

Readability Tests

Gunning Fog Index or FOG Readability Formula http://www.readabilityformulas.com/gunning-fog-readability-formula.php

Flesch Reading Ease Readability Formula www.readabilityformulas.com/flesch-reading-ease-readability-formula.php

(SMOG) www.readabilityformulas.com/smog-readability-formula.php

Suitability of Materials (SAM) Instrument (Doak & Doak, 1996)

build a patient's motivation and readiness to change. MI has been used in many health care decision domains; however, it is most successfully used in promoting healthy diet, exercise, diabetes management, and oral health behaviors (Martins & McNeil, 2009).

Ready-to-use print and web-based health promotion and patient education resources are in abundance and often available free of charge (Tables 14.2 & 14.3). Whether free or fee-based resources are used, the materials are reviewed by a multidisciplinary program planning team that includes clinicians, patients and families for final selection. Furthermore, the use of EHR and secure, personalized patient portals has expanded technology-based opportunities to provide tailored health promotion and disease management information to patients. Federally promulgated EHR guidelines provide quality assurance for patient reminders, security and confidentiality, and seek practices to assure that patients not only can view their medical record, but define plain language standards to ensure understanding. Patient engagement requirements of EHRs are expected to increase (Silow-Carroll, Edwards, & Rodin, 2012).

The Medicare and Medicaid EHR Incentive Program provides financial incentives to meaningfully use EHRs to improve the quality of care, reduce medical errors, and improve efficiency. The "Meaningful Use" guidelines not only provide for capturing health information in a standardized fashion, but advise using that information to provide patients and families access to their health information and support their engagement in their care. Meaningful Use criteria states that certified EHR technology must be used to identify patient-specific education resources and provide those resources to the patient if appropriate. It also defines specific measures of patient utilization for each stage. For example, the Stage 2 measure to achieve

Table 14.3   Health Promotion and Patient Education Resources Available from the Federal Government

Agency for Healthcare Research and Quality
www.ahrq.gov

Centers for Disease Control and Prevention
www.cdc.gov

Centers for Medicare and Medicaid Services
www.cms.gov

Department of Defense (Health Affairs)
www.dod.gov

Indian Health Service
www.ihs.gov

National Institutes of Health
www.nih.gov

National Library of Medicine
www.nlm.gov

U.S. Department of Veteran Affairs www.va.gov

Health Promotion and Patient Education Resources Available from Health Professional Organizations

American Hospital Association
www.aha.org

American Medical Association
www.ama.org

American Nurses Association
www.ana.org

Institute for Patient and Family-Centered Care
www.ifpcc.org

National Patient Safety Foundation
www.npsf.org

Society for Public Health Education
www.sophe.org

World Health Organization
http://www.who.org

higher-level EHR certification requires providing education resources to more than 10 percent of all unique patients seen by the health care provider (Centers for Medicare and Medicaid Services, 2016).

Once the assembly of needs assessment data, the design of the educational program, and the selection of the resources is complete, the interdisciplinary committee is well situated to contribute marketing and communication suggestions. Members can serve as spokespersons promoting and recruiting participation in the new program, including writing influential articles promoting the program for their organization's publications.

Table 14.4   Evaluating Health Promotion Tools in Health Care Settings

Questions to consider asking when you are evaluating whether a specific educational tool is right for a particular audience:

- Do the teaching tools that accompany the program enhance the content or reinforce key messages being conveyed by the program instructors?
- Can the patient demonstrate a specific self-care skill such as, how to change wound dressings for safe care at home?
- Can the family member describe their role in supporting the care of the patient at home, such as what steps they need to take to ensure meals meet the dietary requirements of the patient?
- Did health promotion program participants adhere to their action plan co-created in the program, such as follow an exercise regime after participating in a program for those at increased risk for heart disease?

After a short period of implementation, program planners conduct evaluations with education program participants to determine if the program objectives have been achieved (Table 14.4). The teach-back method of evaluation is used as best practice in health care settings. It is a way to confirm in one-on-one instruction that you have taught the patient in a way that they understand. Patient understanding is confirmed when the patient explains to the clinician, in their own words, what they learned. The method is especially valuable because it gives the individual staff member immediate feedback about what is being understood or misunderstood by their patient (Institute for Healthcare Improvement, 2016).

Challenges for Programs in Health Care Organizations

Implementing effective health promotion programs within a health care organization is dependent on numerous factors: the support and engagement of administrative and clinical leadership, interdisciplinary health care providers, patients and their families, a department or program with responsibility and adequate resources for planning and conducting health promotion and patient education programs, and a commitment to quality performance improvement, collaboration, and continual evaluation. Although the benefits to offering health-promoting activities within a hospital, clinic, or physician's office seem quite obvious, there are many challenges, especially within the context of a health care delivery system that is driven by demands to manage patients with multiple comorbidities or chronic conditions, reduce per capita costs of care, treat and care for an increasingly diverse patient population, and utilize evidence-based practices in support of improved quality and patient safety. Recent shifts in health care policy and payment reform have focused on reducing fee-for-service financial barriers that have historically impeded health organization adoption of highly effective preventive services and the promotion of promising innovations strengthening alliances between clinical care and public health services to support population health (Centers for Medicare & Medicaid Services, 2016).

Health care organizations differ from other settings in that their core mandate is restoring, maintaining, and promoting health through the application of clinical services and the collaboration of both medical and public health staff members. Additionally, health care organizations deal with life-threatening situations on a daily basis, an element that doesn't have to be considered when implementing health promotion programs in workplace and school settings. Since health care organizations are subject to many clinical service-driven regulations, restrictions, and guidelines, it is important for those responsible for health promotion program planning to understand and be responsive to these organizational policies and procedures that influence their programs.

An important challenge for anyone responsible for the implementation of health promotion programs within a health care setting is the presence of multiple stakeholders—patients and families; medical professionals; administrators of health service institutions; insurance companies; payer groups; large employers and government-sponsored research, regulatory, and policy-making entities—and their diverse and dynamic priorities and recommendations on how to manage and improve the care experience with limited resources. Professional practice conflicts have emerged showcasing the divergent priorities of clinicians focused on preventing disease and clinicians whose work and income is based on expensive treatments of disease. In addition, responsibility for informing and educating patients and families, once considered to be the sole responsibility of physicians and nurses, is increasingly provided by multidisciplinary teams of professionals with varying degrees of training in educational principles, behavior change, and counseling. In the past decade, many professional societies such as the American Academy of Family Physicians, the American Nurses Association, and the National Association of Social Workers have introduced patient education curriculum guidelines for their members, including those in training. These professional groups recognize that as health care practices become increasingly patient centered, patient involvement in the health care decision-making process through patient education is necessary and will lead to improvements in health outcomes and patient satisfaction.

With changing demographics nationwide, health care professionals whether working in large systems or small office practices must have the

Table 14.5   Strategies for Sharing Best Practices in a Health Care Setting

- Create forums for staff collaboration to bolster programming.
- Encourage staff and patients to share their stories profiling positive experiences with health promotion programs within the health care system community.
- Engage staff and patients in processes to integrate health promotion programming in clinical workflow and the design of plans to disseminate information and spread innovations.
- Engage staff to support the selection of valid and reliable instruments or design measurement systems for monitoring impact and improvements (for example, use of the Assessment of Chronic Illness Care Survey (Acton et al., 1993, 1995) to address the basic elements for improving chronic illness care at the community, organization, practice, and patient level (http://www.ihi.org/resources/Pages/Tools/default.aspx).

knowledge and skills to assess and provide tailored educational interventions for many different patient populations, as described earlier in this chapter. Health care organizations are continually challenged to identify practitioners who represent these diverse patient groups and to create educational systems that will support and sustain a culturally competent workforce. Health promotion program leadership also need to develop in-person and as appropriate, technology-based staff training and coaching programs that are integrated in the organization's competency training curriculum to strengthen staff skills and knowledge to deliver quality health promotion services. These staff development strategies will need to fit institutional staff development schedules, such as a commitment to repeated offerings across two to four staff shifts for settings that provide 24-hour care.

Although often challenging to orchestrate, interdisciplinary collaborations that support patients, families, and medical staff have proven to be effective in providing health promotion services and programs in health care organizations (Table 14.5). Furthermore, without collaboration, programs often cannot be sustained. Collaboration enhances credibility and engages staff in all steps of the planning and implementation process. While it might be time consuming, the initial investments of time or resources has long-term benefits.

A team of researchers at the University of Oregon has led the movement to develop patient activation measures to assess levels of activation, and their work needs to be closely followed for its potential to strengthen patient and family collaboration with their health care providers. The time it takes to build these partnerships and acquire appropriate knowledge and skills for collaboration will eventually be repaid several times over. When administrators, clinicians, consumers, and families have a shared understanding of and respect for what each brings to the health care experience, the stage is set for mutually beneficial relationships. With programming tailored to a patient's activation threshold and defining shared priorities and goals, there is promise that time will not be wasted on repetitive, ineffective, or counterproductive activities. When patients are active and involved in the management of their care, their health care outcomes are improved. The possibility of misunderstanding, dissatisfaction, and even medical error will be greatly diminished (Hibbard, Stockard, Mahoney, & Tusler, 2004).

Since many health professionals have not received specific training on how to work as a member of a team, staff training and in-service education challenges exist within the health care setting. Courses need to be offered that include content areas such as communication, conflict management and negotiation, team roles, and leadership.

While collaboration is important, administrative and clinical champions are essential to support health promotion programs in health care organizations. Champions, ideally individuals who are viewed as role models and opinion leaders by their peers, need to be engaged to advocate for health promotion programs within their organizations. Champions serve on the committees and task forces that design and support these programs; optimally these leaders are managers, clinicians, and support staff with an interest in or knowledge about health promotion programs.

Sustaining health promotion programs in a medical care setting also requires building the credibility of programs through evaluation and reporting back to stakeholders. Frequent and varied program communication and program materials for both health care organization employees who are program participants and to program staff need to be an ongoing part of program operations.

Career Opportunities

Money Magazine named health and wellness educators as the fastest-growing, high-paying career for the future (Bortz, 2015) and the profession is projected to have faster than average job growth through 2022. The traditional venues for careers and employment in the health care field include hospitals, clinics, physicians' offices, group practices, and home health agencies. Many other opportunities have opened up in IT for website and course design, pharmaceutical and health education companies for health promotion products' development, teaching, training and evaluation as well as other new direct service settings like fitness and health coaching in the community or online. Traditional venues for careers include hospitals, public health offices, and so on (Table 14.6).

An increasing number of health care organizations now offer many opportunities for a career in health promotion. At the same time, career connections and opportunities in a number of other organizations and

Table 14.6   Traditional and Emerging Job Titles for Health and Wellness Professionals

Health education specialist	Patient- and family-centered care coordinators
Health educator	Family educator
Patient educator	Patient relations coordinator
Health promotion specialist	Community relations specialist
Dietician	Community education specialist
Tobacco educator	Program specialist/coordinator
Patient navigator	Public health officer
Patient advocate	
Community health worker	

fields related to health and medicine are now more plentiful and available (Table 14.6). Physicians, nurses, health educators, counselors, psychologists, and individuals trained in the allied health professions may find health promotion-related positions in their specific professional fields. Health promotion and wellness professionals work in a variety of settings:

- **Traditional health care settings.** Health care settings include hospitals, clinics, health centers (community and federally qualified); rehabilitation services, long-term care facilities, home health care agencies; tribal, state, and local health departments.

- **Consumer groups and interest groups.** Interest groups are voluntary associations with specific and narrowly defined goals. Probably the most common among the health-related interest groups are those focused on a particular health condition, such as the American Cancer Society, American Diabetes Association, American Lung Association, and American Heart Association. All these groups have large health promotion program operations that work at both the national and local levels. The Cystic Fibrosis Association is an example of a leading association that integrates patient engagement with their health promotion operations. It recognizes exceptional hospital partnerships with patients and families with a Cystic Fibrosis Foundation's Quality Care Award: Recognizing Outstanding QI Processes and Accomplishments (https://www.cff.org/). Some interest groups may represent one segment of the public (such as retired people or students), or they may focus on promoting values such as patient engagement led by such organizations as the Institute for Patient- and Family-Centered Care, Planetree, World Health Organization, or the Institute for Healthcare Improvement. And patient or consumer-led groups include National Organization for Rare Disorders, Patient Power, and Cystic Fibrosis Parent Advocacy Group.

• **U.S. government.** The U.S. government offers numerous career opportunities for health education specialists, from entry-level to senior positions. The Department of Health and Human Services employs many health educators both at its headquarters in Washington, D.C., and throughout the nation in state and regional offices. Operating divisions such as the Centers for Medicare and Medicaid Services, the National Institutes of Health, the CDC, the Agency for Healthcare Research, and many other governmental agencies have relied on health educators for decades. In addition, the Indian Health Service, Department of Defense, and the Veterans Administration have well-organized health care systems that employ health educators and patient- and family-centered care coordinators. Specific job announcements are found at http://www.usajobs.opm.gov.

• **Medical technology, pharmaceutical, genetics, and biologics companies.** Medical technology is the diagnostic or therapeutic application of science and technology to improve or manage health conditions. Technologies can encompass any means of identifying the nature of health conditions in order to allow intervention with devices or with pharmacological, biological, or other methods for the purpose of increasing life span or improving quality of life. Many of these organizations have websites and offer print materials that provide information, feedback, personal coaching, and support of health promotion activities related to particular medical conditions.

• **Professional associations focused on medicine, public health, and wellness.** A professional association is an organization, usually nonprofit, whose purpose is to further a particular profession and to protect both the public interest and the interests of the professionals. Almost all health and medical professions have associations. Many are involved in development and monitoring of professional education programs and the updating of professional skills and professional certifications. Examples below include organizations health promotion programs include the following:

  • American Academy of Family Physicians (http://www.aafp.org/online/en/home.html)

  • American Nurses Association (http://nursingworld.org/)

  • American Public Health Association's Public Health Education and Health Promotion Section (www.apha.org/membergroups/sections/aphasections/phehp)

  • Cancer Patient Education Network (www.cancerpatienteducation.org)

- Health Care Education Association (http://www.hcea-info.org)
- Medical Library Association (https://www.mlanet.org/)
- National Association of Social Workers (http://www.naswdc.org/)
- Society for Public Health Education (www.sophe.org)

- **Nonprofit and private publishers of educational materials and programs for patients and family members.** Information—whether print, multimedia, or electronic—is at the core of health promotion programs. Education and health publishers and, more recently, IT organizations recruit staff members with knowledge and expertise in health education and health communications to apply health literacy tenets and provide content, design, and testing of integrated media before they become final products.

- **Health insurance or managed care organizations.** Increasingly, the health insurance industry has embraced health promotion programming as a vehicle for lowering health risks and medical care costs. Many employer's health insurance benefit packages include health promotion programs and opportunities as a strategy to lower overall health insurance costs. Often employers will provide incentives for their employees to participate in such activities.

- **Academic health and medical career education programs.** Colleges, universities, and training programs prepare and train people to work in health care organizations. Universities have schools of medicine, nursing, global public health and allied health, as well as programs in school health, community health, health communications, health education, health promotion, and information management schools. Many other institutions prepare individuals to work as medical assistants, community health workers, and other medical support staff. Careers as professors and instructors in these institutions require advanced degrees; however, there are increasing numbers of opportunities for individuals with health promotion training and experience to work in professional preparation programs and support research efforts.

Summary

Today's health care organizations have broadened their focus on caring for the sick to embracing health-promoting activities for their patient populations, as well as health care providers and other professionals. As illustrated in this chapter, the wide range of health promotion programs available within the hospital, clinic, or office setting is enhanced by the use of innovative teaching approaches and information technologies. The leaders of health care organizations recognize the value of promoting the active engagement of patients and their families with health care providers in the design and delivery of both patient education and health promotion programs. When health care providers partner with patients and have patient-centered care interactions, patient adherence and patient health status improves, and care coordination and efficiency (fewer tests and referrals) increase. Health education specialists are trained and poised to advocate and facilitate patient engagement and activation.

For Practice and Discussion

1. One way to begin working with patients and families in planning for improvement of a health literate health care organization is to explore a clinical care setting through the eyes of patients and their families. Visit a doctor's office, your student health services, a community health clinic, or a local hospital to capture observations, flow, and interactions of a typical care encounter. As you walk through the reception area or waiting room and through the examination rooms, identify features or opportunities to strengthen the health literacy of the organization. Check for health promotion materials and information (e.g., brochures, posters, handouts, videos, Internet services). Visit the organization's website and ask staff about how they use technology to communicate with their patients and their family members. Using your observations, develop a short report to share with the staff to reinforce current best practices and recommendations to improve health literacy practices.

2. Think about the ways in which eHealth tools and technology are currently being used by health care organizations to encourage and promote consumers in their own health management. Using your cell phone as a technology platform, describe how you might create a new service to support consumers as they evaluate, choose, and use eHealth tools to derive benefits for themselves and those they care for.

3. Select one or more health care systems from the Institute for Patient- and Family-Centered Care's Profiles for Change website (http://www .ipfcc.org/profiles/index.html) and identify at least five strategies that demonstrate patient engagement in health promotion programs.

4. Go to Healthtalk.org's website section on healthcare decision making (http://www.healthtalk.org/peoples-experiences/improving-health-care/shared-decision-making/topics) and listen to three stories to understand why people want to take part in decision making, what information needs to be exchanged, and the role of values and

personal choices. What desired qualities and features of the health care interaction are important to these individuals, and how would you incorporate these messages in clinical staff training or coaching on health promotion communications?

5. A hospital is advertising a new job, seeking an individual to plan, implement, and evaluate patient engagement strategies for health promotion programs. To evaluate job candidates, prepare a list of interview questions requesting specific "real life" examples of how the candidate behaved in situations that would demonstrate the competencies sought for this position.

KEY TERMS

Electronic health record (EHR)	Patient and family-centered care
Evidence-based practices	Patient and family education
Health literacy	Patient engagement
Motivational interviewing (MI)	Patient safety
Patient activation	Teach-back

References

Acton K., Valway S., Helgerson S., Huy J.B., Smith K., Chapman V., Gohdes D. *"Improving Diabetes Care for American Indians."* Diabetes Care. 1993; *16*(1): 372–5. [PubMed]

Acton, K., Bochenski, C., Broussard, B., Gohdes, D., Hosey, G., Rith-Najarian, S., Stahn, and R., Stacqualursi, F. (1995). *Putting Integrated Care and Education to Work for American Indians/Alaska Natives Manual of the Indian Health Services Diabetes Program.* Albuquerque NM: Department of Health and Human Services.

Agency for Healthcare Research and Quality. (2013). *Guide to patient and family engagement in hospital quality and safety.* Retrieved from http://www.ahrq .gov/professionals/systems/hospital/engagingfamilies/index.html

American Academy of Family Practice. (2016). *Patient-centered medical home.* Retrieved from https://www.acponline.org/practice-resources/business-resources/payment/delivery-and-payment-models/patient-centered-medical-home

American Hospital Association. (2004). *Strategies for leadership: Patient- and family-centered care.* Retrieved from http://www.aha.org/advocacy-issues/quality/strategies-patientcentered.shtml

American Hospital Association. (2013). *Workforce roles in a redesigned primary care model* (White Paper). Retrieved from http://www.aha.org/aha_app/index .jsp

Banerjee, M., MacDougall, M., & Lakhdar, A. F. (2012). Impact of a single one-to-one education session on glycemic control in patients with diabetes. *Journal of Diabetes, 4*(2), 186–190.

Bortz, D. (2015). The 5 best jobs you've never heard of. *Money*. Retrieved from http://time.com/money/3661833/new-job-titles-2015/

Cancer Patient Education Network. (2013). *Guidelines for establishing comprehensive cancer patient education services*. Retrieved from http:// www.cancerpatienteducation.org/members/Resources/Educator_Resources/ CPENStandardsofPractice.Nov14.pdf

Centers for Disease Control and Prevention. (2010). *Health risk appraisals*. Retrieved from http://www.cdc.gov/nccdphp/dnpao/hwi/programdesign/ health_risk_appraisals.htm

Centers for Medicare and Medicaid Services. (2016). *Electronic health records (EHR) incentive programs*. Retrieved from https://www.cms.gov/Regulations- and-Guidance/Legislation/EHRIncentivePrograms/index.html

Davenport-Ennis, N., Cover, M. T., Ades, T. B., & Stovall, E. (2002). An analysis of advocacy: A collaborative essay. *Seminars in Oncology Nursing, 18*(4), 290–296.

Doak, C., & Doak, L., (1996). *Teaching patients with low literacy skills* (2nd ed.). Philadelphia, PA: Lippincott.

Edgman-Levitan, S., Brady, C., Howitt, P. (2013). Partnering with patients, families, and communities: a global imperative. Doha: World Innovation Summit for Health (WISH).

Elwyn, G., O'Connor, A., Stacey, D., Volk, R., Edwards, A., Coulter, A., . . . Whelan, T. (2006) Developing a quality criteria framework for patient decision aids: Online international Delphi consensus process. *BMJ, 333*(417).

Greene, S. M., Tuzzio, L., & Cherkin, D. (2012). A framework for making patient- centered care front and center. *Permanente Journal, 16*(3), 49–53.

Haas, L., Maryniuk, M., Beck, J., Cox, C. E., Duker, P., Edwards, L., . . . Youssef, G. (2014). National standards for diabetes self-management education and sup- port. *Diabetes Care, 37*(Suppl. 1), S144–S153.

Hesse B. W., Nelson D. E., Kreps G. L., Croyle R. T., Arora N. K., Rimer B. K., & Viswanath K. (2005). Trust and sources of health information: The impact of the Internet and its implications for health care providers: Findings from the first Health Information National Trends Survey. *Archive of Internal Medicine, 165*(22), 2618–2624.

Hibbard, J., Stockard, J., Mahoney, E., & Tusler, M. (2004). Development of the Patient Activation Measure (PAM): Conceptualizing and measuring activation in patients and consumers. *Health Services Research, 39*(1), 1005–1026.

Indian Health Service. (n.d.). *Health education program.* Retrieved from http://www.ihs.gov/HealthEd/index.cfm?module=pepc

Institute for Healthcare Improvement. (2016). *Always use teach-back!* Retrieved from http://www.ihi.org/resources/Pages/Tools/AlwaysUseTeachBack!.aspx

Institute for Patient- and Family-Centered Care. (2015), Patient and family resource centers. Retrieved from http://www.ipfcc.org/advance/topics/pafam-resource.html

Institute of Medicine, Committee on Quality of Health Care in America. (2001). *Crossing the quality chasm: A new health system for the 21st century.* Washington, DC: National Academies Press.

Jack, B. W., Chetty, V. K., Anthony, D., Greenwald, J. L., Sanchez, G. M., Johnson, A. E., & Culpepper, L. (2009). A reengineered hospital discharge program to decrease rehospitalization: A randomized trial. *Annals of Internal Medicine, 150*(3), 178–187.

Johnson, B., Abraham, M., Conway, J., Simmons, L., Edgman-Levitan, S., Sodomka, P., . . . Ford, D. (2008). *Partnering with patients and families to design a patient- and family-centered health care system.* Bethesda, MD: Institute for Patient- and Family-Centered Care. Retrieved from http://www.ipfcc.org/pdf/PartneringwithPatientsandFamilies.pdf

Joint Commission (2015). *Hospital national patient safety goals.* Retrieved from http://www.jointcommission.org/assets/1/6/2015_HAP_NPSG_ER.pdf

Krueger, R., & Casey, M. (2014). *Focus groups: A practical guide for applied research* (5th ed.). Thousand Oaks, CA: Sage.

Kruis, A. L., Smidt, N., Assendelft, W. J., Gussekloo, J., Boland, M., Rutten-van Mölken, M., & Chavannes, N. H. (2013). Integrated disease management interventions for patients with chronic obstructive pulmonary disease. *Cochrane Database of Systematic Reviews 2012*(10). doi:10.1002/14651858.CD009437.pub2

Martins, R., & McNeill, D. (2009). Review of motivational interviewing in promoting health behaviors. *Clinical Psychology Review, 29*(1), 283–293.

O'Connor, A. M., Stacey, D., Entwistle, V., Llewellyn-Thomas, H., Rovner, D., Holmes-Rovner, M. et al. Decision aids for people facing health treatment or screening decisions. *Cochrane Database of Systematic Reviews, 2003*(1). doi: 10.1002/14651858.CD001431.pub3

Silberman, P., Ricketts T. C., & Cohen Ross, D. (2008). The U.S. healthcare system and the need for patient advocacy. In J. Earp, E. French, & M. Gilkey (Eds.), *Patient advocacy for health care quality: Strategies for achieving patient-centered care* (pp. 29–58). Sudbury MA: Jones & Bartlett.

Silow-Carroll, S., Edwards, J., & Rodin, D. (2012). *Using electronic health records to improve quality and efficiency: The experiences of leading hospitals.* Retrieved from http://www.commonwealthfund.org/publications/issue-briefs/2012/jul/using-ehrs-to-improve-quality-and-efficiency

Smith, D. (2011) Health care consumer's use and trust of health information sources. *Journal of Communication in Healthcare, 4*(3), 200–210.

Stewart, M., Brown, J. B., Donner, A., McWhinney, I. R., Oates, J., Weston, W., & Jordan, J. (2000). The impact of patient-centered care on outcomes. *J Family Practice, 49*(9), 796–804.

U.S. Preventive Services Task Force. (2015). *Recommendations for primary care practice.* Retrieved from http://www.uspreventiveservicestaskforce.org/Page/Name/recommendations

CHAPTER 15

HEALTH PROMOTION PROGRAMS IN WORKPLACE SETTINGS

Laura Linnan and Anna Grummon*

Workplace Health Promotion—A Brief History and Current Trends

More than 60% of U.S. adults over age 18 are employed, and they spend a majority of their waking hours at work (Bureau of Labor Statistics, 2015). Thus, the workplace is an important place to reach the U.S. adult population with health information and services. The workplace environment exerts an independent influence on the health of employees as well. Specifically, the physical and social environment at work; the pace of work; and exposures to noise, chemicals, repetitious movement, hazardous conditions, harassment, or abuse can influence employee health. When the work environment and work conditions support health, include opportunities to access health-related information and services, and offer screening services with appropriate follow-up and education, employees are more productive and are better positioned to achieve and maintain positive health outcomes and improved quality of life. Nearly all private and public organizations employ individuals. Regardless of the size or type of organization, employees, as well as their dependents and the larger community, can benefit from comprehensive workplace *health promotion* programs. The most effective workplace health promotion efforts also take place within a community where health is valued and promoted in the larger social, political, economic, and physical environment. Thus, promoting health in the workplace, and

LEARNING OBJECTIVES

- Discuss the benefits of offering health promotion programs and services at the workplace.

- Describe a brief history of workplace health promotion, highlighting at least three trends over the past three decades.

- Explain how the changing nature of work, changing demographics of the population, and changing health care environment will influence workplace health promotion programs.

- Describe resources and materials available for developing and implementing effective workplace health promotion programs.

- Describe the type of skills required to have a career in the field of workplace health promotion.

creating a health-supportive workplace and community, represents an important public health priority.

Most historical reviews of health promotion efforts at workplaces in the United States begin in the 1970s, when a handful of employers developed executive fitness programs (Reardon, 1998). Companies began offering such programs in an attempt to reduce the likelihood of premature death among key executives, and to provide a company "perk" to help recruit and retain top management. As evidence grew of the positive health outcomes experienced by executives, and the related economic benefits to the company's bottom line, health promotion programs were expanded beyond fitness programming to general *wellness* and were offered to the entire workforce.

At the same time that program designers shifted from a fitness focus to a wellness focus, they also began to direct attention to prevention rather than treatment of high-risk conditions. Until the mid-1980s, executive fitness programs typically included a physical examination in order to identify leaders who were at high risk for cardiovascular disease—the leading cause of premature death then, as now. The idea was that top leaders at high risk could be referred into intensive treatment programs focused on reducing blood pressure and improving physical activity and diet. As the public health community began to emphasize the importance of primary prevention, workplace health promotion interventions followed suit. However, it was not practical or affordable for an employer to offer complete physical examinations for the entire workforce. Moreover, multisession, clinic-oriented treatment programs for high blood pressure, high blood cholesterol, smoking cessation, and weight loss required significant staffing and resources and pulled employees away from work. As a result, many employees were unable to participate. To address this dilemma, employers and other service providers (e.g., voluntary health agencies, private vendors, and health insurers) developed minimal-intensity interventions that were less costly to create and deliver, accommodated the schedules of more employees, and were feasible to implement throughout an entire workplace (Reardon, 1998). For example, intensive, multisession classes on smoking cessation were replaced with self-help or other web-based cessation programs, clean air campaigns and policies to reduce exposure to smoke, and contests to motivate individuals to quit smoking with minimal help.

The early 1990s represented a time of unprecedented growth for workplace health promotion. Even as the U.S. economy stagnated, research on workplace health promotion programs was funded at greater levels

(Stokols, Pelletier, & Fielding, 1996). Employers began to realize that the social and physical environment of a workplace can have both direct and indirect influences on employee health, and also came to understand that employee health is closely linked to organizational health. For example, employers learned that creating a policy change leading to a smoke-free work environment both increased the actual cessation rates and reduced cleaning and insurance costs. Employers began experimenting with discounting low-fat food choices in vending machines, making healthier food options available in the cafeteria and vending machines, and developing nutrition education programs.

As workplace health promotion moves into the 21st century, the pace of change has begun to accelerate and several new trends are note-worthy. First, there is increasing recognition that "comprehensive" workplace health promotion programming is necessary for achieving the maximum benefits from these programs. A comprehensive program includes offering health education programs; a supportive social and physi-cal environment; health screenings with appropriate education, follow-up, and treatment; administrative supports including staffing and budget; and linkages with other related programming such as safety, *employee assistance programs*, and other benefits. A second trend is that workplace health programs are increasingly integrating efforts to both protect and promote health (Pronk, 2013). U.S. labor unions have long fought for workers' rights, safe work environments, and access to health benefits/health care for their members. Yet trained personnel, budget, and programming for creating safe work conditions are often completely separate from resources allocated for health promotion. The National Institute for Occupational Safety and Health (NIOSCH) launched the Total Worker Health Program, which provides support for research and advocacy related to integrating occupational safety and *health protection* with health promotion (National Institute for Occupational Safety and Health, 2014) to help bridge this gap.

A third recent trend is the increasing demand for *accountability* for the results of workplace health promotion and health protection efforts. Increasingly, evaluators must be specific about the value that a work-place health and safety program will provide to an organizational sponsor. New metrics are helping to uncover previously unstudied benefits of offering comprehensive safety and health programs, such as employee well-being, vitality, productivity, satisfaction, and retention/turnover, which may represent significant "hidden" costs (or cost savings) for employers. Additionally, more employers are using value-based benefit design, which emphasizes the use of incentives to encourage certain behaviors (University of Michigan Center for Value-Based Insurance Design, n.d.). For example, incentives are used to nudge employees to a preferred provider or preventive service or a preferred pharmaceutical, or to encourage employees to complete a health risk assessment, participate in certain types of health or screening services, or to adopt (or relinquish) certain health behaviors. The overall evidence of incentives programs remains mixed (Dudley, Tseng, Bozic, Smith, & Luft, 2007; O'Donnell, 2010; O'Donnell, 2013; Paul-Ebhohimhen & Avenell, 2008; Seaverson, Grossmeier, Miller, & Anderson, 2009; Volpp et al., 2008; Volpp et al., 2009), but most agree that incentives work to increase participation even if the results are less clear about changing health behaviors over the long term (Volpp et al., 2009). State and local governments, which employ a large number of employees in all states, have emerged as key proponents of value-based benefit design (University of Michigan Center for Value-Based Insurance Design, n.d.). Taken together, these trends in workplace health promotion are identifying new methods, strategies, and approaches for supporting the health of workers and creating healthy workplaces.

Leading by Example: Workplace Success Stories

To support the efforts of employers, the U.S. Chamber of Commerce and Partnership for Prevention have united to share employers' success stories about improving the health and productivity of their workforce. *Leading by Example: Leading Practices for Employee Health Management* provides examples and strategies for improving employee health from employers of every size (Partnership for Prevention & U.S. Chamber of Commerce, 2007). In addition, the Wellness Council of America (WELCOA) and the Health Project each sponsor award programs for employers who submit applications and meet certain criteria for excellence (WELCOA, 2015; The Health Project, 2015).

Here, we highlight one organization that exemplifies many of the trends and also demonstrates positive outcomes. Lincoln Industries is a medium-sized manufacturing company that was recognized in *Leading by Example* and was an Innovation in Prevention Award recipient for its efforts in promoting healthy lifestyles in its community (Partnership for Prevention, 2007). Table 15.1 provides a case example of Lincoln Industries, which offers a comprehensive program and has created and sustained a culture of wellness and health that has been recognized with a myriad of state and national awards.

Table 15.1   Workplace Health Promotion at Lincoln Industries: Comprehensive Programming at a Small to Medium-Sized Employer

Location: Lincoln, Nebraska

Type of industry: Manufacturing

Number of employees: 450

Company belief statement: "Wellness and healthy lifestyles are important to our success."

Program vision: "Lincoln Industries Wellness encompasses the body, mind, and spirit. We support our people in making smarter, healthier lifestyle choices. We encourage balance between work, home, and personal goals. We believe that supporting our people's health and wellness interests is a sound investment in our company, and the most important asset of the company is the people."

Comprehensive program components

Health interventions

Free on-site, on-the-clock tobacco cessation and weight management interventions for employees and their family members

More than 10 major health interventions

Supportive social and physical environment

Tobacco-free campus

Wellness mentors

Recognition of wellness (incentives include free trip to Colorado to climb 14,000-foot mountain)

Linkage to related programs

Health reimbursement account with credits for being tobacco-free

Wellness presented in concert with all other company benefits and business strategies at the onset of employment

Integration of health program into organizational structures

Wellness objectives, set by all employees, tied to overall performance and pay

Departmental wellness champions

Company-sponsored wellness events

Wellness integrated into Lincoln's strategic plan, business initiatives, and employee development

Workplace screening programs

Mandatory quarterly health screenings and individual coaching

Results:

Go! Platinum received several national wellness program awards.

Health care costs are 50% below national average.

Workers compensation costs average less than 1% of payroll.

CEO statement: "Too often, companies look at wellness as just another benefit. We have fully integrated wellness into every aspect of our company's culture. It's a source of pride and reflects how we care for one another. As a result, wellness has become a critical element of our success."

The Future of Workplace Health Promotion

The Changing Landscape

The future of workplace health promotion programs must take into account several important demographic changes in the U.S. population (Figure 15.1). First, the overall population is aging, as is the working population. By 2050, 22% of Americans will be over the age of 65, compared to just 13% in 2010 (Colby & Ortman, 2015). This trend has important implications, as some of these older Americans will remain in the workforce past the traditional retirement age. Chronic disease incidence increases with age. New intervention strategies will be required to address the epidemic of chronic diseases in the face of the aging workforce. Second, women continue to outnumber men in the U.S. population, and the ratio of women to men is expected to increase over the next several decades. In addition, the percentage of working women overall and of working women with children are increasing (Juhn & Potter, 2006). Third, there is a significant increase in the prevalence of nonwhite workers. The aggregate minority population is expected to become the majority by about 2043 (Ortman, Velkoff, & Hogan, 2014). The Hispanic population is expected to double between 2012 and 2060; by the end of this period, nearly one in three U.S. residents are expected to be Hispanic, compared to about one in six today. The Asian population is expected to more than double by 2060, and will make up about 8.2% of the total population, compared to 5.1% today (U.S. Census Bureau, 2012). The largest source of new workers in the United States is expected to be Hispanic workers, who by 2022 are expected to account for almost 20% of the labor force, up from 15.7% in 2012 (Bureau of Labor Statistics, 2013a). See Figure 13.1 for projected changes in the labor force.

What do these demographic shifts mean for health promotion efforts at workplaces? Employers will need to develop health programs and services that are culturally and programmatically appropriate for a diverse set of workers. For example, an aging workforce may require programs and services to prevent or treat arthritis or other chronic health conditions that are more prevalent in older workers.

In addition to dramatic demographic shifts, we are also in the midst of changes in the work environment that will influence workplace health promotion programs. For example, during the 20th century, work in the United States changed from primarily farming, manufacturing, or production work to service-oriented work. Nearly 40% of the workforce in 1900 had a farm-related job, while less than 2% of workers were in farm-related jobs in 2012, while today more than three-quarters of Americans work in the service sector (National Research Council, 1999; Bureau of Labor

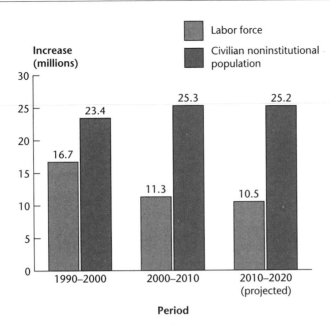

Figure 15.1   Changes in the U.S. Labor Force and Population 1990 to 2020 (Projected)
Source: Bureau of Labor Statistics, 2013a.

Statistics, 2013b). There are also more contingent workers and individuals who work multiple part-time jobs. According to national estimates, just over 40% of U.S. workers are now considered "contingent" (i.e., not in traditional full-time work, including temporary workers, part-time workers, and independent contractors) compared with 30.6% in 2005 (Murray & Gillibrand, 2015). Contingent workers are more likely to experience job instability, lower pay, experience higher poverty rates, and lack health insurance—factors that place individuals at higher risk of experiencing health problems and make it challenging to reach them with workplace health programming. The design and development of future workplace interventions will undoubtedly need to account for the growing number of contingent workers, as well as full-time workers who work at home for all or part of their workday.

To keep pace with the changing work environment, health promotion programs will be needed for workers at nontraditional workplaces, with adaptations for workers who are not based in a single organizational setting or who have less direct contact with their co-workers. For example, more "workplace" health promotion programs may need to be via the web or cell phones. And, while many employees receive access to health promotion services through health benefits offered by an employer, an increasing number of lower-wage workers, part-time, or contingent workers receive no health insurance benefits, and may not have access to any type of health promotion program or service at work. In this case, employees will need information about how to best access free or low cost health services, health clinics, and prevention programs in the local community. Employers, at a minimum, could provide information or discount access to these resources.

The passage of the Affordable Care Act (ACA) in 2010 is also changing the landscape of workplace health promotion. In 2014, the average annual health plan covering a family of four averaged $16,834 (Kaiser Family Foundation, 2014). As a result of these high costs, fewer employers offer health insurance, and employees have less access to health care, including both treatment and preventive services. With the passage of the ACA, millions of previously uninsured Americans gained access to affordable health care via private health care exchanges. By March 2015, more than 10.2 million Americans had paid their premiums and were covered through ACA health insurance exchanges (U.S. Department of Health and Human Services, 2015). As more Americans gain coverage, more individuals have access to free preventive services such as colonoscopy screening, Pap smears, mammograms, well-child visits, and flu shots. The ACA, via Medicaid expansion and subsidies to employers, has also led to increased access to insurance among low-wage workers and employees working in smaller workplaces. Finally, and although no funds have yet been appropriated for this component, the ACA authorizes grants for small employers (less than 100 employees) to offer comprehensive workplace health promotion programs.

How will changes in the health care environment influence those who are planning and delivering health promotion programs at work? Better access to care improves the health of everyone, yet the role of employer-sponsored health insurance and health promotion services is likely to change. Over the past several decades, employers relied heavily on their health insurance providers for the health promotion and disease management programs offered to their employees (Linnan et al., 2008). It's not yet clear whether employers will continue to offer health insurance for their employees, or instead provide subsidies and ask employees to purchase their insurance through a health care exchange. Estimates currently range from 7%–60% of employers who will consider major changes in their coverage plans, including the idea of moving to a public or private exchange (Singhal, Stueland, & Ungerman, 2011; Accenture, 2013). It's also not clear what effect insurance changes will have on workplace health promotion programs—some employers, motivated by improved employee morale, productivity, job satisfaction, or reduced absenteeism, may continue to offer programs and services; some employers may leave preventive health services to outside providers. In any case, we expect that individuals who know how to plan, implement, and evaluate comprehensive workplace health promotion program will be in demand, though they are providing services in new venues and with new partners.

Selecting, Designing and Implementing Workplace Health Promotion Initiatives: Challenges and Opportunities

Several features are critically important when selecting or designing a workplace health promotion initiative. First, programs are evidence based. For example, Weight Watchers is a proven weight loss program that is implemented in a group or online format (Dansinger, Gleason, Griffith, Selker, & Schaefer, 2005). Rather than developing or using an untested weight loss campaign or program, an employer could provide access to Weight Watchers for free or at a discounted rate to employees. One challenge to selecting evidence-based programs is that practitioners don't always have access to the most current research results. Thus, forming strategic partnerships to increase information sharing about research results, and then accelerating the pace at which evidence-based programs get into practice, is a worthwhile goal. Partnerships between employers of all sizes, voluntary health organizations, federal/state and local health departments, and researchers could facilitate getting evidence-based programming in place. For example, the CDC-funded Workplace Health Research Network (http://www.workhealthresearchnetwork.org/) has established a national research agenda to accelerate research to practice results, build strategic partnerships, and act as a catalyst for positive health change in workers and their workplaces.

Workplace health promotion initiatives need to be theory-guided and tailored to the employees and sponsoring organization. Programs take into account the particular culture, needs, and assets of the workplace and its employees (Linnan, Jeffries, & Eastman, 2014). For example, promoting employee health at a manufacturing setting is different than offering programs at a hospital or university setting. In larger organizations, there are differences by department or location. Workplace health promotion programs are more likely to be successful when they are grounded in behavior change theory (Goetzel & Ozminkowski, 2008). Theory is integrated into a comprehensive workplace health program in a variety of ways. For example, the U.S. Community Guide indicates that offering employees *health risk appraisals* along with feedback and appropriate educational programming has "sufficient evidence" of success for promoting behavior change. Program planners can use theory to develop the feedback employees receive, and to create effect follow-up outreach. For example, a program planner might use the transtheoretical model (Prochaska, Redding, & Evers, 2008) to tailor an employee's feedback and counseling sessions to his or her stage of change for different behaviors: a first follow-up coaching call could focus on the behavior that an employee is "mostly ready to change"; and subsequent calls would be designed to move an individual along the pathway to successful behavior change.

In addition to integrating theory, workplace health promotion initiatives recognize the role of the work environment in ensuring employee health and safety. The work environment, including work pace, work demands, and exposure of employees to violence, harassment, discrimination, noise, repetitive strains, hazards, and chemicals, can present significant harm to employees. Employers address these potentially harmful environmental conditions. Unions and other organized employee groups will often advocate for supportive health conditions. As union membership has decreased to 12% in the United States, it is even more important that integrated safety and health approaches like Total Worker Health are adopted and implemented (Bureau of Labor Statistics, 2008).

And while management support is necessary, it is not sufficient for long-term program success—programs must also be integrated into the organizational structure and culture of a workplace if they are to be sustained. Program planners will benefit from understanding the challenges to offering these programs. For example, small employers are less likely to offer all types of programs and services, a problem that has persisted for more than three decades (Harris, Hannon, Beresford, Linnan, and McClellan, 2014). Specifically, small employers are less likely to offer programs, policies, and environmental supports, and the most common barriers or challenges to offering health promotion programs reported by employers of all sizes and industry types were lack of interest among employees, lack of staff resources, lack of funding, and lack of management support (Linnan et al., 2008). Especially among small to mid-sized organizations which employ low-wage workers, lack of capacity to offer workplace programming can reduce the likelihood of program adoption and make program implementation challenging (Hannon et al., 2012).

Even when workplace health promotion programs are offered, employees often face challenges to participating in such programs. First, not all employees have equal access to programs at work. Grosch, Alterman, Petersen, and Murphy (1998) found that laborers, men, and minorities report less access to health promotion programs at work. Employees may also choose not to participate in workplace health promotion programs because they are concerned about privacy, face negative peer pressure, are juggling competing work and time demands, or feel they lack the support of their supervisor. These challenges are anticipated and addressed when health promotion is supported by all levels of management and when programs are developed through a systematic planning effort that engages employers and employees in the process.

There is a growing interest in interventions that influence multiple levels of the Social Ecological Framework (SEF), including intrapersonal, interpersonal, organizational, community, and policy levels (Golden & Earp, 2012; Linnan, Sorensen, Colditz, Klar, & Emmons, 2001; McLeroy, Bibeau, Steckler, & Glanz, 1988). Programs at the intra- and interpersonal levels (e.g., self-help or peer support programs), organizational (campaigns for the entire workplace), community (referrals and/or discounts for employees who join the YMCA), and policy (regulations about smoke-free spaces or taxes on sugar-sweetened beverages) can all work to support individual employees who want to make a health change at work, home, and in the community. Within the SEF, health educators can choose up to five levels of intervention, multiple interventions, and let different theories guide the selection of intervention strategies at each level. Table 15.2 describes the different levels of the SEF and gives examples of theories at each level.

Table 15.2   Behavior Change Theories at Different Levels of the Social Ecological Framework (SEF)

Level of Influence	Intervention Target	Relevant Theories and Concepts
Intrapersonal	Characteristics of individuals (knowledge, attitudes, beliefs, motivations, intentions, self-efficacy, skills)	• Health Belief Model • Theory of Planned Behavior • Transtheoretical Model
Interpersonal	Relationships between individual and others including family, friends, neighbors, co-workers, and supervisors	• Social Support Theory • Social Network Theory
Organizational	Characteristics of organizational settings (e.g., structures, policies, rules, norms, processes of workplaces, schools, institutions)	• Organizational Development Theory • Social Norms • Stage Theory of Organizational Change
Community	Relationships that exist between organizations, institutions, and other formal networks	• Community Organizing • Social Action model • Political Economy of Health
Policy	Public or social policy, legislation, regulations	• Political Economy of Health

Finally, future workplace health promotion program trends include a strong emphasis on more sustainable workplace interventions. As employers and employees become more environmentally conscious, "green" intervention strategies become more prevalent at work. For example, offering vouchers or incentives for bicycling to work might also promote physical activity. Local farmers may provide healthy, locally grown food products to employees directly or as part of cafeteria offerings. Future workplace health and safety programs are likely to become more environmentally and ecologically conscientious, with an eye toward sustainability for both the organization and the planet.

Career Opportunities in Workplace Health Promotion

Professionals with expertise in planning, developing, implementing, and evaluating health promotion programs at workplaces currently come from a variety of fields and/or specialties, including exercise physiology, health education, public health, health promotion, nutrition, and organizational development. Given that dedicated staff is the single most important predictor of having a comprehensive workplace health promotion program, it is useful to consider the amount and type of specialized training program that might be beneficial for those who want to manage workplace health promotion programs in the future (Peabody & Linnan, 2007). Despite the fact that no consensus training approach exists, a growing number of universities offer undergraduate or graduate training programs in workplace health promotion (see, for example, East Carolina University, 2015) or a master's degree in health promotion with a concentration in workplace wellness (see, for example, Maryland University of Integrative Health, 2015). One of the newest training option includes the CDC-sponsored Work@Health Train-the-Trainer or a Work@Health Wellness Champions option (Centers for Disease Control and Prevention, 2015). Another option includes the Certified Worksite Wellness Specialist and Program Manager certification programs offered by the National Wellness Institute (National Wellness Institute, n.d.). Additionally, the Chapman Institute (Chapman Institute, 2015) offers WelCert, a wellness program certification program for practitioners at one of four levels: Certified Wellness Program Coordinator, Certified Wellness Program Manager, Certified Wellness Program Director, and Certified Worksite Wellness Program Consultant.

Health educators are familiar with theory-grounded approaches for individual and organizational-level health changes. They know how to identify evidence-based programs and adapt them for a particular workplace setting and workforce. Program evaluation skills, including quality improve-ment efforts, are essential. Ability to tailor interventions to the unique needs of an individual employee and a workplace environment are important (Linnan, Jeffries, & Eastman, 2014).

Various paths are available to someone who is interested in a career in workplace health promotion. Potential employers include companies with existing workplace wellness programs, insurance companies, for-profit ven-dors of health promotion programs, national/state and local government agencies, voluntary health agencies, or research institutions. Workplace health professionals employed by vendors are involved in program devel-opment, sales, customer relations, or evaluation. Government agencies will typically hire staff to manage or offer programming for their employ-ees or constituents. New training programs for integrating occupational safety with health promotion are also available through the NIOSH-funded occupational safety and health educational research centers (http://niosh-erc.org/).

Voluntary health agencies such as the American Heart Association, American Cancer Society, American Lung Association, and American Red Cross all hire workplace health professionals. Jobs with these organizations are at the local, state, regional, or national level. For example, field staff from the American Cancer Society (American Cancer Society, 2015) are hired to implement Active for Life, a workplace health promotion program that encourages people to become more physically active in order to reduce their risk of cancer and other chronic diseases.

Some health promotion professionals are more interested in joining a university-based research team that manages or delivers workplace health promotion programs. For example, the Carolina Collaborative for Research on Work at the University of North Carolina, Chapel Hill, sponsors a monthly journal club, speaker series, and meetings designed to stimu-late interdisciplinary research that will improve worker and workplace health (University of North Carolina at Chapel Hill, n.d.). Individuals can obtain the necessary preparation to enter a career in workplace health promotion through various forms of academic training or advanced, specialized training. Health professionals who work in this field may have undergraduate or graduate training in nutrition, health education, health promotion, public health, social work, exercise science, organiza-tional behavior, business, and/or psychology. It is advantageous to pursue one degree (undergraduate or master's) that provides generalist training (for example, in health education) and a second degree that provides con-tent expertise (for example, in nutrition, exercise science, or psychology) that moves beyond the generalist training. For example, an individual with an undergraduate degree in health education (generalist) and a master's degree in exercise physiology (specialist) broadens her career options in several directions. Pursuing graduate-level training is highly desirable in the field of workplace health promotion.

Resources and Tools

An increasing number of resources are available to help those who wish to plan, implement, and evaluate health promotion programs at workplaces. Most of these resources have been developed in the past 25 years in order to address a wide range of health issues and problems.

Healthier Worksite Initiative

In 2002, the Centers for Disease Control and Prevention (CDC) developed the Healthier Worksite Initiative (HWI) for its own employees, with the vision of making the CDC a workplace where healthy choices are easy choices and sharing the lessons learned with other federal agencies (Centers for Disease Control and Prevention, 2010). In the years since its inception, HWI has worked on a number of demonstration projects, policies, and environmental changes that affect the entire CDC workforce. The HWI website offers lessons learned from these projects, suggestions for new and revised policies, and step-by-step instructions for implementing similar programs at other workplaces (http://www.cdc.gov/nccdphp/dnpao/hwi/). The website serves as a one-stop shop for individuals and organizations looking to implement their own workplace wellness programs.

The Guide to Community Preventive Services, "The Community Guide"

The Centers for Disease Control and Prevention Community Preventive Services Task Force was established in 1996 to identify interventions that have been scientifically shown to improve health and quality of life and increase lifespan (The Community Guide, 2015). The Community Guide website provides a collection of the official findings of the Task Force. A section of the website focuses specifically on workplace health promotion programs, highlighting the importance of this topic. Table 15.3 shows the worksite (workplace) health promotion interventions currently recommended by the Task Force as having sufficient evidence of effectiveness

Table 15.3 Evidence-Based Workplace Health Promotion Programs

Topic	Recommended Interventions
Workplace Recommendation	
Promoting seasonal influenza vaccinations among health care workers	• Interventions with on-site, free, actively promoted vaccinations
Promoting seasonal influenza vaccinations among non-healthcare workers	• Interventions with on-site, reduced cost, actively promoted vaccinations
Assessment of health risks with feedback (AHRF) to change employee health	• AHRF plus health education with or without other interventions
Related Recommendations	
Obesity prevention	• Programs to control overweight and obesity
Skin cancer prevention	• Interventions in outdoor occupational settings
Physical activity promotion	• Point-of-decision prompts to encourage use of stairs
	• Creation of or enhanced access to places for physical activity combined with informational outreach
Reducing tobacco use and secondhand smoke exposure	• Smoke-free policies
	• Incentives and competitions when combined with additional interventions

Source: Adapted from www.thecommunityguide.org

(see www.thecommunityguide.org/worksite for more information). The website also provides recommendations on where to offer programs, what type of activities tend to be most effective, the average cost of programs, and potential barriers to implementing the recommended programs.

HERO

HERO is a national nonprofit, membership-based organization organized to advance the health and well-being of employees, families and communities through workplace based research, education, and policy. HERO has been in existence as an organization for more than years and is dedicated to identifying and sharing best practices in the field of workplace health and well-being to improve the health and well-being of workers, their spouses, dependents, and retirees by sharing best practices, advocating for improvements in the field, and providing practical solutions for employers who share our commitment to supporting health and well-being for employees, families, and communities. HERO convenes "think tanks," holds annual meetings, has established a research council, and publishes a wide array of documents designed to support employer-based decision making that improves employee health and well-being.

Guide to Developing a Workplace Injury and Illness Prevention Program with Checklists for Self-Inspection

The California Occupational Safety and Health Administration created the Guide to Developing a Workplace Injury and Illness Prevention Program with Checklists for Self-Inspection (State of California, 2005). The online manual is intended to help employers offer their employees protection from injury and to reduce the damages that result from accidents and injuries. The guide is used as a first-step resource for organizations that are putting a new program in place or for ensuring the ongoing success of existing programs.

Total Worker Health Approach

The National Institute for Occupational Health and Safety (NIOSH) in 2004 initiated the WorkLife Initiative to improve overall worker health through better work-based programs, policies, practices, and benefits. The WorkLife Initiative supports addressing worker health and well-being by taking into account the physical and organizational work environment while at the same time addressing the personal health-related decisions and behaviors of individuals. The workplace is viewed as a site to implement programs and policies to prevent both work-related risks and chronic illnesses and injuries that are linked to employee choices. As part of the initiative, Centers of Excellence to Promote a Healthier Workforce were established to create new research in this area, effectively demonstrating the impact of improved and integrated approaches to health protection and health promotion on the improvement of worker health and safety, and defining critical elements of health-supportive workplaces.

Employee Health Services Handbook

The *Employee Health Services Handbook* (U.S. Office of Personnel Management, n.d.) provides policy guidance to assist agency managers and program administrators in developing and administering comprehensive employee health services programs. The handbook uses a question-and-answer format to address issues including providing physical fitness programs; administering employee assistance programs; federal program resources;

a list of employee health resources available on the Internet; and examples of surveys, contracts, and forms.

Essential Elements of Effective Workplace Programs and Policies for Improving Worker Health and Well-Being

This document describes 20 key aspects of a comprehensive workplace-based health promotion and health protection program developed by the National Institute for Occupational Safety and Health (NIOSH; 2008) with substantial input from experts in occupational safety and health promotion which includes a focus on organizational culture and leadership; program design; program implementation and resources; and program evaluation. The document is a framework that will be enhanced by links to resource materials intended to assist in the design and implementation of workplace programs and offer specific examples of best and promising practices. An update will be released on the original 2008 edition in 2016 with a focus on integrated approaches using the Total Worker Health focus.

Centers of Excellence to Promote a Healthier Workforce

NIOSH funds four Centers of Excellence that focus on research efforts to promote the integration of worker and workplace health, safety, and well-being. The Centers of Excellence test policies and programs, develop and distribute best practice guides and toolkits, research the cost and benefits of integrated workplace health programs, develop strategies to improve adoption of comprehensive workplace health interventions, and assist in the delivery of these interventions.

California Nutrition Education and Obesity Prevention Branch Worksite Program

This state-led initiative (www.cdph.ca.gov/programs/cpns/Pages/Worksite Program.aspx) focused on increasing fruit and vegetable consumption and physical activity among low-income workers. The program offers a "Fit Business Kit" with tools and resources for employers looking to improve workplace environments and culture to support healthy eating and physical activity among employees. The tools in the kit include assessment tools, information on starting *wellness committees* and farmers' markets, and guidance for offering healthy meetings, dining options, and work environments supportive of physical activity and breastfeeding, among other resources.

Business Responds to AIDS/Labor Responds to AIDS (BRTA/LRTA)

The Business Responds to AIDS/Labor Responds to AIDS (BRTA/LRTA, www.cdc.gov/hiv/workplace/index.html) Program draws on public and private partnerships, including collaboration between businesses, trade associations, and labor organizations, to offer resources and technical assistance for developing comprehensive workplace and workforce HIV/AIDS programs and policies. BRTA/LRTA offers guidance on employee education, workplace policies, and community service and volunteering opportunities for employers and businesses.

Summary

The workplace remains an important setting for promoting health and reaching a large percentage of the U.S. adult population. Workplace health interventions will be most successful when they address the concerns of individual employees, the interactions between employees and co-workers or supervisors, the physical and social environment at the workplace, policies within the workplace, and the larger social context in which workplaces are embedded. In this chapter, we have acknowledged the importance of workplace health promotion and improving employee well-being, reviewed a brief history of workplace health promotion efforts, and discussed important trends that will influence program planning, implementation, and evaluation efforts such as the changing workforce demographics, the changing nature of work, and a changing health care environment. We share examples of challenges and opportunities for promoting worker health and safety in the future. Finally, we offered an overview of ways to pursue a wide range of career opportunities in workplace health promotion.

For Practice and Discussion

1. List three challenges that employers face when planning and/or implementing workplace health promotion programs, and how you would overcome each one.

2. Small employers are much less likely than large employers to offer any type of workplace wellness program. Name three strategies that small employers might consider to promote and/or support the health of their employees.

3. Think about the growing diversity of employees at most workplaces. In a workplace with mostly young, Hispanic women, what type of health programs or services would you consider offering?

4. Debate this question: Employers need access to employee medical information? Why or why not?

5. Review the job description for a workplace health promotion program director in Table 15.4. How do the skills of a typical health educator match up with the requirements of this job?

Table 15.4   Job Description—Director of Workplace Health Promotion

The **Workplace Health Promotion** Director oversees the selection, delivery/implementation, and evaluation of programs and services designed to promote employee health and well-being. The director will oversee day-to-day operations, including monthly and quarterly budgets; supervise full-time and part-time staff; identify appropriate evidence-based health education and screening programs and services to prevent or treat leading chronic diseases; lead marketing/promotion efforts; and conduct rigorous program evaluation. The director will report to organization leadership, including regular updates and status reports. She/he will lead the planning, implementation, and evaluation of all new and existing center health promotion programs and tailor these to the unique needs and demographics of the workforce. The director collaborates with all other medical, safety, human resource, employee assistance personnel to create a healthy, safe, violence-free, and drug-free work environment, and with the Food Services Director on employee food and nutrition services to ensure healthy food options are available.

Position Requirements

B.S. degree in health promotion, health education, public health, wellness, exercise physiology, allied health, nursing, or related field

Master's degree in related field is preferred

Eight to 10 years of experience in the health and wellness industry; experience in promoting corporate wellness is a must

Minimum of 5 years of experience with supervision and a proven track record of hiring, scheduling, training, evaluation, and other supervisorial duties

CHES, MCHES, CPH, or ACSM (American College of Sports Medicine) credential preferred

CPR, AED (automated external defibrillator), and First Aid certifications

Experience in budgetary and fiscal management

Expertise in marketing and program evaluation

Direct experience in high-quality customer service delivery and development

Advanced skills in computer technology

The director must possess excellent professional and interpersonal skills. The director must appreciate organizational decision making and behavior change. A strong background in administration, planning, organization, and supervising, as well as the ability to teach others, is desirable. The director must be willing and able to explore creative and new approaches in health promotion programming, policies, and services that will be effective and stay within budget.

KEY TERMS

Comprehensive workplace health
  promotion

Employee assistance programs
  (EAPs)

Health protection

Health risk appraisal

Policy change

Wellness

Wellness committee

References

Accenture. (2013). *Are you ready? Private health insurance exchanges are loom-ing*. Retrieved from https://www.accenture.com/us-en/insight-private-health-insurance-exchanges-looming-summary.aspx

American Cancer Society. (2015). *Active for life*. Retrieved from https://www.activeforlife.org/

Bureau of Labor Statistics. (2008). *Union members in* 2007. Retrieved from http://www.bls.gov/news.release/union2.nr0.htm

Bureau of Labor Statistics. (2013a). Labor force. *Occupational Outlook Quarterly, 57*(4): 24–28.

Bureau of Labor Statistics. (2013b). Industry employment and output projects to 2022. *Monthly Labor Review*. Retrieved from http://www.bls.gov/opub/mlr/2013/article/industry-employment-and-output-projections-to-2022.htm

Bureau of Labor Statistics. (2015). *The employment situation: March 2015*. Retrieved from http://www.bls.gov/news.release/empsit.toc.ht

Centers for Disease Control and Prevention. (2010). *Healthier Worksite Initiative: About us*. Retrieved from http://www.cdc.gov/nccdphp/dnpao/hwi/aboutus/index.htm

Centers for Disease Control and Prevention. (2015). *Work@Health*. Retrieved from http://www.cdc.gov/workathealth/

Chapman Institute. (2015). *Does your wellness program work?* Retrieved from https://www.chapmaninstitute.com/

Colby, S. L., & Ortman, J. M. (2015). *Projections of the size and composition of the U.S. population: 2014 to 2060* (Current Population Reports, P25-1143). Washington, DC: U.S. Census Bureau. Retrieved from http://www.census.gov/content/dam/Census/library/publications/2015/demo/p25-1143.pdf

The Community Guide. (2015). *What is the Community Guide?* Retrieved from http://www.thecommunityguide.org/about/index.html

Dansinger, M. L., Gleason, J., Griffith, J. L., Selker, H. P., & Schaefer, E. J. (2005). Comparison of the Atkins, Ornish, Weight Watchers, and Zone diets for weight loss and heart disease risk reduction: A randomized trial. *Journal of the American Medical Association, 293*(1), 43–53.

Dudley, R. A., Tseng, C., Bozic, K., Smith, W. A., & Luft, H. S. (2007). *Consumer financial incentives: A decision guide for purchases.* Rockville, MD: Agency for Healthcare Research and Quality.

East Carolina University. (2015). *The College of Health & Human Performance: Department of Health Education and Promotion.* Retrieved from http://www.ecu.edu/cs-hhp/

Goetzel R. Z., & Ozminkowski, R. J. (2008). The health and cost benefits of work site health-promotion programs. *Annual Review of Public Health, 29*(1): 303–323.

Golden S. D., & Earp, J. A. L. (2012). Social ecological approaches to individuals and their contexts: Twenty years of health education & behavior health promotion interventions. *Health Education & Behavior, 39*(3), 364–372.

Grosch, J. W., Alterman, T., Petersen, M. R., & Murphy, L. R. (1998). Worksite health promotion programs in the U.S.: Factors associated with availability and participation. *American Journal of Health Promotion, 13*(1), 36–45.

Hannon, P. A., Garson, G., Harris, J. R., Hammerback, K., Sopher, C. J., & Clegg-Thorp, C. (2012). Workplace health promotion implementation, readiness, and capacity among midsize employers in low-wage industries: A national survey. *Journal of Occupational and Environmental Medicine, 54*, 1337–1343.

Harris, J., Hannon, P., Beresford, S., Linnan, L., & McClellan, D. (2014). *Health promotion in small workplaces.* Ann Rev Public Health. *35*, 327–342.

The Health Project. *Winning programs, 2015.* Retrieved from http://thehealth project.com/winning-programs/

Hunt, M. K., Barbeau, E. M., Lederman, R., Stoddard, A. M., Chetkovich, C., Goldman, R., . . . Sorensen, G. (2007). Process evaluation results from the Healthy Directions–Small Business Study. *Health Education & Behavior, 34*(1), 90–107.

Juhn, C., & Potter, S. (2006). Changes in labor force participation in the United States. *Journal of Economic Perspectives, 20*(3), 27–46.

Kaiser Family Foundation. (2014). *2014 employer health benefits survey: Summary of findings.* Retrieved from http://kff.org/report-section/ehbs-2014-summary-of-findings/

Linnan, L., Sorensen, G., Colditz, G., Klar, N., & Emmons, K. M. (2001). Using theory to understand the multiple determinants of low participation in worksite health promotion programs. *Health Education & Behavior, 28*(5), 591–607.

Linnan, L., Bowling, M., Bachtel, J., Lindsay, G., Blakey, C., Pronk, S., . . . Royall, P. (2008). Results of the 2004 National Worksite Health Promotion Survey. *American Journal of Public Health, 98*(8), 1503–1509.

Linnan, L., Jeffries, J., & Eastman, M. (2014). Tailoring worksite-based interventions at the individual and organizational levels. In M. O'Donnell (Ed.), *Worksite health promotion* (3rd ed., pp. 377–405). New York, NY: Springer.

Maryland University of Integrative Health. (2015). *Master of science in health promotion*. Retrieved March 29, 2016 from http://www.muih.edu/academics/masters-degrees/master-science-health-promotion

McLeroy, K. R., Bibeau, D., Steckler, A., & Glanz, K. (1988). An ecological perspective on health promotion programs. *Health Education Quarterly, 15*(4), 351–377.

Murray, P., & Gillibrand, K. (2015). *Contingent workforce: Size, characteristics, earnings, and benefits*. Washington, DC: U.S. Government Accountability Office.

National Institute for Occupational Safety and Health. (2008). *Essential elements of effective workplace programs and policies for improving worker health and wellbeing*. Retrieved from http://www.cdc.gov/niosh/twh/essentials.html

National Institute for Occupational Safety and Health. (2014). Total worker health. Retrieved from http://www.cdc.gov/niosh/TWH/

National Research Council. (1999). *The changing nature of work: Implications for occupational analysis*. Washington, DC: National Academies Press.

National Wellness Institute. (n.d.). *NWI certificate options*. Retrieved from http://www.nationalwellness.org/?page=Certifications

O'Donnell, M. P. (2010). Integrating financial incentives for workplace health promotion programs into health plan premiums is the best idea since sliced bread. *American Journal of Health Promotion, 24*(4), iv–vi.

O'Donnell, M. (2013). Does workplace health promotion work or not? Are you sure you really want to know the truth? *American Journal of Health Promotion. 28*(1): iv–vii.

Ortman, J. M., Velkoff, V. A., & Hogan, H. (2014). An aging nation: The older population in the United States (Current Population Reports, P25-1140). Washington, DC: U.S. Census Bureau.

Partnership for Prevention and the U.S. Chamber of Commerce. (2007). *Leading by example: Leading practices for employee health management*. Retrieved from http://www.prevent.org/initiatives/leading-by-example.aspx

Paul-Ebhohimhen, V., & Avenell, A. (2008). Systematic review of the use of financial incentives in treatments for obesity and overweight. *Obesity Reviews, 9*(4), 355–367.

Peabody, K., & Linnan, L. (2007). Careers in worksite health promotion. *Eta Sigma Gamma: The Health Education Monograph Series, 23*(2), 18–21.

Prochaska, J. O., Redding, C. A., & Evers, K. E. (2008). The transtheoretical model and stages of change. *In Health behavior and health education: Theory, research, and practice* (4th ed, pp. 97–122). San Francisco: Jossey-Bass.

Pronk, N. P. (2013). Integrated worker health protection and promotion programs: Overview and perspectives on health and economic outcomes. *Journal of Occupational and Environmental Medicine, 55*(12 Suppl.), S30–S37.

Reardon, J. (1998). The history and impact of worksite wellness. *Nursing Economics, 16*, 117–121.

Seaverson, E. L., Grossmeier, J., Miller, T. M., & Anderson, D. R. (2009). The role of incentive design, incentive value, communications strategy, and worksite culture on health risk assessment participation. *American Journal of Health Promotion, 23*(5), 343–352.

Singhal, S., Stueland, J., & Ungerman, D. (2011). *How US health care reform will affect employee benefits.* Retrieved from http://www.mckinsey.com/insights/health_systems_and_services/how_us_health_care_reform_will_affect_employee_benefits

State of California. (2005). *Guide to developing a workplace injury and illness prevention program with checklists for self-inspection.* Retrieved from https://www.dir.ca.gov/dosh/dosh_publications/IIPP.html

Stokols, D., Pelletier, K., & Fielding, J. (1996). The ecology of work and health: Research and policy directions for the promotion of employee health. *Health Education Quarterly, 23,* 137–158.

University of Michigan Center for Value-Based Insurance Design. (n.d.). *State employee health plans.* Retrieved August 21, 2016, from http://vbidcenter.org/initiatives/state-employee-health-plans/

University of North Carolina at Chapel Hill. (n.d.). *Carolina collaborative for research on work and health.* Retrieved August 24, 2016, from http://sph.unc.edu/ccrwh/carolina-collaborative-for-research-on-work-and-health/

U.S. Census Bureau. (2012). *U.S. Census Bureau projections show a slower growing, older, more diverse nation a half century from now.* Retrieved from https://www.census.gov/newsroom/releases/archives/population/cb12-243.html

U. S. Department of Health and Human Services. (2015). *The Affordable Care Act is working.* Retrieved from http://www.hhs.gov/healthcare/facts/factsheets/2014/10/affordable-care-act-is-working.html

U.S. Office of Personnel Management. (n.d.). *Employee health services handbook.* Retrieved January 22, 2016, from https://www.opm.gov/policy-data-oversight/worklife/reference-materials/employee-health-services-handbook/

Volpp, K. G., John, L. K., Troxel, A. B., Norton, L., Fassbender, J., & Loewenstein, G. (2008). Financial incentive–based approaches for weight loss: A randomized trial. *Journal of the American Medical Association, 300*(22), 2631–2637.

Volpp, K. G., Troxel, A. B., Pauly, M. V., Glick, H. A., Puig, A., Asch, D. A., . . . Audrain-McGovern, J. (2009). A randomized, controlled trial of financial incentives for smoking cessation. *New England Journal of Medicine, 360*(7), 699–709.

Wellness Council of America. (2015). *Well workplace awards.* Retrieved from https://www.welcoa.org/services/recognize/well-workplace-awards/

*The authors acknowledge Jennifer Weiland and Kimberly Peobody for their help in preparation of a previous version of this chapter.

CHAPTER 16

PROMOTING COMMUNITY HEALTH: LOCAL HEALTH DEPARTMENTS AND COMMUNITY HEALTH ORGANIZATIONS

Michael T. Hatcher, Diane D. Allensworth, and Frances D. Butterfoss

Brief History of Community Health Organizations

Both *local health departments* and *community health organizations* have their roots in public health. Life expectancy was less than 50 years in 1900. The crude death rate at the beginning of the 20th century was 17.2 deaths per 1,000 people per year, and the infant mortality rate was approximately 120 per 1,000 births. The top three causes of death in 1900 were infectious diseases. By the end of the 20th century, life expectancy had increased to 77 years, while the annual death rate had dropped to 8.7 per 1,000 and the annual infant mortality rate had dropped to 6.9 per 1,000. Heart disease, cancer, and stroke were the top causes of death at the beginning of the 21st century (Ward & Warren, 2007).

A number of public health innovations were responsible for the shift in causes of mortality from infectious disease to chronic disease during the past century. The top 10 public health achievements during the 20th century, as identified by the Centers for Disease Control and Prevention (2013), were (1) immunizations; (2) control of infectious diseases through sanitation and antimicrobial therapy; (3) motor vehicle safety (improved engineering and seat belt use); (4) workplace safety; (5) recognition of tobacco as a health hazard; (6) decline in deaths from

LEARNING OBJECTIVES

- Describe the history of health departments as well as the history of voluntary health organizations in the United States.

- Describe the functions of your local health authority and the impact of its structure on its staffing, the services provided, and the percentage of the population served.

- Identify tools and resources to plan, implement, and evaluate health promotion programs in local communities.

- Discuss the challenges of engaging a community in public health promotion efforts, campaigns, and services.

- Describe administrative, clinical, and programmatic careers in local or state health departments.

heart disease and stroke as a result of smoking cessation and lowering of the mean blood pressure of the U.S. population; (7) safer and healthier food, which has virtually eliminated nutritional deficiency diseases; (8) healthier mothers and babies as a result of improvements in nutrition, advances in clinical medicine, and improvements in access to health care; (9) increased availability of family planning and contraceptive services as restrictive policies and laws affecting family planning were largely replaced by legislative and funding support for family planning services; and (10) fluoridation of drinking water to prevent tooth decay.

Although a few cities that experienced severe health problems from infectious disease established local health departments during the colonial period, it was not until a major epidemic of typhoid fever occurred in 1910 and 1911 that a federal recommendation prompted the organization of local health departments. By the mid-1930s, more than a quarter of the counties in the United States provided public health services (Novick, 2001). The services provided by local health departments have expanded over the past century to include prevention of epidemics and the spread of disease, protection against environmental hazards, prevention of injuries, prevention of health risk behaviors, disaster response and recovery assistance, and ensuring the quality and accessibility of health services. Local health departments have the authority to protect, promote, and enhance the health of people living in a specific geographic area. The extent of public health services as well as their relationship to the state department of health varies across the nation. Some local health departments (LHDs) are state governed, others are governed locally and some share governance with local and state authorities (NACCHO, 2015). Tax dollars fund local health departments, and their staff members are government employees.

Both the recession of 2008 and passage of the Patient Protection and Affordable Care Act (ACA) in 2010 stimulated new challenges and opportunities for public health departments. Since 2008, local health departments have lost approximately 51,700 employees, which reduced their capacity to provide some services. The implementation of the ACA has resulted in some individuals, who now have insurance, to choose other health care providers instead of the LHD. However, 38 percent of local health departments reported in 2015 that they are now serving more patients with health insurance and billing third party payers. The provision of clinical services also appears to be shifting. More LHDs reported reducing clinical services, immunizations, diabetic screenings, and maternal and child services than reported expanding those services, while other health departments reported expanding services such as obesity prevention and tobacco, alcohol, and other drug use prevention (NACCHO, 2015). The ACA also has stimulated new opportunities for local health departments to join in collaborative partnerships with nonprofit hospitals since both need to complete community needs assessments. The ACA requires tax-exempt hospitals to complete a community assessment every 3 years, while those local health departments who would like to become nationally accredited are required to complete a community assessment every 5 years. The launching of a system of national voluntary accreditation for local health departments by the Public Health Accreditation Board just happened to coincide with passage of the ACA.

At the same time that local health departments were developing, the first voluntary health organizations were formed. These organizations were designed to address specific health problems and were run primarily by volunteers. For example, the National Association for the Study and Prevention of Tuberculosis was established in 1902, and the American Cancer Society was founded in 1913. The March of Dimes, another voluntary health organization, which was founded in 1938 to address polio was instrumental in eliminating the disease from the United States. Following that success, the organization now focuses on preventing birth defects.

A large number of diverse health organizations have developed over the past hundred years. Today, many are large, well-run national organizations with state and local chapters that are managed by a professional staff. Many small, local organizations also have a professional staff and solid funding. Illustrative examples of the types of community health organizations that address local health concerns such as diabetes, physical inactivity, substance abuse, and clean water are found in Table 16.1. Community health organizations go by many names but their common bond is their operation by community members trying to ameliorate a local health problem. Many community organizations are nonprofit and are not owned by an individual; by law, they are governed by boards of directors who have responsibility for their operation. They are recognized as exempt from paying federal, state, and local taxes, in accordance with section 501(c)(3) of the U.S. Internal Revenue Code (26 U.S.C. 501(c)). Tax-exempt status also has implications for how organizations conduct advocacy efforts (see Chapter 7). Health care organizations such as hospitals and medical clinics (discussed in Chapter 13) may have the same organizational structure as community organizations (nonprofit) but have a broader mission that includes medical treatment.

The positive benefits of public health and community health services are continuing in this century. For example, improvements in the age-adjusted annual death rates for heart disease, cancer, and stroke occurred in the population between 2005 and 2011. The decline on mortality over the

Table 16.1 Types of Community Health Organizations

Health and mental health programs (treatment and counseling)

Environmental health programs (clean food, water, soil, and air)

Voluntary health agencies (for example, organizations focusing on cancer, heart, or lung diseases)

Human or social service programs (for example, child protection, homeless shelters)

Community primary health care clinics

Recreation and fitness programs

Nutrition programs

Health coalitions and collaborations

Safety and disaster preparedness programs

Faith-based organizations and their child, family, and/or elder programs

Youth development programs (for example, Boys and Girls Clubs, YWCA, and YMCA)

Senior service programs

Neighborhood policing and safety programs

Labor unions' health programs

Urban planning agencies (built environment and land use issues)

Brownfield programs (industrial site redevelopment)

Community health foundations

6-year period was 3.54% for heart disease, 1.44% for cancer, and 3.77% for stroke. Infant mortality continued to improve falling to 6.1 per 1,000 births in 2011. Life expectancy during this period also improved with infants born in 2010 having a life expectancy of 78.7 years for an annual increase during this period of 0.3% (CDC, 2014).

Local Health Department Services

The size of the population served by a LHD influences the size of the department's staff as well as the scope of the services provided. For example, although approximately 2,800 LHDs exist in the United States, the population that they serve ranges from less than 1,000 to nearly 10 million. Five percent of LHDs, which serve large jurisdictions of over a half a million people or more, actually serve about half of the U.S. population (49%). Most LHDs (61%) are small and serve less than 50,000 residents. These departments, in general, have about 18 employees, while health departments with jurisdictions serving over a million people have approximately 470 employees (NACCHO, 2015).

The 2013 National Profile of Local Health Departments (NACCHO, 2015) identified 87 different public health programs and services offered by LHDs, but only seven of these services are provided by more than three quarters of all LHDs nationwide. Categories of services include immunization; screening and treatment for various diseases and conditions, particularly tuberculosis, STD, and HIV; maternal and child health services including Women, Infants and Children (WIC) programs and maternal-child health home visits; surveillance services; primary prevention services; environmental health services including prevention, protection, and educational services; regulation, inspection, or licensing services; and a variety of others including vital records, enrollment for medical insurance, and school health. The types and variety of services provided in a particular LHD depends on numerous factors, including state laws, community needs and priorities, funding, and the lack of availability of similar services from other agencies in the community. See Table 16.2 for examples of services provided nationwide in both jurisdictions serving a population

Table 16.2   Illustrious Examples of Services of Local Health Departments, by Size of Population Served (Percentages)

Services and Activities	All Departments (%)	Population of Fewer Than 25,000 (%)	Population of More Than 500,000 (%)
Adult immunizations	90	87	92
Child immunizations	90	85	95
Communicable disease surveillance	91	86	96
Tuberculosis screening	83	75	90
Food service regulation	78	67	91
Food safety education	72	63	78
Environmental health surveillance	78	69	82
Tuberculosis treatment	76	67	91
Chronic disease prevention	69	60	86
WIC clinics	65	58	77
Maternal child home visits	60	53	78
School health services	36	34	44
Behavioral risk factor surveillance	36	28	55
School-based clinics	27	31	27
Oral health	24	14	50
Injury surveillance	27	21	48
Primary care	11	7	20

Note: Some local health departments that served populations between 25,000 and 500,000 provided more services than departments that served populations below 25,000 and above 500,000.
Source: NACCHO, 2015.

Table 16.3   Percent of Local Health Departments (LHDs) Providing Primary Prevention Services, by Population Served (Percentages)

Primary Prevention Services	All LHDs	Populations Under 25,000	Populations 25,000– 49,999	Populations 50,000– 99,999	Populations 100,000– 499,999	Populations Over 500,000
Nutrition	69	60	68	72	83	86
Tobacco	68	60	72	72	77	80
Physical Activity	52	44	53	57	61	68
Chronic Disease Programs	50	42	48	54	60	72
Unintended Pregnancy	49	42	50	50	56	69
Injury	38	35	37	39	43	50
Substance Abuse	24	19	27	29	28	30
Violence	21	16	21	21	27	38
Mental Illness	12	9	12	13	18	17

Source: NACCHO, 2014.

of under 25,000 and those serving populations from 100,000 to 500,000 (NACCHO, 2015).

Almost all of the services provided by a LHD have implications for health promotion. The scope of services delivered generally increases with population size. However, even in small health departments, health promotion activities are a priority. Table 16.3 identifies the percent of health departments providing primary prevention services including the prevention of unintended pregnancy, injury, substance abuse, violence, mental illness, and/or the promotion of nutrition and physical activity to prevent chronic diseases. One source of guidance for health promotion in local health departments was the development in 1995 of the *10 essential public health services* (EPHS) by the Public Health Functions Steering Committee of the U.S. Department of Health and Human Services (2008). The 10 essential services (outlined in Table 16.4) define public health practice and are performed within local health departments in collaboration with their community partners. Many of these services are invisible to the public and are only recognized when a problem develops (for example, when an outbreak of disease occurs). However, effective performance of these services facilitates health promotion efforts and is crucial in safeguarding the health of a community.

Tackling the health implications of modern lifestyles such as tobacco use; consumption of high-calorie, high-salt foods; and physical inactivity, as well as the threat of globally spreading infectious diseases, requires the availability of a well-trained public health workforce. Having fewer public health staff means fewer screenings and immunizations. Not having

Table 16.4 Ten Essential Public Health Services

1. Monitor health status of the population to identify and solve community health problems.

2. Diagnose and investigate health problems and health hazards in the community.

3. Inform, educate, and empower people about health issues.

4. Mobilize community partnerships and action to identify and solve health problems.

5. Develop policies and plans that support individual and community health efforts.

6. Enforce laws and regulations that protect health and ensure safety.

7. Link people to needed personal health services and ensure the provision of health care when otherwise unavailable.

8. Ensure a competent public health and personal health care workforce.

9. Evaluate effectiveness, accessibility, and quality of personal and population-based health services.

10. Conduct research to discover new insights and innovative solutions to health problems.

enough epidemiologists makes it harder to respond to food-borne outbreaks or to track emerging infectious diseases like drug-resistant staph infections (MRSA). Hurricane Katrina made clear the importance of local health department workers in responding to natural disasters. Given the growing complexity of public health challenges, more specialists need to be trained in additional public health subdisciplines. Furthermore, in the era of globalization, the U.S. public health workforce needs to be adequately prepared to prevent and handle health threats that often arise from beyond U.S. borders. Two such threats are Ebola, which could have escalated in 2014 to become a threat in the United States and the Zika virus that emerged in 2015 and 2016 as a threat to the U.S. population, especially pregnant women and their developing fetuses.

The structure of a local health department typically includes a local board of health and a health commissioner. Laws may prescribe who is a health commissioner (for example, a physician, dentist, or someone who holds a doctorate in public health). If the health commissioner is not a physician, then the department will probably have a health officer who is a physician who provides medical guidance and support to the department through a consulting relationship. The health commissioner is appointed by the board of health. Boards of health are elected city or county government officials or elected officials appoint the board of health.

Community Health Organization Services

Community health organizations are typically nonprofit organizations that have been created by individuals in a community to address a specific health issue. They are local affiliates of a national organization or organizations unique to the community. The issues addressed by community health organizations are numerous. Community health organizations are usually started in order to raise money for research, educate professionals, serve individuals affected by a disease or health problem, and/or advocate for beneficial government policies and procedures. However, almost all of these organizations have health promotion and disease prevention of the disease that is the focus of their mission.

The numbers and types of community health organizations engaged in health promotion programs also are directly related to the population size and the diversity of the health needs of the community. Compared with the focus of a local health department, the focus of a community health organization is generally more tailored and fitted to that priority population. This tighter focus on a particular population provides an opportunity to develop in-depth expertise on the health concerns of that priority population. For example, Table 16.5 lists the services of a community organization that is focused on the mission of positively influencing the experience of the elderly within the community. The organization's goals are for individuals aged 60 and older to (1) stay active and healthy, (2) maintain independence, (3) pursue interests, and (4) make new friends.

Recently funders of community health programs (for example, *United Way*, foundations, and local government) have placed more emphasis on community health program outcomes; this has been accompanied by changes in policy and an increase in general public concern about accountability. Pressure for results has intensified, and organizations are increasingly being asked to demonstrate that specified goals have been achieved. For example, the U.S. Government Performance Results Act (Office of Management and Budget, 1993) specifies that organizations funded by the federal government must set program outcome goals and publicly report on progress toward achieving those goals. Community health organizations are asked to demonstrate outcomes, including the achievements of their health promotion programs, and report those outcomes during their annual budget cycles.

Resources and Tools

A number of unique resources can help health promotion specialists in planning, implementing, and evaluating community health promotion programs. Most of the organizations listed in this section provide tools, technical assistance, and other resources needed to address the range of

Table 16.5   Services of a Community Health Organization That Promotes the Health of Senior Citizens in the Community

Health risk assessments: assessments that evaluate the health status of an individual comparing chronological age to health age

Routine health screening: screenings for certain diseases or conditions, which may include hypertension, glaucoma, high cholesterol, cancer, impaired vision, impaired hearing, memory problems, diabetes, and inadequate nutrition

Fitness activities: organized activities that promote the physical health of older adults, incorporating cardiovascular exercise, muscle toning, and agility improvement

Nutrition counseling: provision of individualized advice and guidance on options and methods for improving nutritional status of those at nutritional risk because of their health or nutritional history, their dietary intake, their use of medications, or chronic illness; performed by a health professional in accordance with state law and policy

Education for individuals or groups: programs to promote better physical or mental health by providing accurate health information and instruction to participants or caregivers in a group or individual setting, overseen by an individual with health-related expertise or experience

Health promotion programs: programs relating to management of chronic disabling conditions (including osteoporosis and cardiovascular disease), alcohol and substance abuse reduction, smoking cessation, weight loss and control, and stress management

Home injury control services: screening of high-risk home environments and provision of educational programs on injury prevention (including fall and fracture prevention) in the home environment

Medication management: oversight of medications by a registered nurse for older adults who have been assessed as requiring management of their medications

Informational programs concerning Medicare benefits: educational programs on availability, benefits, and appropriate use of preventive health services covered by Medicare

Senior center: an attractive center that provides a wide variety of activities and programs (for example, arts and crafts, social engagement and sponsored outings, and exercise) for seniors

Adult day care: the time demands of caring for an older adult require many family care providers to make sacrifices in their professional and personal lives. At some point, they simply need some help. Adult day care programs provide assistance in caring for a dependent adult family member.

issues that health promotion specialists are asked to address in their work at health departments and community organizations.

Area Health Education Centers

The mission of area health education centers (AHECs) is to improve the supply, distribution, diversity, and quality of the health care workforce in medically underserved communities (U.S. Department of Health and Human Services, n.d). The long-term educational strategy of the AHECs is to form academic and community partnerships in order to train health care providers at sites and in programs that are responsive to state and local health workforce needs. Programs to interest K–12 students in health careers and recruit them for those careers are also emphasized. AHECs link the resources of university health science centers with local planning, educational, and clinical resources. This network of health-related institutions provides multidisciplinary educational services to students, faculty, and local practitioners and works extensively in the planning, implementing, and evaluating of health promotion programs emphasizing community collaborations and the elimination of health disparities. Fifty-six AHEC programs and 235 affiliated AHECs operate in 46 states. There are no AHECs in Delaware, Iowa, Minnesota, and Mississippi (National AHEC Organization, 2015).

America's Health Rankings

This site (http://www.americashealthrankings.org/) ranks health disparities, and rates of obesity, tobacco use, and diabetes by state. Want to see how all states stack up on a certain measure? Or maybe compare your state to another? America's Health Rankings employs a unique methodology, developed and periodically reviewed by a panel of leading public health scholars, which balances the contributions of various factors such as smoking, obesity, sedentary lifestyle, binge drinking, high school graduation rates, children in poverty, access to care, and incidence of preventable disease, to the health of the inhabitants in a state. The easy to use, web-based report is based on data from the U.S. Departments of Health and Human Services, Commerce, Education, Justice and Labor; U.S. Environmental Protection Agency; U.S. Census Bureau; the American Medical Association; the Dartmouth Atlas Project; and the Trust for America's Health.

Children's Safety Network

The Children's Safety Network (CSN; http://www.childrenssafetynetwork .org), funded by the Maternal and Child Health Bureau of Health Resources and Services Administration, seeks to prevent injuries and violence among children and adolescents by strengthening the staff and organizational capacity for injury prevention of state maternal and child health programs. It is a source for funding, resources, current research, and legislative updates and regulations. CSN also works with national organizations and federal agencies that are responsible for promoting child and adolescent health and safety.

County Health Roadmaps

The County Health Roadmaps (http://www.countyhealthrankings.org/) show what we can do to create healthier places to live, learn, work, and play.

The Robert Wood Johnson Foundation collaborates with the University of Wisconsin Population Health Institute to bring this groundbreaking program to cities, counties, and states across the nation.

Community Commons

With the advent of the Community Commons website (http://www .communitycommons.org/about/), community groups can now use data templates and support from other groups nationwide to tackle critical health issues in ways that were not imagined a few years ago. Assessment data is converted into maps that help community members to better understand the problem. The website is organized into six channels that capture the breadth and depth of community issues: economy, education, environment, equity, food, and health. Each channel provides accessible resources for peer learning via articles, webinars, stories, map templates, technical assistance, data integration, and collaboration tools that support the community health promotion specialists.

CHANGE Tool

The Community Health Assessment and Group Evaluation (CHANGE): Building a foundation of knowledge to prioritize community needs (http:// www.cdc.gov/nccdphp/dch/programs/healthycommunitiesprogram/tools/ change/downloads.htm) helps community coalitions develop their community action plan. This tool guides team members through the assessment process and helps define and prioritize possible areas of improvement. The tool developed by the Centers for Disease Control and Prevention assesses current policy, systems, and environmental change. The tool provides eight action steps and provides guidance for engaging the community at large, community organizations, health care sector, schools, and the worksite sector.

Community Tool Box

The Community Tool Box (CTB) is the world's largest online resource for free information on essential skills for building healthy communities (http:// ctb.ku.edu/en). The CTB has been continuously updated since 1994 and provides over 7,000 pages of practical, step-by-step guidance on specific community-building skills, along with key tasks, examples, and support for developing and performing 16 core public health competencies that promote community health and development. The University of Kansas hosts the CTB team within the Work Group for Community Health and Development. The national and international partners of the CTB team have identified what community members need to know to build healthier and more equitable communities.

MAP-IT: A Guide to Using *Healthy People 2020* in Your Community

Healthy People (http://www.healthypeople.gov/2020/tools-and-resources/ Program-Planning) is based on a simple but powerful model: (1) establish national health objectives; and (2) provide data and tools to enable states, cities, communities, and individuals across the country to combine their efforts to achieve them. Use the MAP-IT framework to help (1) mobilize partners; (2) assess the needs of your community; (3) create and implement a plan to reach *Healthy People 2020* objectives; and (4) track your community's progress.

National Association of County and City Health Officials

The National Association of County and City Health Officials (NACCHO) represents approximately 3,000 local health departments. NACCHO supports local health efforts by calling for strong national policy, developing useful resources and programs, promoting health equity, and supporting effective local public health practice and health system performance. NACCHO provides assistance in four key areas: (1) conducting health promotion and preventive disease initiatives within communities; (2) promoting human health by building safe environments that address the relationship between people's health and their environments; (3) helping local health departments perform their core governmental functions and the 10 essential public health services; and (4) enhancing local health departments' readiness to respond to emergencies. As part of its services, NACCHO has created a public health toolbox on the web (http://www.naccho.org/toolbox). This is a free service available for public use, intended to promote public health objectives including health promotion.

National Public Health Performance Standards Program

The CDC National Public Health Performance Standards Program (NPH-PSP) is a partnership initiative that was formed with national public health organizations in order to work collaboratively to establish national performance standards (http://www.cdc.gov/od/ocphp/nphpsp). The standards identify the optimal level of performance for state and local public health systems and local governing boards. The NPHPSP provides a framework for assessing the capacity and performance of a public health system and seeks to ensure that strong, effective public health systems are in place to deliver the 10 essential public health services. The standards provide a foundation for state and local health departments to plan, implement, and evaluate health promotion programs.

National Public Health Accreditation Board

The goal of the voluntary national accreditation program is to improve and protect the health of the public by advancing the quality and performance of tribal, state, local, and territorial public health departments. The accreditation standards define the expectations for all public health departments that seek to become accredited. National accreditation has been developed to improve service, value, and accountability to public health stakeholders. The EPHS and the capacity to meet the complexity of contemporary public health go hand-in-hand with accreditation of local public health agencies. In late 2011, the National Public Health Accreditation Standards were released. The first 10 domains of the accreditation standards aligned with the 10 essential public health services, and the 11th domain addresses management and administration, whereas Domain 12 addresses governance (Bender, Kronstadt, Wilcox, & Lee, 2014). In March 2016, 117 public health departments within 39 states and the District of Columbia had been awarded national accreditation status. Those accredited departments collectively serve 154 million people, or 50 percent of the U.S. population (Nicolaus, 2016).

Public Health Foundation

The Public Health Foundation (PHF) (http://www.phf.org), which is dedicated to achieving healthy communities through research, training, and technical assistance, is a national nonprofit organization that creates new information and helps public health agencies and other community health organizations access and more effectively use information in order to manage and improve performance, understand and use data, and strengthen the competencies of the public health workforce. The foundation is a resource and support for creating innovative health promotion programs for diverse populations and settings. PHF also has created TRAIN, a web-based learning resource for health professionals that allows users to find current local, regional, and national training opportunities, many of them offered via the Internet (https://www.train.org/DesktopShell.aspx).

A Practical Playbook

The resources offered at the Practical Playbook site are responsive to the challenges of integration of public health and health care (https://www.practicalplaybook.org/principles-of-integration). This site provides tools and resources to assist public health and health care organizations to develop infrastructures and strategies to manage *community engagement;* improve decision making and health planning; and support delivery of effective community-level interventions (Hatcher, 2015).

United Way

Over 1,300 United Ways operate in the United States via a coalition of local nonprofit organizations that pool efforts in fundraising support (http://www.liveunited.org). The focus of United Way is identifying and resolving pressing community issues, as well as making measurable changes in communities through partnerships with schools, government agencies, businesses, organized labor, financial institutions, community development corporations, voluntary and neighborhood associations, the faith community, and others. The issues that United Way offices address are determined locally, out of respect for the diversity of the communities served. United Way organizations raise money in numerous ways—most notably, through workplaces, where employees can authorize automatic payroll deductions for United Way.

What Works for Health

Developed by experts at the University of Wisconsin Population Health Institute, this is an online tool used to find effective policies and programs to improve the many factors that affect one's health (http://www.countyhealthrankings.org/roadmaps/what-works-for-health/using-what-works-health). Each of the included programs is given an evidence rating and the highest rated programs and policies have been shown to work. Just choose a health factor of interest (i.e., tobacco use, employment, access to health care, environmental quality, etc.) and browse through the evidence ratings for particular programs, policies, or system changes that address this health factor.

Challenges

Health promotion in communities depends on effective community engagement. Engaging community members and organizations in community health promotion work presents many challenges. Lack of trust or respect often exists among local health departments and community health organizations that may have experienced few direct benefits from their community-level participation. The unequal distribution of information, formal education, income, and power in communities reflects underlying social inequalities of economic class, race, ethnicity, age, and gender. These may, in turn, affect whether community members feel they will have influence over decisions and whether they want to engage and participate in community-based activities. Differences in community organizations' perspectives, priorities, assumptions, values, beliefs, and languages also may make engagement difficult and conflict more likely. Finally, because of resource competition or turf issues between community groups (Israel, Schultz, Parker, & Becker, 1998), challenges may arise over the extent to which community organizations represent and reflect the "real" community. Ultimately, participation is influenced by whether community members believe that the benefits of participation outweigh the costs. Overcoming the challenges to community engagement depends on successful community assessment and community self-empowerment, as well as attention to the general conclusions about community building that are detailed in this section. In order to bring about desired changes, community engagement efforts address multiple levels of the social environment and health determinants within the community rather than only specific individual behaviors.

A focus on continuous improvement of ongoing action planning can identify specific community and system changes that influence or compel widespread behavior changes and make community health improvements more likely (Butterfoss, 2013; Roussos & Fawcett, 2000). Health behaviors are influenced by culture. To ensure that engagement efforts are culturally and linguistically appropriate, they must be developed from an understanding and respect for the culture of the community being served. While a sense of empowerment cannot be externally imposed on a community, engendering the ability for individuals to take action, influence, and make decisions on critical issues is crucial for successful engagement efforts. Coalitions and partnerships, when adequately supported, are useful to mobilize community assets for decision making and action on health issues.

Community mobilization and self-determination frequently need nurturing. Before individuals and organizations can gain control and influence and become partners in making decisions and acting on community health issues, they frequently need training to develop additional knowledge, leadership skills, and resources in order to exert their power. Health professionals and community leaders can use their understanding of perceived costs associated with health issues in order to develop appropriate incentives for participation. Such incentives might include fostering a sense of community, choosing relevant issues, and making the process and organizational climate of participation open and supportive of community members' right

Table 16.6   Factors That Contribute to the Success of Community Engagement Efforts

Environment
A history of collaboration or cooperation exists in the community.
The collaborating group (and its member agencies) is seen as a leader in the community.
The political and social climate is favorable.

Membership
Partners have mutual respect, understanding, and trust.
Partners represent an appropriate cross-section of the community.
Engagement is perceived as being in partners' self-interest—the benefits of engagement offset the costs.
Partners are willing to compromise.

Process and Structure
Partners have ownership—that is, share a stake in both the process and the outcome.
Every level of each organization in the collaborating group participates in decision making.
The collaborating group has flexibility.
Roles and guidelines are clear.
Partners can sustain collaboration in the midst of changing conditions.

Communication
Open and frequent interaction, information, and discussion occur.
Informal and formal channels of communication exist.

Purpose
Goals are clear and appear realistic to all partners.
Partners have a shared vision.
The purpose is unique to the effort (that is, it is at least, partly different from the mission, goals, or approaches of the member organizations).

Resources
The effort has sufficient funds.
The effort has a skilled convener.

to have a voice in the process. Based on the social science literature and the principles discussed in this section, Table 16.6 summarizes some specific factors that can positively influence the success of community engagement efforts. Additional review of community engagement literature is available in the publication *Principles of Community Engagement,* 2nd edition (http://www.atsdr.cdc.gov/communityengagement/). Table 16.7 highlights specific barriers to community participation and some suggestions for how to overcome them.

Career Opportunities

Local health departments and community health organizations are where people work and develop careers in community health promotion programming. However, government agencies and community organizations operate under different personnel rules. *Civil service* or other personnel

Table 16.7 Barriers to Community Engagement and Potential Solutions

Problem	Solution
Organization is cautious about engaging.	Consistency about opportunities and incentives for participation.
Organization faces administrative challenges (for example, staff are unavailable to answer phone or work irregular hours).	Consistency and patience in communication with organization. Flexibility: meeting staff when and where they are available.
Organization needs help with capacity building.	Suggesting ways to help the organization maximize strengths and work around its challenges. Offers to share effective practices that have worked for other programs or organizations. Step-by-step analysis through the organization's processes or procedures to highlight areas of inefficiency.
Organization lacks access to information.	Invitation of the organization to partnership and networking opportunities. Introduction of the organization's staff to new and different sources of information.
Organization has language barriers or uses words in ways that differ from other organization's uses.	Clarification of questions and definition of terms. Provision of translation services
Organization is protective of its programs and perceives other programs may potentially take money, volunteers, or other resources away from its already limited capacity.	Discuss how the new activity or partnership will support the organization's mission and use its resources to benefit the community. Ensure that the organization has both the benefits and the responsibilities of full partnership.

hiring rules bind government agencies at the local, state, and federal levels to prescribed hiring practices. Historically, the civil service has used job classifications and competitive examinations to fill vacant positions. Civil service or other government personnel systems have formal procedures for announcing and filling position vacancies. Vacancy announcements describe a job, including the title, salary, duties, qualifications and requirements, closing date, and application procedures. There is no universal format for vacancy announcements. Each government personnel system independently manages its vacancy announcement and hiring practices. Typically, vacancy announcements include a section with directions called "How to Apply." Because application procedures vary across government agencies, following the directions provided within each vacancy announcement is essential. Failure to do so could result in rejection of an application.

Jobs in community health organizations often have less rigorous application processes and may require only submission of a résumé. Many types

Table 16.8 Community Health Organizations That Post Health Promotion Jobs

Community health centers

Faith-based organizations or groups based in places of worship such as churches, synagogues, or mosques (for example, Catholic Charities, Council of Jewish Women)

Community action and consumer advocacy organizations

Local housing and homeless coalitions

Organizations that focus on children and families (for example, Boys and Girls Clubs)

Organizations that address birth defects and developmental impairments (for example, March of Dimes)

Senior service and senior advocacy groups (for example, Area Agencies on Aging)

Mental health, drug, and alcohol programs (for example, MADD)

Organizations that address the health needs and protect the rights of people of color (for example, local chapters of the NAACP, Council of La Raza)

Organizations that address the health needs and protect the rights of women (for example, YWCA, Big Sister Association)

Organizations that address the health needs and protect the rights of gays and lesbians (for example, Gay Men's Health Crisis, AIDS Action)

Disability rights organizations (for example, National Alliance for the Mentally Ill)

Health service organizations and health reform advocacy organizations

Organizations that address specific diseases or groups of diseases (for example, American Cancer Society, American Heart Association, American Lung Association)

Primary health care clinics

Hospitals

Hospital and health care associations (for example, American Hospital Association, American Health Care Association)

Professional societies and associations (for example, those that represent pediatricians, nurses, health educators, nurse midwives, or physician assistants)

Immigrant or migrant worker health rights groups (for example, Migrant Health Network)

Agricultural extension offices

Youth development (for example, Youth Empowered Solutions [YES!], Peer Health Exchange)

of community organizations hire individuals who are skilled in health promotion. Table 16.8 lists examples of community organizations that typically advertise health promotion positions. The job title may not fully describe the responsibilities and tasks involved in a position. Therefore, reading the job description closely and talking with the agency's human resource officer, the person who will supervise the position, and people in similar jobs is critical. Some jobs require staff members to work in an office, clinic, or storefront, while others require staff members to visit people at their homes or work sites. Local or overnight travel is required in some jobs. Public speaking, preparing health communication materials, maintaining electronic correspondence, and working with people in small and large groups are common and key to working successfully in community health promotion settings.

Careers in local health departments and community health organizations are demanding. Although the work is rewarding, community organizations and health departments often have difficulty recruiting and retaining well-qualified staff. Geographic locations, budget constraints, low salaries, demanding workloads, and complex work tasks may create challenges, but staff members often have opportunities to develop, implement, and sometimes direct programs early in their career. Work is readily available at the local level and provides excellent career development opportunities. To retain and develop staff, directors and supervisors in community organizations and health agencies provide supervision that is informative, instructive, and supportive. They offer flexible schedules, staff development, and training events (for example, participation in conferences, professional associations, and online learning), and opportunities for leadership.

Other factors that may help a person obtain employment opportunities and a successful career in health departments or community organizations include cultural competence, personal values that align with the mission of a perspective employer, and networking skills. Individuals who work in community health promotion interact and serve people of diverse cultural and ethnic backgrounds. Such interactions require knowledge, skill, and appreciation of the assets, strengths, and differences among people of different cultures and ethnicities. Staff members of community organizations often become community leaders who serve as champions and advocates for the communities they serve. Having a passion for serving others and empathy for community members who need assistance builds support for health programs and those who work in them. Likewise, networking skills that help to build relationships with stakeholders and funders can create opportunities that contribute to effective programs and successful professionals. Empathy, passion, and connecting with others contribute to health promotion professionals being recognized, valued, and recruited for their work capabilities.

Summary

Communities are the site for many health promotion programs. Programs focus on individuals, families, and populations that reside in the community, or programs focus on the environment in order to ensure safe and healthy living conditions. Local health departments and community health organizations employ people to plan, implement, and evaluate community health promotion programs. Local health departments and their partners perform the 10 essential public health services. Community health organizations focus their efforts on the unique needs and service gaps within communities. The key to effective community health promotion programs in these settings is community engagement and empowered community actions. Careers in community-level health promotion are demanding but offer many opportunities to develop as a health promotion professional. To get the most out of early job opportunities, seek out organizations that provide informative, instructive, and supportive supervision and offer continuing education opportunities.

For Practice and Discussion

1. Visit your local health department. What health issues are being addressed, and how is the department working to promote those health issues among local citizens?

2. Rural communities are often less able than urban communities to offer access to public health services for their community members. Name three strategies for enabling rural communities to develop and offer access to public health services.

3. Forming a coalition or partnership takes a lot of work, time, and energy. Can you identify times in your life when you felt that working with other people was problematic and that you would rather have worked alone (for example, on a class team project in which team members did not share the work evenly)? If working with people is difficult, why do you think that forming and supporting health coalitions is so important? Why not just let each person take care of himself or herself?

4. Think about the ways in which technology currently is being used to promote health for your family and friends in the community where you attended high school. Using your cell phone as the technology platform, create a new health promotion service to improve the health of your family and friends in that community.

5. Visit a local organization that is working to promote the health of community members. What is the organization's focus (for example, cancer, heart disease, alcoholism, violence)? Who participates in the organization's programs, and what are the programs? How does the organization know whether the programs are effective?

KEY TERMS

Barriers to community engagement

Civil service

Community empowerment

Community engagement

Community health organizations

Local health departments

Ten essential public health services (EPHS)

United Way

References

Bender, K., Kronstadt, J., Wilcox, R., & Lee, T. (2014). Overview of the Public Health Accreditation Board. *Journal of Public Health Management & Practice, 20*(1), 4–6. doi:10.1097/PHH.0b013e3182a778a0

Butterfoss, F. D. (2013). *Ignite! Getting your community coalition "fired up" for change.* Bloomington, IN: AuthorHouse.

Centers for Disease Control and Prevention. (2013). *Ten great public health achievements in the 20th century.* Atlanta, GA: Author. Retrieved from http://www.cdc.gov/about/history/tengpha.htm

Centers for Disease Control and Prevention. (2014). *CDC National Health Report: Leading Causes of Morbidity and Mortality and Associated Behavioral Risk and Protective Factors—United States, 2005–2013.* MMWR Supplements October 31, 2014 / 63(04); 3-27.

Hatcher, M. T. (2015). A commentary on drivers of community health needs assessment. *Journal of Public Health Management and Practice, 21*(1), 31–33.

Israel, B. A., Schultz, A. J., Parker, E. A., & Becker, A. B. (1998). Review of community-based research: Assessing partnership approaches to improve public health. *Annual Review of Public Health, 19,* 173–202. NACCHO. (2014). *2013 National Profile of Local Health Departments.* Retrieved from http://nacchoprofilestudy.org/wp-content/uploads/2014/02/2013_National_Profile021014.pdf

NACCHO. (2015). *The changing public health landscape: Findings from the 2015 Forces of Change Survey.* Retrieved from http://nacchovoice.naccho.org/2015/06/11/the-changing-public-health-landscape-findings-from-the-2015-forces-of-change-survey/

National AHEC Organization. (2015). *About us.* Retrieved from http://www.nationalahec.org/about/AboutUs.html

Nicolaus, T. (2016, March 14). *Public health accreditation board awards accreditation status to eight more health departments.* Retrieved from http://www.phaboard.org/wp-content/uploads/PressReleaseFinalMarch2016-1.pdf

Novick, L. F. (2001). Defining public health: History and contemporary developments. In L. F. Novick & G. P. Mays (Eds.), *Public health administration: Principles for population-based management* (pp. 3–33). Gaithersburg, MD: Aspen.

Office of Management and Budget. (1993). *Government Performance Results Act of 1993*. Retrieved from http://www.whitehouse.gov/omb/mgmt-gpra/gplaw2m .html

Roussos, S., & Fawcett, S. (2000). A review of collaborative partnerships as a strategy for improving community health. *Annual Review of Public Health, 21,* 369–402.

U.S. Department of Health and Human Services, Health Resources and Services Administration. (n.d.). *Area health education centers*. Retrieved from http:// bhpr.hrsa.gov/grants/areahealtheducationcenters/

U.S. Department of Health and Human Services, Public Health Functions Steering Committee. (2008). *Public health in America*. Retrieved from http://www .health.gov/phfunctions/public.htm

Ward, J. W., & Warren, C. (2007). *Silent victories: The history of public health in twentieth-century America*. New York, NY: Oxford University Press.

GLOSSARY

501(c)(3) Tax-exempt nonprofit organizations having the following purposes: charitable, religious, educational, scientific, literary, testing for public safety, fostering amateur sports competitions, or preventing cruelty to children or animals.

Access People's ability to use health care services that are available, acceptable, and affordable.

ACHA–National College Health Assessment The American College Health Association's survey of student behaviors assessing health risk behaviors.

Action objectives Needed changes in actions or behaviors of the priority population. Behavioral objectives are developed during program planning and are often assessed as part of the impact evaluation.

Action plan A document that guides an organization's development of a health promotion program, including a mission statement, overall program goal, measurable objectives, marketing plan, evaluation plan, budget, and timeline.

Activities The types of programming that a health promotion program provides to program participants.

Adaptation The degree to which an intervention undergoes change in its implementation to fit the needs of a particular delivery situation.

Advisory boards Groups of key stakeholders who come together to provide program support, guidance, and oversight. They have a genuine interest in the setting or program. Also see *Wellness committee.*

Advocacy The process by which individuals or groups attempt to effect social or organizational change on behalf of a particular health goal, program, interest, or population.

Advocacy agenda An advocacy strategy statement that articulates the problem to be addressed and the participants, audience, action steps, and advocacy procedures to be employed.

Affordable Care Act (ACA) See *Patient Protection and Affordable Care Act* (ACA).

Alignment When all components of a health promotion program and its evaluation design (i.e., mission, goals, objectives, program activities, measures, data collection methods, and data analysis methods) are tightly linked with one another in a bidirectional supportive relationship.

Appropriations Legislation that designates funding for a program.

Audience segmentation The division of a target population into subgroups that share similar qualities or characteristics, such as geographic, demographic, or psychographic traits or behaviors.

Authorizations Legislation that sets policies or programs.

Balance sheet A snapshot of an organization's financial condition (also called a *statement of financial position*); assets and liabilities are listed as of a specific date, such as the end of a financial year.

Barriers to community engagement Obstacles that block citizen's access and participation in health promotion programs.

Behavior Any overt action, conscious or unconscious, with a measurable frequency, intensity, and duration.

Bill A proposed law presented for approval to a legislative body.

Big data A set of information and data so large and complex that it becomes difficult to process using conventional database management tools.

Big data challenges Integration of disparate sources, consistency/standardization, data fragmentation, trustworthiness, and protection.

Board members' fundraising responsibilities Board members can provide input on a fundraising plan, identify and cultivate new funding prospects, ask peers for donations, or accompany staff members on key visits to funders.

Budget A financial document used to project future income and expenses. The budgeting process is used to estimate whether the organization can continue to operate with its projected income and expenses.

Capacity assessment Part of a needs assessment at a site that determines what resources are available as well as what gaps and needs in resources need to be filled in order to address the identified health concerns and problems.

Cash flow statement A financial statement that shows how changes in balance sheet and income accounts affect cash and cash equivalents; it analyzes the cash flows into operating, investing, and financing activities.

CDC evaluation framework A six-step framework for health promotion programs that is promulgated by the Centers for Disease Control and Prevention.

Certified Health Education Specialist (CHES) A health educator who has successfully completed the competency-based exam given by the National Commission for Health Education Credentialing, Inc.

Certified in Public Health (CPH) A credential created in 2005 to ensure that graduates of institutions accredited by the Council of Education for Public Health have the knowledge and skills to be successful in the field of public health.

Champion An important program stakeholder who provides the leadership, passion, and emotion for a program. A champion knows the setting, health problem, and priority population affected by the health problem. Also see *Key informant.*

Change The process or the result of individuals' and environments' altering, modifying, transforming, or transitioning from one health status, condition, or phase to another, which health promotion programs need to accommodate.

Channels The media or routes through which a health message is transmitted to its intended audience.

Client fees The amounts that individuals pay (also known as *fees for services*) to receive a service or participate in a program.

Climate The environment or mood of a particular group that emanates from their cultural background and the tenor of the group's official and unofficial leaders. It also refers to the meaning that people attach to the interrelated bundles of experiences at a site.

Civil service Employment in federal, state (or provincial), or local governmental agencies that are responsible for the public administration of the government in a country.

Collaboration The mutually beneficial association of two or more parties who are working to achieve a common goal.

Collaborations and cooperative agreements Legal instruments, distinct from contracts, between two or more organizations that are substantially involved in carrying out specific funded activities.

Collective impact The commitment of a group of actors from different sectors to a common agenda for solving a specific social problem, using a structured form of collaboration.

Commitment to quality performance, improvement, and evaluation An element of effective patient-focused health promotion programs in health care organization.

Communication objectives The intended goals and outcomes of a health promotion program.

Communication theories Theories that focus on message production, content, context, design and production, and amount and type of channels in order to impact individuals and groups.

Communities One of the four major settings for health promotion programs, communities are usually defined as places where people live. Communities are also groups of people who come together for a common purpose.

Community empowerment A multidimensional social process where people in a community act in their own self-interest in making decisions and taking actions to benefit their well-being.

Community empowerment A multidimensional social process that helps people gain control over their own lives. It is a process that fosters peoples' capacity to implement actions or change in their own lives, in their communities, and in their society through acting on issues that they define as important.

Community engagement Process of working collaboratively with and through groups of people affiliated by geographic proximity, special interests, or similar situations to address issues affecting their well-being.

Community health organizations Organizations created by community members and rooted in local community health concerns, issues, and problems. The term *community health organization* is synonymous with the terms *community agency, program, initiative, human services,* and *project*.

Community health workers (CHWs) Members of a community who are chosen by community members or organizations to provide basic health and medical care to their community.

Community involvement A WSCC component encouraging schools to create partnerships with community groups, organizations, and local businesses to share resources that will support student learning and development.

Community mobilization Individuals or groups that organize around specific community issues to develop community-based strategies that empower communities to create change and solve problems.

Community organizing Working with and through constituents to achieve common goals, it emphasizes changing the social and economic structures that influence health.

Community readiness model A nine-stage model used to assess community readiness and to determine the intervention (or interventions) that best align with each stage.

Comprehensive workplace health promotion Workplace health program covering five elements: education programs, supportive social and physical environment, integration into organizational structure, linkage to related programs, and on-site screening.

Concept A primary component of a theory.

Concept development The process of using the health communication plan and formative research to generate ideas that can be tested and used in developing material.

Consensus building A process for achieving general agreement among program participants and stakeholders about a particular problem, goal, or issue of mutual interest.

Construct A defining element of a theory that has been adopted, developed, and tested over time.

Content validity Refers to the extent to which a measure represents all facets of a given social construct. (Also known as *logical validity*.)

Counseling, psychological, and social services A WSCC component promoting prevention and intervention services supporting mental, behavioral, and social-emotional health of students.

Cross-cultural staff training Training that focuses on developing competencies to serve people of diverse cultural, linguistic, and social backgrounds and critical awareness of the self, others, and the world.

Cultural relevance When the evaluation methods and materials are developed to take into consideration the traits of the priority population regarding all facets of culture.

Cultural sensitivity The acknowledgment that cultural differences affect individuals' health status and health care.

Culturally appropriate Conforming to a culture's acceptable expressions and standards of behavior and thoughts. Interventions and educational materials are more likely to be culturally appropriate when representatives of the intended priority audience are involved in planning, developing, and pilot testing them.

Culture The art and other manifestations of human intellectual achievement regarded collectively in the workplace.

Data mining The process of modeling large amounts of data to discover previously unknown patterns or relationships.

Delphi technique A primary data collection method that was originally conceived as a way to obtain the opinions of experts without necessarily bringing them together face to face.

Demand for big data Three factors contribute to demand for big data in health promotion programs: supply, technology, and government.

Demography The study of statistics such as births, deaths, income, or the incidence of disease, which illustrate the changing structure of human populations.

Developmental evaluation An evaluation approach that focuses on innovative programs in the early stages of development and considers complex and changing environments.

Diffusion of innovations model A community-level (or setting-level) health theory that focuses on the dissemination of new ideas and their adoption by people in a systematic manner.

Direct lobbying Communication with a legislator or his or her staff member that conveys a viewpoint about specific legislation.

Disability The Americans with Disabilities Act (ADA) gives people with disabilities the same protection from discrimination as other minority groups. It is a factor that can be a determinant of health disparities.

Diversity Individual differences along the dimensions of race, ethnicity, gender, sexual orientation, socioeconomic status, age, physical abilities, religious beliefs, political beliefs, health or disease, status, or other conditions or ideologies. The concept of diversity encompasses acceptance and respect and an understanding that each individual is unique.

Early Care and Education Center Preschool facility for children providing educational and health opportunities for children prior to their enrollment in elementary school.

Ecological perspective A perspective that emphasizes the interaction between the interdependence of factors within and across three levels of influence for health-related behaviors and conditions: (1) the intrapersonal or individual level; (2) the interpersonal level; and (3) the community or setting level, which includes institutional or organizational factors, community factors, and public policy factors.

Education A factor that can be a main determinant of health disparities.

Education entertainment The blending of core communication theories and fundamental entertainment pedagogy to guide the preparation and delivery of health communications.

eHealth The use of digital information and communication technologies to improve people's health and health care.

Electioneering The persuasion of voters in a political campaign.

Electronic Health Record (EHR) An electronic version of a health record that is maintained and updated by an individual for himself or herself; a tool that individuals can use to collect, track, and share past and current information about their health or the health of someone in their care.

Elevator speech A concise statement, usually 15 or so seconds long, that highlights program features such as mission, goals, setting, and outcomes.

Employee assistance programs (EAPs) Services provided free of charge to employees through outside agencies to allow confidential assessment, referral, and short-term counseling for personal problems.

Empowerment To give power or authority to a person in terms of health-related matters.

Environmental factors A cause of racial and ethnic disparities. Examples include exposure to toxins, viral or microbial agents, poor or unsafe physical and social environment, inadequate access to nutritious food and exercise, and community norms that do not support protective behaviors.

Epidemiology The branch of medicine that deals with the incidence, distribution, and possible control of diseases and other factors relating to health.

Equity Full and equal access to opportunities that enable all people to lead healthy lives. Lack of equal opportunities result in health disparities among minority groups.

Ethics Moral principles that govern a person's or group's behavior.

Ethnicity A social group that shares a common and distinctive culture, religion, language, or the like; can be a determinant of health disparities.

Evaluation costs The expense of conducting an evaluation, which is related to the complexity of the program being evaluated, the program's time frame, the program's internal resources and expertise, and the credentials and experience of the program evaluator.

Evaluation design The characteristics of an evaluation that must be carefully chosen in order to achieve the evaluation's purpose and meet the needs of the users who will receive the results.

Evaluation ethics Ethics that relate to safeguarding and protecting program participants' rights.

Evaluation report A report on the outcomes and results of a health program evaluation.

Evidence-based interventions Programs evaluated as effective to address a specific health-related condition, in the context of a particular ethnicity or culture, that use health theory both in developing the content of the interventions (e.g., activities, curriculum, or tasks) and evaluation (e.g., the measures and outcomes).

Evidence-based practices Health promotion program activities and strategies based on sound science and theory; a logic model that matches the science and theory to the intended outcomes of interest for a particular priority population at a setting.

Face validity A subjective assessment of the degree to which an assessment covers the concept that is supposed to be measured.

Family engagement A WSCC component asking school staff to utilize families as partners in the educational process of their child(ren) in order to improve learning outcomes.

Fidelity The extent to which the delivery of a health intervention conforms to the curriculum, protocol, or guidelines for implementing that intervention.

Fiscal management The maintaining of sound records and procedures in order to safeguard and maximize a program's money, assets, and resources, which protects the program's sustainability.

Fiscal year The dates that establish a program's funding year; may or may not coincide with the calendar year.

Focus group A qualitative data collection technique in which a small group of individuals meet to share their views and experiences on some topic.

Formative evaluation The gathering of information and materials to aid program planning and development when the program is being formed.

Formative research (or consumer research) Research focused on the intended audience: who they are, what is important to them, what influences their behavior, and what will enable them to engage in a desired behavior.

Foundations Entities that are established as nonprofit corporations or charitable trusts with the principal purpose of making grants to unrelated organizations or institutions or to individuals for scientific, educational, cultural, religious, or other charitable purposes.

Fundraising The process of soliciting and gathering money or in-kind gifts by requesting donations from individuals, businesses, charitable foundations, or governmental agencies. Some organizations have staff members who are dedicated solely to fundraising.

Fundraising field The field advances philanthropy through advocacy, research, education, and certification programs.

Gantt chart A visual depiction of the schedule for completing a program's objectives—that is, a timeline for program implementation.

Gender Personal identification of one's own gender based on an internal awareness. It denotes the social and cultural role of each sex within a given society, and a factor that may contribute to discrimination and health disparities.

Geographic information system (GIS) A technique used in needs assessment data analyses and reporting. A GIS uses computer software to capture, store, analyze, manage, and present data that are linked to location, allowing people to view, understand, question, interpret, and visualize data in ways that reveal relationships, patterns, or trends in the form of maps, reports, and charts.

Geographic location A factor that can be a determinant of health disparities; may be defined by geometry or human or social attributes of place identity and sense of place.

Goal A statement of a program's direction and intent. Program goals clarify what is important in a health promotion program and state the end results of the program.

Grants Sums of money that are awarded to finance a particular activity or program. Generally, these grant awards do not need to be paid back.

Grassroots lobbying Any attempt to indirectly influence legislation by motivating members of the public to express their views to legislators and legislative aides.

Health A resource for everyday life, not the object of living. It is a positive concept that emphasizes social and personal resources as well as physical capabilities.

Health belief model An individual-level health theory that attempts to explain and predict health behaviors by focusing on the attitudes and beliefs of individuals.

Health care organizations One of the four major settings for health promotion programs, including hospitals, health centers, physician's offices, clinics, rehabilitation centers, skilled nursing and long-term care facilities, and home health and other health-related entities.

Healthcare Effectiveness Data and Information Set (HEDIS) Consists of 75 measures across eight domains of care. It is now possible to mine the various data sets available to health promotion programs to help uncover problems and focus on areas of improvement identified using this method.

Health communication The study and use of communication strategies to inform and influence individual decisions that enhance health.

Health communication plan A plan that guides and develops information exchange between and among a health program's staff, stakeholders, and participants so that a program can deliver clear messages to achieve its goals and objectives.

Health disparities Differences among populations in health status, behavior, and outcomes due to gender, income, education, disability, geographic location, sexual orientation, and race or ethnicity.

Health education A WSCC component promoting a discipline with formal, structured lessons providing students the opportunity to acquire information and skills students need to make quality health decisions.

Health education A discipline with a distinct body of knowledge, code of ethics, skill-based set of competencies, rigorous system of quality assurance, and system of credentialing health education professionals.

Health informatics A scientific field that utilizes computer technology in the advancement of medicine. It applies information technology in health care for knowledge creation and management.

Health information management Management of personal health information in hospitals or other health care organizations enabling the delivery of quality health care to the public.

Health information technology (HIT) The application of information processing involving both computer hardware and software that deals with the storage, retrieval, sharing, and use of health care information, data, and knowledge for communication and decision making.

Health insurance Insurance that provides protection against the costs of hospital and medical care or against lost income arising from an illness or injury.

Health literacy The capacity of an individual to obtain, interpret, comprehend, and assess health information and services in order to make informed health decisions and take individual and collective health-enhancing actions.

Health promoting universities Postsecondary institutions that adopt goals of integrating health into the university's culture, structure, and processes and lead health promotion actions locally and globally.

Health promotion The planned change of health-related lifestyles and life conditions through any combination of health education and related organizational, economic, or environmental supports for behavior of individuals, groups, or sites that is conducive to health.

Health promotion policies Operating rules for health promotion programs that specify people's rights and responsibilities as well as spell out the rights and responsibilities of the organization in regards to its stakeholders (for example, students, employees, clients, or members).

Health promotion programs Programs that provide planned, organized, and structured activities and events over time that focus on helping individuals make informed decisions about their health. In addition, health promotion programs promote policy, environmental, regulatory, organizational, and legislative changes at various levels of government and organizations.

Health protection The provision of safe work conditions, particularly through limiting hazardous exposures.

Health risk appraisal An assessment of employees' or other beneficiaries' health risks, interest in participating in specific programs, and readiness to change unhealthy lifestyle habits.

Health services A WSCC component promoting services that intervene with actual and potential health problems and provide emergency care as well as management of chronic conditions.

Health status The overall evaluation of an individual's degree of wellness or illness with a number of indicators, including morbidity, impairments, mortality, functional status, and quality of life.

Healthy People 2020 A strategic plan for public health practitioners and policymakers that sets measurable objectives at the national level.

Hook In advocacy work, an anecdote, statistic, or fact used to capture the reader or listener's attention about a particular health topic.

Impact evaluations An evaluation that measures the immediate effects of a health promotion program and the extent to which program objectives and goals were met. The primary question in an impact evaluation is what the immediate effect on the program's participants has been.

Implementation challenges Challenges often encountered when moving through a program's implementation stages, especially program installation, initial implementation, and full operation.

Implementation stages The phases in the process of creating a health promotion program, moving from exploration of the idea through program operation.

Implementation science The scientific study of methods to promote the uptake of research findings.

Improvement science Discipline with a focus on learning from strong research and evaluation designs, which can then be used in a timely manner to make an impact on the population of interest.

Income Earnings. Education, distribution of wealth, and sociopolitical circumstances affect income and well-being and may determine health disparities.

Income statement A statement that shows the financial performance of an organization over a specified time period—typically a year.

Indicated preventive strategies Interventions that target high-risk individuals who have detectable signs or symptoms but have not reached the diagnostic criteria for a particular health problem.

Individual and behavioral factors Intrapersonal-level factors that may result in health disparities. One example of such a factor is participating in high-risk behaviors such as smoking, not wearing a seat belt, choosing a sedentary lifestyle, and eating poorly.

Individual-level certification and licensure Credentials issued by a recognized professional credentialing body to individuals who meet specified criteria.

Infrastructure (operating, core, or hard) funding Monies that an organization obtains in order to operate its infrastructure before offering any program, activities, or services.

Institutionalized racism Differential access to goods, services, resources, and opportunities by race.

Intended audience The audience for whom the health communication is developed—that is, the intended receivers and users of a health communication.

Integrative model An expansion of the theory of planned behavior that includes both distal and proximal factors that influence intention and behavior.

Intermediate outcomes In a logic model, the results that may or may not be seen after a single activity but that are expected to happen (and be evaluated) in the future.

Internalized racism The acceptance by individuals of negative messages from others about their worth and abilities as members of a stigmatized race.

Interpersonal level The facet of the ecological health perspective that focuses on the influences of interpersonal processes and primary groups that provide social identity, support, and role definition (for example, family, friends, and peers).

Intervention Any set of methods, techniques, activities, or processes designed to effect changes in behaviors or the environment.

Intervention mapping A six-step model that provides health promotion program planners with a framework for effective decision making at each stage of intervention planning, implementation, and evaluation.

Intrapersonal level The facet of the ecological health perspective that focuses on individual characteristics that influence behavior, such as knowledge, attitudes, beliefs, and personality traits.

Jakarta Declaration An agreement signed at the World Health Organization's Fourth International Conference on Health Promotion, which was in Jakarta in1997, gave prominence to the concept of the health setting as the place or social context in which people engage in daily activities in which environmental, organizational, and personal factors interact to affect health and well-being.

Key informant An individual who possesses unique and important information that can provide insights into the health issues at a site.

Key informant interviews A primary data collection data method that uses structured and unstructured interviews to collect qualitative data from key informants.

Lalonde report Titled *A New Perspective on the Health of Canadians*, this report was produced in Canada in 1974 and is considered the first modern government document in the Western world to acknowledge that our emphasis on a biomedical health care system might be misplaced and that the governments need to look beyond the traditional health care system in order to improve the health of the public.

Law In federal government, a bill passed by both houses of Congress and signed by the president (or passed by Congress through overriding a presidential veto).

Letter to the editor Letter addressed to an editor in which the opinions of the author or authors is (are) expressed. Typically, the letter does not exceed 250 words. Also see *Op-ed*.

Levels of analytics Three widely accepted levels of generalization (or abstraction) to help understand highly complex problems in world health. They are the individual, state (or society), and the international system.

Local health departments Local (city and county government) public agencies responsible to protect health, support healthy lifestyles, and create healthy environments. Responsibilities include sanitation, disease surveillance, and monitoring of environmental risks (for example, lead or asbestos poisoning) and ecological risks (for example, air and water pollution).

Logic model A visual depiction of the underlying logic of a planned program. It shows the relationships between the program's resources (inputs), its planned activities (outputs), and the changes that are expected as a result (outcomes).

Long-term outcomes In a logic model, the results that represent the ultimate extension of a program's impact. If the program's activities are effective and achieve both the short-term and intermediate outcomes, it specifies related long-term results that might be reasonably expected.

Master Certified Health Education Specialist (MCHES) A health educator who has successfully completed the competency-based exam given by the National Commission for Health Education Credentialing, Inc.

Mastering change A process of supporting and engaging people and resources in the context of an evolving and dynamic environment.

Matching funds, cost sharing, and in-kind contributions Monies and resources that are provided by one group or organization to another organization for its operations or programs. Matching funds are monies paid concurrently with the expenditure funds for the operation of a program. Cost sharing applies to monies that must be spent by the time a program concludes. In-kind contributions are noncash contributions (for example, materials, equipment, vehicles, or food) used to operate programs or services.

Measures The information or data needed by the program evaluator to accurately measure whether each program objective was met and to accurately measure the impact of the program.

Media advocacy The strategic use of news media and, when appropriate, paid advertising in order to support community organizing to advance a public policy initiative.

Medical care factors Health care system–based factors can be a cause of racial and ethnic disparities. Examples include lack of access to health care, lack of quality health care, and providers who lack cultural competence.

Message concepts Health communication messages intended to present ideas to an audience as a starting point for developing health communications.

Mission A brief (usually one sentence) statement as to why the health promotion program exists. This statement clearly and simply declares the program's core purpose and priority population.

Mixed methods The combination of qualitative and quantitative methods in an evaluation.

Model Draws on two or more health theories to address a specific health problem, event, or situation.

Mothers Against Drunk Driving (MADD) Advocacy organization recognized for raising awareness about the dangers of drunk driving, providing impetus for stricter laws, and reducing alcohol-related traffic fatalities.

Motivational interviewing A method that works on facilitating and engaging intrinsic motivation within the client in order to change behavior.

National Association for the Education of Young Children A professional organization that promotes excellence in early childhood education.

National Partnerships for Action to End Health Disparities A partnership created by the Office of Minority Health in the U.S. Department of Health and Human Services as part of its strategic framework for eliminating health disparities.

National Registry of Evidence-Based Programs and Practices (NREPP) A searchable database of interventions for the prevention and treatment of mental and substance use disorders, established by the Substance Abuse and Mental Health Services Administration.

Need The difference between "what is" at the present time and "what should be" under more ideal circumstances.

Needs assessment The process of obtaining information about individuals' health needs and a site's available support and resources for the purpose of planning, implementing, and evaluating a program.

Needs assessment The process of obtaining information about individuals' health needs and a site's available support and resources for the purpose of planning, implementing, and evaluating a program.

Needs assessment report The final product of a needs assessment. The report is often used as a resource during a program's implementation and evaluation.

Networking The process of building alliances to address a health problem or concern; it involves deliberate action to get to know people, resources, and organizations.

Nutrition services A WSCC component promoting healthy food services' meeting nutrition standards of the National School Lunch and Breakfast Programs as well as foods sold outside of the school meal programs.

Objectives The specific steps that need to be completed in order to attain program goals. An objective statement specifies who, what, when, and where and clarifies by how much, how many, or how often.

Office of Minority Health An agency established in 1986 by the U.S. Department of Health and Human Services (DHHS). Its mission is to improve and protect the health of racial and ethnic minority populations through the development of health policies and programs that will eliminate health disparities.

Op-ed A newspaper article appearing on the editorial page that expresses the opinions of a named writer who is usually unaffiliated with the newspaper's editorial board.

Ordinance A local statute or regulation, usually enacted by a city government.

Ottawa Charter An agreement developed at the first International Conference on Health Promotion, held in Ottawa, Canada, in 1986 that identified the prerequisites for health; methods of achieving health promotion through advocacy, enabling, and mediation; and five key strategies.

Outcome evaluation Assessment of the longer-term (typically greater than 6 months) impact of an intervention.

Outcome objectives The specific, measurable long-term accomplishments (targets) of a health promotion program.

Outreach Sharing health promotion program information with specific individuals and groups for the purpose of educating them about the program and for developing support for program participants.

Partnerships Mutually beneficial relationships between organizations, built on trust and commitment, to extend the reach and effectiveness of a health promotion program.

Pathways of evaluation Five evaluation objectives to guide predictive and prescriptive analyses: right living, right care, right provider, right value, and right innovation.

Patient activation measure A commercial product that assesses an individual's knowledge, skill, and confidence for managing one's health and health care.

Patient and family-centered care An approach to the planning, delivery, and evaluation of health care that is grounded in mutually beneficial partnerships among health care patients, families, and providers and built on the four core concepts of dignity and respect, information sharing, participation, and collaboration.

Patient engagement One strategy to achieve the triple aim of improved health outcomes, better patient care, and lower costs.

Patient Protection and Affordable Care Act or Affordable Care Act (ACA) An act passed in 2010 to decrease the number of uninsured Americans and reduce the overall costs of health care by providing a number of mechanisms, strategies, policies, and initiatives.

Patient safety Efficient service delivery and improved working conditions that protect and promote individuals' health when receiving health care services.

PDCA/PDSA cycle A process of continuous quality improvement through the steps of plan, do, study/check, and act.

PEARL score An approach to making decisions about interventions in health promotion programs. The model considers five exterior feasibility factors that have a high degree of influence in determining how a particular problem can be addressed.

Performance evaluation A way for program directors and supervisors to evaluate staff on a continual basis. Such ongoing evaluation starts with staff goals that are formulated in partnership with supervisors and that meet staff, program, and organizational needs.

Personally mediated racism Discrimination in which the majority racial group treats members of a minority group as inferior and views the minorities' abilities, motives, and intents through a lens of prejudice based on race.

Physical education and physical activity A WSCC component promoting (1) a discipline within the school with a distinct body of knowledge and skill-based set of competencies as well as (2) increasing physical activity within the school day.

Physical environment A WSCC component addressing ventilation, temperature, noise, and lighting within the school as well as protecting occupants from physical threats (e.g., crime, violence, traffic) and biological and chemical agents.

Plain language Also called *plain English*, this refers to communication your audience can understand the first time they read it or hear it.

Policies Operating rules that provide a program's stakeholders (for example, students, employees, clients, and members) with their organizational rights and responsibilities. Effective policies clearly state the health values and priorities of the organization and are tailored to the unique requirements and needs of the setting and stakeholders.

Policy change An intervention approach to reducing disease that focuses on enacting policies (e.g., laws, regulations, or formal or informal rules) or environmental change.

Population level The facet of the ecological health perspective that focuses on institutional or organization factors, social capital factors, and public policy factors.

Power analysis An analysis to ensure having an adequate number of people participating in a needs assessment (that is, a survey) in order to be able to generalize the findings from the sample to the population.

PRECEDE-PROCEED model A model that consists of eight phases that guide planners in developing health promotion programs, beginning with more general outcomes and moving to more specific outcomes.

Pretesting A process of systematically gathering target audience reactions to messages and materials for a health communication program before they are finalized.

Primary prevention Taking action prior to the onset (new incidents) of a health problem to intercept its causation or to modify its course before people are involved.

Priorities The intervention points and strategies of a health promotion program that are derived from analyzing the collected data of a needs assessment. Approaches to establishing priorities from data include the nominal group process and the PEARL model.

Priority population A defined group of individuals who share some common characteristics related to the health concern being addressed. Frequently the term *program participants* is synonymous with *priority population*.

Process evaluation An evaluation intended to learn why and how an intervention worked or did not work and for whom it worked best and worst.

Process objectives The specific, measurable outcomes that identify needed changes or tasks in the administration of a program (for example, hiring staff, providing professional development for staff, or seeking additional funding). This type of objective is used to evaluate progress in the implementation of the program (process or formative evaluation).

Professional Fundraisers Individuals who advance philanthropy through responsibilities that include writing grant proposals, researching requests for proposals from foundations and corporations, overseeing and implementing fundraising plans and strategies, and establishing structures for effective fundraising.

Program evaluation An evaluation that involves systematically collecting information about a health promotion program in order to answer questions and make decisions about the program.

Program Program supports that are drawn from the program policies; they address program logistics and day-to-day operating details such as program participant rights, protection, recruitment, retention, and recognition. Also see *Standard operating procedures*.

Program sustainability The likelihood that a program will remain viable and available over a period of time.

Public funds Tax dollars collected and spent by the government to provide the infrastructure for the systems and organizations that operate national, state, and local health and human services.

Public service announcements (PSAs) Noncommercial radio or television advertisements intended to modify public attitudes by raising awareness about specific issues. The most common PSA topics are health- and safety-related.

Qualitative data Data that are more narrative than numerical, derived more from perceptions than statistical measures.

Qualitative methods Methods of research that involve gathering non-numerical data, including program descriptions that often include the perspectives and experiences of program participants themselves.

Quality improvement The systematic and continuous activities that are conducted that result in measurable improvement for a priority population.

Quality rating and improvement system A national, systematic approach to assess, improve, and communicate the level of quality in early and school-age care and education programs.

Quantitative data Statistical information and measures, such as percentages, means, or correlations.

Quantitative methods Methods of research that involve gathering and analyzing numerical data.

Race A biological classification and social construct that can be a determinant of health disparities. These disparities are generally driven by differences in education and employment opportunities as well as housing and neighborhood segregation.

Racism The belief that race is the primary determinant of human traits and capacities and that certain characteristics produce an inherent superiority of a particular race. Three types of racism affect health outcomes: institutionalized racism, personally mediated racism, and internalized racism.

Random selection A technique that involves selecting members of a population in such a way that each member has an equal chance of being selected to participate (to receive a survey questionnaire, for example).

REACH Communities that are participating in the Centers for Disease Control and Prevention's Project REACH (Racial and Ethnic Approaches to Community Health), which engages minority groups and communities directly in addressing health issues.

RE-AIM evaluation framework An evaluation framework with five dimensions: reach, effectiveness, adoption, implementation, and maintenance, which recognizes the importance of both external and internal validity.

Referral The process of connecting a person to a health promotion program.

Reliability The ability of an evaluation instrument (for example, a needs assessment survey) to provide consistent results each time it is used.

Reliability The ability of an evaluation instrument to provide consistent results.

Research-tested Intervention Programs (RTIPs) A searchable database of evidence-based health promotion interventions developed as a resource to help people, agencies, and organizations implement research-tested programs and practices in their communities, established by the National Cancer Institute.

Response bias Bias that occurs when the people who respond to a survey (for example, as part of a needs assessment) are different in their health beliefs or behaviors from those who do not respond to the survey.

Root causes of health disparities Systemic institutionalized sources of health disparities that have been many decades or even centuries in the making. The relationships among the root causes of health disparities are multidirectional and cyclical, exacerbating one another and calling for intervention at every level.

Sample The group of individuals who are the primary data source in a survey or intervention (for example, in a needs assessment).

Sampling bias Bias that occurs when the sample is selected in a manner that omits people who have unique characteristics (for example, race or ethnicity, health beliefs or behaviors, or socioeconomic status), which results in final survey responses that are uncharacteristic of the population.

School Health Index A planning tool to improve the school health program by assessing the components' strengths and weaknesses with respect to safety, physical activity, nutrition, tobacco use, and asthma.

School Health Policies and Programs Study A survey of state departments of education and a representative sample of districts, elementary, middle, and high schools components of the school health program.

School Health Profiles A biannual survey conducted by the Centers for Disease Control and Prevention to assess secondary schools' programs, services, and policies related to various components of the WSCC.

Schools One of the four major sites for health promotion programs including child care centers; preschools; kindergarten; elementary, middle, and high schools; 2-year and 4-year colleges; universities; and vocational and technical education programs.

Secondary data Data that already exists because they were collected by someone for another purpose. These data may or may not be directly from the individual or population that is currently being assessed.

Secondary prevention Interrupting problematic behaviors among those who are engaged in unhealthy decision making and perhaps showing early signs of disease or disability.

Selective preventive strategies Interventions that target individuals or a subgroup of the population whose risk of developing illness or disorders is significantly higher than average.

Settings The sites of health promotion programs.

Sexual orientation Individuals' personal awareness of identity. Sex-based social structures such as gender roles and gender power can be determinants of health disparities.

Short-term outcomes In a logic model, effects that can be expected as an immediate result of each of the planned activities.

SMART An approach to writing program objectives developed by the Centers for Disease Control and Prevention. The mnemonic SMART indicates that objectives should be specific, measurable, achievable, realistic, and time-bound.

SMART objectives The specific, measurable, attainable, relevant, and time-bound objectives of a health promotion program that form the basic foundation for program evaluation.

Social and emotional school climate A WSCC component that creates and sustains a healthy school environment by promoting the psychosocial aspects of students' educational experience.

Social media Websites and applications that enable users to create and share content or to participate in social networking.

Staff members' fundraising responsibilities These responsibilities can include writing grant proposals, researching foundation and corporation requests for proposals, overseeing and implementing fundraising plans and strategies, and working to establish structures for effective fundraising.

Stakeholders The people and organizations that have an interest in the health of a specific group, community, or population. Stakeholders have a legitimate interest (a stake) in what kind of health promotion program is planned, implemented, and evaluated.

Standard operating procedures A commonly used label for program procedures that are drawn from program policies. Also see *Program procedures*.

Structured A specialized format for organizing and storing data. General data structure types include the array, the file, the record, the table, the tree, and so on. Any data structure is designed to organize data to suit a specific purpose so that it can be accessed and worked with in appropriate ways.

Social capital The degree to which relationships and social networks help a society to function effectively.

Social cognitive theory An interpersonal-level health theory, based on the reciprocal determinism between behavior, environment, and person, where their constant interactions influence human action.

Social determinants of health The conditions in which people are born, grow, live, work, and age. These circumstances are shaped by the distribution of money, power, and resources at global, national, and local levels.

Social marketing A strategy that uses commercial marketing techniques to influence the voluntary behavior of target audience members for a health benefit.

Social network and social support theory An interpersonal-level health theory that recognizes that social ties and levels of support influence health status and behaviors.

Societal factor A socially rooted cause of racial and ethnic disparities. Examples include poverty, racism, economics, health literacy, limited education, and educational inequality.

Staff diversity A way to boost the representation of minorities in the health care workforce and a strategy for reducing health disparities.

Stages of change model See *Transtheoretical model.*

Summative evaluation An evaluation intended to measure the short- and long-term outcomes from a health promotion program.

Survey questionnaires The most common means of gathering data for a needs assessment (for example, information about perceptions, behaviors, and issues). Questionnaires can be administered in four ways: as mail surveys, as telephone surveys, face to face, or as electronic surveys.

Sustainability An evaluation of a program that is ongoing through providing a feedback loop to participants and decision makers.

Teach-back method Also known as the *show-me method*, this is a communication confirmation method used by health care providers to verify whether a patient (or caretakers) understands what is being explained to them. If a patient understands, they are able to "teach back" the information accurately.

Tertiary prevention Improving the lives of individuals currently in treatment for a medical or health problem or individuals with chronic illness.

The 10 Essential Public Health Services (EPHS) A guiding framework for the responsibilities of local public health systems, defining public health practice within local health departments and in collaboration with community partners.

Theory A "set of interrelated concepts, definitions, and propositions that present a systematic view of events by specifying relationships among variables in order to explain and predict the events of situations" (F. N. Kerlinger, *Foundations of Behavioral Research*, 3rd ed. [New York: Holt, Rinehart & Winston, 1936], p. 25).

Transtheoretical model An individual-level health model proposing that behavior change occurs in stages (stages of change) and that people move through these stages in a specific sequence as they change.

Universal preventive strategies These interventions target the general public or a population that has not been identified on the basis of individual risk.

Unstructured data Refers to information that either does not have a predefined data model or is not organized in a predefined manner. Unstructured information is typically text-heavy, but may contain data such as dates, numbers, and facts as well.

Validity The degree to which an instrument or procedure (for example, a needs assessment survey, evaluation questionnaire, or key informant interview) accurately reflects or assesses the specific concept that the program staff, stakeholders, or participants are attempting to measure.

Variable A construct (also called an indicator) that is operationally defined and can be measured.

Visual mapping A mix of objective knowledge and subjective perceptions: precise knowledge about the location of geographic features as well as impressions of places and connections between places or objects.

Volunteers Individuals who serve an organization or cause without compensation for services rendered. In health promotion programs, volunteers perform many tasks from direct service delivery to service on boards of directors or as program advocates.

Wellness Physical well-being, often obtained through healthful lifestyles (e.g., regular exercise, nutritious diet).

Wellness committee A group of employees from key departments or subgroups within an organization that have an interest in or commitment to workers' health and safety.

Workplaces One of the four major settings for health promotion programs including any setting where people are employed—in business or industry (small, large, or multinational) as well as in government (for example, in the armed services; local, state, or federal civil service; or offers of elected officials) or in the non profit sector.

World Health Organization The directing and coordinating authority for health within the United Nations system. It is responsible for providing leadership on global health matters, shaping the health research agenda, setting norms and standards, articulating evidence-based policy options, providing technical support to countries, and monitoring and assessing health trends.

Youth Risk Behavior Survey The biannual national school-based survey conducted by the Centers for Disease Control and Prevention to assess health-risk behaviors of youth.

Zone of drastic mutation The point after which further modification of a program to fit a target population other than the one it was designed for will compromise the program's integrity and effectiveness.

Page references followed by *fig* indicate an illustrated figure; followed by *t* indicate a table.